Medical Intelligence Unit

Immunotherapy of Cancer with Sensitized T Lymphocytes

Alfred E. Chang
Suyu Shu

University of Michigan Medical Center
Ann Arbor, Michigan, U.S.A.

R.G. Landes Company
Austin

MEDICAL INTELLIGENCE UNIT

IMMUNOTHERAPY OF CANCER WITH SENSITIZED T LYMPHOCYTES

R.G. LANDES COMPANY
Austin

CRC Press is the exclusive worldwide distributor of publications of the Medical Intelligence Unit.
CRC Press, 2000 Corporate Blvd., NW, Boca Raton, FL 33431. Phone: 407/994-0555.

Submitted: June 1994
Published: September 1994

Please address all inquiries to the Publisher:
R.G. Landes Company, 909 Pine Street, Georgetown, TX 78626
or
P.O. Box 4858, Austin, TX 78765
Phone: 512/ 863 7762; FAX: 512/ 863 0081

ISBN 1-57059-049-4
CATALOG # LN9049

Library of Congress Cataloging-in-Publication Data

Immunotherapy of cancer with sensitized T lymphocytes / [edited by]
Alfred E. Chang, Suyu Shu.
p. cm. --(Medical intelligence unit)
Includes bibliographical references and index.
ISBN 1-57059-049-4 (hardcover)
1. Cancer--Immunotherapy. 2. T cells. 3. Lymphocyte
transformation. I. Chang, Alfred E. II. Shu, Suyu. III. Series.
[DNLM: 1. Neoplasms--therapy. 2. Immunotherapy. 3. T
-lymphocytes--immunology. QZ 266 I3478 1994]
RC271.I451467 1994
616.99'406--dc20
DNLM/DLC
for Library of Congress 94-23037
CIP

While the authors, editors and publisher believe that drug selection and dosage and the specifications and usage of equipment and devices, as set forth in this book, are in accord with current recommendations and practice at the time of publication, they make no warranty, expressed or implied, with respect to material described in this book. In view of the ongoing research, equipment development, changes in governmental regulations and the rapid accumulation of information relating to the biomedical sciences, the reader is urged to carefully review and evaluate the information provided herein.

To Our Readers

R.G. Landes Company publishes four book series: *Medical Intelligence Unit, Molecular Biology Intelligence Unit, Neuroscience Intelligence Unit,* and *Biotechnology Intelligence Unit.* Our goal is to publish the most recent information in biomedical science for sophisticated researchers and physicians.

To achieve this goal we have accelerated our publishing program to conform to the fast pace in which information grows in biomedical science. Most of our books are published *within 90 to 120 days of receipt of the manuscript.*

As you might expect, this causes a few problems for us; sometimes it makes our office more like a big city newspaper than a scholarly publisher. So as you look through this book you may see something that isn't just right. Please let us know. Or if you have an idea for improving our books, we'd like very much to hear from you. If the problem you describe hasn't already been discovered or if your idea is provocative enough to promote a discussion here, we'll give you a free book of your choice. Just list three titles in order of preference and we'll send you one, based on availability—with our thanks. Our address is printed on the copyright page of each of our books.

Carol Harwell
Publications Director
R.G. Landes Company

CONTENTS

EDITORS

Alfred E. Chang, M.D.
Professor of Surgery
University of Michigan
Ann Arbor, Michigan
Chapters 1 and 12

Suyu Shu, Ph.D.
Professor of Surgery
University of Michigan
Ann Arbor, Michigan
Chapters 1 and 12

CONTRIBUTORS

Peter M. Anderson, M.D., Ph.D.
Assistant Professor of Pediatric Hematology/Oncology
University of Minnesota
Minneapolis, Minnesota, U.S.A.
Chapter 5

Atsushi Aruga, M.D., Ph.D.
Research Fellow
University of Michigan
Ann Arbor, Michigan, U.S.A.
Chapter 12

Richard J. Barth, Jr., M.D.
Assistant Professor of Surgery
Dartmouth-Hitchcock Medical Center
Lebanon, New Hampshire, U.S.A.
Chapter 6

Harry D. Bear, M.D., Ph.D.
Associate Professor of Surgery
Medical College of Virginia
Richmond, Virginia, U.S.A.
Chapter 3

Arie S. Belldegrun, M.D.
Associate Professor of Surgery
Division of Urology
UCLA School of Medicine
Chapter 11

Ronald M. Bukowski, M.D.
Staff, Department of Hematology & Medical Oncology
The Cleveland Clinic Foundation
Cleveland, Ohio, U.S.A.
Chapter 9

Ulrike L. Burger, M.D.
Chapter 2

CONTRIBUTORS

Mark J. Cameron, M.S.
Research Associate
University of Michigan
Ann Arbor, Michigan, U.S.A.
Chapter 12

Peter A. Cohen, M.D.
Senior Investigator
Surgery Branch
National Cancer Institute
Bethesda, Maryland, U.S.A.
Chapter 4

Brendan D. Curti, M.D.
Division of Cancer Treatment
Biological Response Modifiers Program
Frederick Cancer Research and Development Center
National Cancer Institute
Frederick, Maryland, U.S.A.
Chapter 5

Linda M. Douville, R.N., B.S.N.
Chapter 2

Timothy J. Eberlein, M.D.
Associate Professor of Surgery
Brigham and Women's Hospital
Harvard Medical School
Boston, Massachusetts, U.S.A.
Chapter 2

Robert A. Figlin, M.D.
Associate Professor of Medicine
Division of Hematology/Oncology
Department of Medicine
UCLA School of Medicine
Chapter 11

James H. Finke, Ph.D.
Staff, Department of Immunology
The Cleveland Clinic Foundation
Cleveland, Ohio, U.S.A.
Chapter 9

Bernard A. Fox, Ph.D.
Assistant Professor of Medicine
Oregon Health Sciences University
Chief, Laboratory of Molecular and Tumor Immunology
Earle A. Chiles Research Institute
Portland, Oregon, U.S.A.
Chapter 7

Peter S. Goedegebuure, Ph.D.
Chapter 2

Jon M. Hain, M.D.
Research Fellow
St. Joseph's Mercy Hospital
Ann Arbor, Michigan, U.S.A.
Chapter 8

Eric Klein, M.D.
Section Head, Urologic Oncology
Department of of Urology
The Cleveland Clinic Foundation
Cleveland, Ohio, U.S.A.
Chapter 9

William C. Kopp, Ph.D.
Clinical Monitoring Laboratory
Biological Response Modifiers Program
Frederick Cancer Research and Development Center
National Cancer Institute
Frederick, Maryland, U.S.A.
Chapter 5

CONTRIBUTORS

John C. Krauss, M.D.
Assistant Professor of Internal Medicine
University of Michigan
Ann Arbor, Michigan, U.S.A.
Chapter 1

Kyung Lee, M.D.
Chapter 2

Hong Li, M.D.
Chapter 2

Dan L. Longo, M.D.
Director, Biological Response Modifiers Program
Frederick Cancer Research and Development Center
National Cancer Institute
Frederick, Maryland, U.S.A.
Chapter 5

Vicki Lorenzi, R.N., B.S.N.
Research Nurse
Cancer Center Experimental Therapeutics Program
The Cleveland Clinic Foundation
Cleveland, Ohio, U.S.A.
Chapter 9

Vikram Mali, B.S.
Medical Student
Michigan State University
East Lansing, Michigan, U.S.A.
Chapter 7

Denise McLain, B.S.
Clinical Research Manager
Cancer Center Experimental Therapeutics Program
The Cleveland Clinic Foundation
Cleveland, Ohio, U.S.A.
Chapter 9

Augusto C. Ochoa, M.D.
Head, Immunotherapy Laboratory
Biological Response Modifiers Program
Frederick Cancer Research and Development Center
National Cancer Institute
Frederick, Maryland, U.S.A.
Chapter 5

Thomas Olencki, D.O.
Assistant Staff, Department of Hematology & Medical Oncology
The Cleveland Clinic Foundation
Cleveland, Ohio, U.S.A.
Chapter 9

John J. Osterholzer, B.S.
Medical Student
University of Michigan
Ann Arbor, Michigan, U.S.A.
Chapter 7

George E. Peoples, M.D.
Chapter 2

William C. Pierce, M.D., Ph.D.
Fellow, Division of Hematology/Oncology
Department of Medicine
UCLA School of Medicine
Chapter 11

Gregory E. Plautz, M.D.
Assistant Professor of Pediatrics
University of Michigan
Ann Arbor, Michigan, U.S.A.
Chapter 1

CONTRIBUTORS

Patricia Rayman, M.S.
Research Technologist, Department of Immunology
The Cleveland Clinic Foundation
Cleveland, Ohio, U.S.A.
Chapter 9

Mark Saxton, M.D.
Immunotherapy Laboratory
Biological Response Modifiers Program
Frederick Cancer Research and Development Center
National Cancer Institute
Frederick, Maryland, U.S.A.
Chapter 5

Mark Schomogyi, M.D.
Research Fellow, Department of Medicine
University of Washington
Seattle, Washington, U.S.A.
Chapter 7

Vernon K. Sondak, M.D.
Associate Professor of Surgery
University of Michigan
Ann Arbor, Michigan, U.S.A.
Chapter 8

Susan S. Strobl
Immunotherapy Laboratory
Biological Response Modifiers Program
Frederick Cancer Research and Development Center
National Cancer Institute
Frederick, Maryland, U.S.A.
Chapter 5

Scott E. Strome, M.D.
Research Fellow, Department of Otolaryngology
University of Michigan
Ann Arbor, Michigan, U.S.A.
Chapter 1

Laurie Tuason, M.S.
Biostatistician, Department of Biostatistics and Epidemiology
The Cleveland Clinic Foundation
Cleveland, Ohio, U.S.A.
Chapter 9

Raymond R. Tubbs, D.O.
Section Head, Immunopathology
Department of Clinical Pathology
The Cleveland Clinic Foundation
Cleveland, Ohio, U.S.A.
Chapter 9

Todd M. Tuttle, M.D.
Research Fellow
Medical College of Virginia
Richmond, Virginia, U.S.A.
Chapter 3

Walter J. Urba, M.D., Ph.D.
Associate Professor of Medicine
Oregon Health Sciences University
Director, Cancer Research
Earle A. Chiles Research Institute
Portland, Oregon, U.S.A.
Chapter 5

CONTRIBUTORS

Theresa L. Whiteside, Ph.D.
Professor of Pathology and Otolaryngology
University of Pittsburgh
Pittsburgh, Pennsylvania, U.S.A.
Chapter 10

Ichiro Yoshino, M.D.
Chapter 2

Arnold H. Zea, M.Sc.
Immunotherapy Laboratory
Biological Response Modifiers Program
Frederick Cancer Research and Development Center
National Cancer Institute
Frederick, Maryland, U.S.A.
Chapter 5

PREFACE

The sentinel observations made by William B. Coley in the 1890s that patients with solid tumors could respond to the intratumoral inoculation of live bacterial organisms lead to the hypothesis that the host immune response is capable of eradicating cancer. Despite these fascinating clinical responses, it has taken nearly one hundred years to understand even the most fundamental mechanisms involved in the establishment of immunity to cancer. The development of current immunologically based therapies of cancer stems from Coley's early observations. Immunologic approaches to the treatment of malignancy can be broadly classified into either active or passive immunotherapies. With active immunotherapy, treatment relies on the in vivo stimulation of the endogenous host immune system to react against tumor antigens with the administration of biological response modifying agents such as bacterial adjuvants, tumor vaccines or cytokines. With passive immunotherapy, treatment involves the delivery of immunologic reagents with demonstrated anti-tumor reactivity such as antibodies or cells. The transfer of immune cells to the host with established malignancy is known as "adoptive immunotherapy" and has become more feasible with our increased understanding regarding immune recognition of immune cells to tumor antigens. The realization that human cancers can be responsive to the manipulation of the cellular component of the immune system has only recently been demonstrated in clinical trials.

This book will highlight several key subjects by investigators in the field of cellular therapy which summarize our current knowledge and identify prospects for future investigations. The principles for much of what we understand about cellular therapy have been derived from experimental animal studies. Utilizing transplantable tumors in inbred animals, researchers have clearly demonstrated that the immune rejection of localized or disseminated tumors can be mediated by the passive transfer of appropriately sensitized lymphoid cells. Moreover, the therapeutic efficacy of these sensitized cells is directly related to the number of cells transferred and requires the cells to be syngeneic to the host. However, unlike experimental animal systems, humans do not have readily available syngeneic counterparts to obtain immune cells. Tumor-reactive lymphoid cells will have to be identified and isolated from the patient with cancer. Furthermore, to generate sufficient quantities of immune cells, in vitro methods to activate and expand these cells while maintaining their immunological reactivities are required to render clinical therapy feasible. Different sources of immune lymphoid cells are described in this book including lymphoid cells infiltrating progressive solid tumors (i.e., tumor-infiltrating lymphocytes) lymphoid cells derived from tumor-draining lymph nodes or vaccine-primed lymph nodes and lymphoid cells derived from the peripheral blood. In addition, several different in vitro methods of activating and expanding these lymphoid cells are described that include the use of cytokines, monoclonal antibodies to T cell epitopes, pharmacologic agents and bacterial superantigens.

The results of clinical trials of cellular therapy from different institutions are also reviewed in this book. Although these efforts represent the "state-of-the-art", the collective experience should also be viewed as "testing the waters" and can only be considered the beginning. Important to improving the success of this approach will be an understanding of the cellular interactions which are required to mediate an effective anti-tumor response. To date, the interactions between T cell subpopulations which can be broadly categorized into "helper" or $CD4^+$ cells versus "cytotoxic" or $CD8^+$ cells are complex and may differ according to the experimental or clinical models as illustrated by these discussions. Another area of interest has been the role of cytokines elaborated by immune lymphoid cells which is reviewed in several chapters and clearly represents an important mechanism leading to successful tumor immunotherapy. Lastly, another phenomenon which is not clearly understood is the existence of tumor-induced immunosuppression that may interfere with the sensitization of lymphoid cells or their ability to mediate anti-tumor effects. Tumor-induced suppression of the immune response appears to be manifested by a variety of mechanisms as described by several investigators. Methods to abrogate these suppression mechanisms may also improve the efficacy of T cell therapies. As this field evolves, it is anticipated that cellular therapy will become an important modality in the treatment of malignancy.

Alfred E. Chang
and
Suyu Shu

CHAPTER 1

Tumor-Draining Lymph Nodes as a Source for Generating Therapeutic Immune T Cells

Suyu Shu, Scott E. Strome, John C. Krauss
Gregory E. Plautz, Alfred E. Chang

INTRODUCTION

Early studies performed in rodents with chemically induced syngeneic transplantable tumors demonstrated that the host immune system had the potential to specifically recognize and reject malignant cells.[1,2] Studies during the ensuing decades elucidated the remarkable heterogeneity of tumor antigens expressed on chemically induced tumor cells, with each individual tumor expressing an apparently unique tumor antigen capable of eliciting recognition of itself but not other similarly induced tumors. It was soon realized that even tumors induced by RNA and DNA oncogenic viruses expressed transplantation antigens.[3] However, unlike chemically induced tumors, virus-induced tumor antigens were shared by neoplasms caused by the same virus and were different from neoplasms caused by different viruses. These demonstrations of the presence of tumor-specific transplantation antigens implied that manipulation of the immune system might prevent and regulate the outgrowth of tumor cells.

Attempts to utilize immunologic manipulations to control neoplastic growth may logically be categorized into two different approaches based on scientific principles and procedures. Active immunotherapy involves the direct stimulation of the host immune system for eliciting an anti-tumor response. In the 1970s, a popular approach focused on attempts to provide nonspecific immune stimulation of the cancer patient

Immunotherapy of Cancer with Sensitized T Lymphocytes, edited by Alfred E. Chang and Suyu Shu.

with the intention to concurrently enhance immunity to the growing tumor. The results of many clinical trials have been published and with the possible exception of the injection of BCG into dermal metastatic lesions of melanoma, this approach has, in general, not demonstrated efficacy for treatment of cancer.[4] A more specific form of active immunotherapy is the use of tumor-associated antigens to immunize a tumor-bearing individual. Although active specific immunotherapy has been attempted for more than two decades with limited clinical success, interest in this form of therapy has been rekindled by the recent development of recombinant DNA technology. The direct modification of tumor cells using cytokine or other genes as a strategy to enhance tumor immunogenicity for active immunization has been intensively studied in animals over the last several years. In many situations, the expression of certain cytokines, notably IL-2 and IFNγ by tumor cells rendered them less tumorigenic and capable of augmenting T cell-mediated immunity.[5] However, vaccination of mice with genetically modified tumor cells to promote the regression of existing tumor has been less successful.

The second category of immunotherapy is termed passive immunotherapy. Passive immunotherapy refers to approaches in which immunologic reagents such as sera, cells, or cell products that are thought to have anti-tumor activities are administered to a tumor-bearing host. The use of immune sera or antibodies for the immunotherapy of malignant disease has been referred to as passive immunization. With the development of monoclonal antibody (mAb) technology, efforts have evolved with the goals of generating specific antibodies to membrane antigens expressed on tumor cells, and modification of these antibodies through conjugation with toxins or radionuclides to render them more effective in tumor cell killing.[6] The subject of immunotherapy with antibodies, however, is outside the scope of this review and will not be discussed further.

Passive immunotherapy with sensitized lymphoid cells, referred to as adoptive immunotherapy, is theoretically attractive as an approach to the treatment of cancer. In animal studies, cell transfer experiments clearly identified the cellular arm of the immune response as crucial in mediating the rejection of syngeneic tumors.[7] However, in most experiments, a common requirement for successful therapy has been the use of syngeneic lymphocytes from animals that have been hyperimmunized to the tumor. This requirement gives little provision for the development of human adoptive immunotherapy because humans usually do not have a syngeneic counterpart available for immunization and cell donation. Recent developments have identified several promising sources of cells obtainable from animals bearing progressively growing tumors which, following in vitro stimulation and expansion, demonstrated potent anti-tumor effects. This chapter describes our efforts to develop an adoptive immunotherapy approach, based on the ability to identify, isolate and expand lymphocytes from tumor-bearing animals. Some of the principles and methodologies established in animal models have been successfully extrapolated to the clinical trials for treatment of metastatic melanoma and renal cell carcinoma.

PRINCIPLES OF ADOPTIVE IMMUNOTHERAPY

The ability to immunize normal, healthy, tumor-free animals against subsequent tumor challenge has had no direct application to the eradication of growing neoplasms in cancer patients, but it has helped dissect important immunologic components involved in the immune response to autochthonous tumors. Early studies with experimental animal tumors have shown that the transfer of tumor immunity with sensitized cells can prevent the outgrowth of an inoculated tumor, but such a transfer is rarely effective as therapy for established tumor masses. Although therapeutic efficacy can be improved with increased numbers of transferred cells or with repeated infusion of immune cells, established tumors are often refractory to the adoptive immunotherapy.[8] It was subsequently discovered that growing tumors could interfere with adoptive T cell therapy by inducing cells and soluble factors that prevented the action of transferred immunity. Many aspects of the suppression phenomenon represent nonspecific biologic effects on the immune system from a metabolically active growing tumor, which in most cases, correlates with the extent of the tumor burden. Another mechanism by which a growing tumor can subvert the expression of adoptively transferred immune cells is through the induction of antigenically specific T suppressor cells. The detrimental effects of suppressor T cells to the transferred tumor immunity has been clearly illustrated by North's studies with many immunogenic tumors.[9] In their studies, the transfer of specific immune T cells into immunologically intact tumor-bearing hosts was not therapeutically effective. However, if tumor-bearing animals were previously rendered T cell deficient by thymectomy followed by lethal irradiation and reconstitution with T-cell-depleted bone marrow cells, adoptive immunotherapy resulted in complete eradication of an established tumor. The significance of suppressor T cells was confirmed in experiments in which the efficacy of the transferred immune T cells in T cell deficient hosts was completely inhibited by the concurrent infusion of T cells derived from tumor-bearing intact animals. Subsequently, it was demonstrated that cyclophosphamide treatment or sublethal irradiation were equally effective in eliminating the function of suppressor T cells in tumor-bearing animals and facilitating adoptive immunotherapy.[10,11]

It thus appears that the elimination of host suppressor cells is crucial for successful therapy. However, close scrutiny of animal tumor model systems in which tumor-induced specific immunologic suppression was documented revealed a common feature associated with all experimental procedures. The tumors to be treated by the adoptive immunotherapy were invariably located in the skin as a result of intradermal or subcutaneous transplantation. In the early 1980s, experimental solid tumor metastases, which typically represented sarcomas, renal cell carcinomas and melanomas that were established by intravenous inoculation and had a tendency to colonize in the lung or liver, gained popularity as a model system for the study of adoptive immunotherapy. We therefore compared the effect of tumor-induced suppression on the adoptive therapy of established visceral tumors to subcutaneous tumors. With the use of two newly-induced immunogenic sarcomas, MCA 105 and MCA 106, we were able to demonstrate and confirm the presence of functional suppressor T cells in animals bearing subcutaneous tumors and the adoptive immunotherapy with specific immune T cells was effective only if the recipient mice were treated with whole-body irradiation (500 cGy) or rendered T cell depletion.[12,13] However, the therapeutic efficacy of the transferred immune cells for the treatment of pulmonary or hepatic metastases was demonstrated in immunologically intact as well as in sublethally irradiated tumor-bearing animals. There were two possible interpretations to these results; the inability of visceral tumor metastases to induce suppressor cells or a lack of influence of the suppresser cells on tumors located in visceral organs. To distinguish between these two possibilities, we initiated subcutaneous and pulmonary tumor growth concurrently in the same animals. In intact tumor-bearing mice, adoptive immunotherapy was capable of eliminating pulmonary metastases, whereas dermal tumor growth was refractory to the transferred immune cells.[13] It thus became apparent that the function of host-derived suppression to adoptive immunotherapy was not a universal phenomenon.

Tumor-induced specific immunologic suppression is obviously an important subject to consider in the development of immunotherapy in general and adoptive immunotherapy in particular. However, in spite of numerous demonstrations of the phenomenon of T cell-mediated suppression in a variety of experimental systems, the lack of definitive cellular markers of suppressor cells and of molecular characterization of suppression makes it difficult to elucidate mechanistic details. Recent demonstration of the interplay between two types of T helper cells, Th1 and Th2, suggests that T cell suppression of a desired response may reflect a preferential activation of the alternate T helper subpopulation.[14]

Clinical therapeutic immunology has had its greatest impact in the prevention of infectious diseases. Investigations into the potential efficacy of immune therapy for established infectious diseases was abruptly curtailed by the development of antibiotics. Therefore, the most obvious question to be asked is "will immunotherapy be effective against clinically relevant tumor burden?" A common proffered answer is that specific immunity can only cope with minimal tumor burdens. In almost all animal tumor models, in spite of the elimination of the host suppressor T cells, there is a close relationship between tumor burden and the number of immune cells needed to observe an anti-tumor response. This quantitative relationship has been best illustrated in immunoprophylaxis studies where inoculation of tumor and infusion of immune cells were performed concurrently. Working with the guinea pig line-10 hepatocellular carcinoma, we have established an in vivo quantitative relationship between the number of infused immune spleen cells and that of tumor cells resulting in 50% cure.[15] To our surprise, the efficacy of tumor eradication by adoptive immunity did not follow an arithmetic ratio but rather appeared to be an exponential function of increasing numbers of immune cells; i.e., a twofold increment of immune cells led to an increased resistance of approximately 6-fold in the tumor challenge doses. While this finding provides some additional optimism to the potential of adoptive immunotherapy it is generally agreed that the greatest therapeutic efficacy may be obtained in the treatment of low tumor burden. Several nonimmunologic approaches may be used to reduce tumor burden to augment the benefit of cellular therapy. For example, surgical resection of large growing primary tumors could facilitate an effective immunotherapy with immune cells. Alternatively, cytoreductive chemotherapeutic drugs may be used in conjunction with adoptive immunotherapy to achieve therapeutic effects.

The principles of adoptive immunotherapy discussed above are mainly established from animal studies in which immune effector T cells can be conveniently generated by hyperimmunization of the syngeneic donor animals. One essential requirement for the development of adoptive immunotherapy for the treatment of human malignancies is therefore, the identification and isolation of tumor immune T cells from cancer patients. Since cancer patients might represent immunologically "pre-selected" groups for whom sufficient tumor reactive T cells have failed to develop, it is anticipated that cells directly isolated from patients might be few in number and weak in tumor reactivity. Therefore, clinical adoptive immunotherapy will likely require the development of in vitro methods for sensitization and expansion of tumor-reactive cells to large enough numbers for therapeutic purposes. The discovery of interleukin-2 (IL-2, previously termed T cell growth factor) seemed to have provided a means for circumventing the obstacle of inadequate cell numbers.[16] In several animal models, addition of IL-2 to the medium allowed the long-term culture of activated T cells with maintenance of their specific immunologic reactivities.[17,18]

In summary, the preponderance of data accumulated over the past decades supports the notion that cellular mechanisms are important and can be exploited for inhibiting tumor growth. The theoretical insights and recent experimental findings have engendered significant enthusiasm for expanded efforts to provide clinical adoptive immunotherapy with tumor-specific T cells. However, there are many important issues to be resolved before adoptive immunotherapy can be made more effective.

These issues include a better understanding of basic T cell immunology in tumor antigen recognition, effector cell generation and immunologic mechanisms underlying in vivo tumor eradication. Investigation of these issues will require the use of animal tumor models in which individual immunologic parameters can be isolated and assessed independently. In the remainder of this chapter, we will review studies—performed mainly in our laboratory—that are relevant to the identification and characterization of the immunologic reactivities of T cells isolated from animals bearing progressively growing tumors. Such model systems likely represent a prototypic approach to the development of clinical adoptive immunotherapy.

CHARACTERISTICS OF IMMUNE EFFECTOR T CELLS ISOLATED FROM LYMPH NODES DRAINING A PRIMARY TUMOR

There are many potential sources of cells readily obtainable from cancer patients that may serve the function of tumor-reactive effector cells. One approach that has received a great deal of attention in the past several years has been the generation of lymphokine-activated killer (LAK) cells from peripheral blood leukocytes incubated in high doses of IL-2.[19] These LAK cells preferentially lyse tumor targets while sparing normal cells. The infusion of autologous LAK cells with concurrent administration of IL-2 into cancer patients has had therapeutic benefit in some patients, but such treatment is frequently toxic and effector cells lack several of the most attractive qualities of T lymphocytes such as immunologic specificity and memory. Clearly, the generation of specific tumor-sensitized T cells is more complicated than that of LAK cells. Studies in animal tumor models have suggested that leukocytes infiltrating a tumor mass (tumor-infiltrating lymphocytes or TIL) may be enriched with tumor-reactive T cells.[20,21] Similarly, TIL from human cancers expanded in vitro, have often demonstrated specific cytotoxicity for autologous tumor cells[22] Several clinical trials which utilized TIL in adoptive immunotherapy for a variety of metastatic cancers, demonstrated the greatest success in the treatment of malignant melanoma.[23]

In the past few years, we have been interested in utilizing the regional draining lymph nodes (LN) as an alternative source for generating tumor-reactive effector cells. Our interest in the local LN stemmed from findings of early studies demonstrating the significance of changes in local lymphoid tissue during the induction of delayed hypersensitivity.[24] In inbred guinea pigs, the induction of contact sensitivity to DNCB was found to be crucially dependent on intact regional draining LN. As late as 4 days after sensitization, removal of the LN prevented the manifestation of sensitization while the area of skin on which a chemical sensitizer had been painted was only necessary for 16-24 hours. The essential role draining LN played was confirmed by the observation that methotrexate was only capable of blocking the development of contact sensitivity if given on or before the fourth day after sensitization, the day the animal began to show the earliest sign of sensitivity. These findings indicate that some major event must have occurred before the development of a generalized state of sensitivity.

Exploiting the selective inhibitory effect of methotrexate on the primary immune response, we established that the development of systemic anti-tumor immunity to the syngeneic line-10 guinea pig hepatoma required at least 8 days because a course of methotrexate started as late as 8 days after initial immunization would block the sensitization.[25] In this animal model, removal of the skin site of immunization 24 hours after immunization had no impact on the development of immunity. However, systemic immunity to the line 10 tumor would not develop when surgical excision of the draining LN was performed up to 8 days after immunization. Single cell suspensions prepared from the nodes draining the immunization site for 8 days were transferred intravenously into normal recipient guinea pigs but no animal developed immunity. These results clearly demonstrated the significance of intact draining LN for the induction of a primary anti-tumor immune response. Although there are some differences in the kinetics, similar findings were also documented in a murine fibrosarcoma, MCA 105.[26]

The lack of induction of protective immunity during progressive growth of an antigenic tumor may be explained by several possible reasons such as insufficient antigen presentation, insufficient cytokine production and the occurrence of inhibitory regulatory circuits. Considering the crucial role that draining LN play in the induction of a primary immune response, it is possible that the tumor-draining LN could be the target site of these deficiencies. We therefore hypothesized that tumor reactive T cells can be isolated from the regional draining LN and the in vivo limitations to their development may be overcome by in vitro stimulation. In addition, conditions can be manipulated to generate large numbers of effector cells with greater efficacy for therapeutic purposes.

To test this hypothesis, we initiated primary tumor growth in the footpad of mice by inoculation with the weakly immunogenic MCA 105 sarcoma cells. Initial experiments were carried out to assess the in vivo anti-tumor reactivity of freshly isolated tumor-draining LN cells. In two experiments (Table 1. 1), the transfer of as many as 6×10^7 draining LN (popliteal) cells to mice with 3-day established pulmonary MCA 105 metastases did not result in a significant reduction of metastatic nodules. The same LN cells were also stimulated in vitro according to the previously described in vitro sensitization (IVS) method with irradiated tumor cells in the presence of IL-2.[27] This method allowed a 3- to 7-fold cell expansion in 9 days of culture and the transfer of these IVS LN cells into mice bearing 3-day pulmonary metastases mediated the regression of tumors (Table 1.2). Treatment with as few as 2×10^7 IVS cells resulted in a significant reduction of metastatic nodules in the lung.[28,29] Since the IVS cells initiated with normal lymphoid cells did not have an anti-tumor effect, the induction of therapeutic lymphocytes reflects a secondary in vitro immune response. These findings suggested the existence of "pre-effector" cells in the regional LN during progressive tumor growth. Although they lack inherent reactivity, these pre-effector cells can differentiate during IVS, into mature effector cells capable of mediating in vivo anti-tumor effects.

Table 1.1. Adoptive immunotherapy of established pulmonary MCA 105 metastases with freshly harvested lymphoid cells from mice bearing progressively growing tumors: lack of therapeutic efficacy

Donor and source of lymphoid cells[a]	Mean no. metastases (SEM)[b] Exp. 1	Exp. 2
–	136 (33)	72 (23)
Normal spleens	127 (37)	72 (28)
MCA 105 immune spleens	2 (1)[c]	5 (1)[c]
11 to 12 day tumor-bearing lymph nodes	102 (28)	26 (12)
14 to 16 day tumor-bearing lymph nodes	86 (26)	27 (12)

[a] C57BL/6 mice were inoculated with 5×10^5 MCA 105 tumor cells into the footpad. Spleens and lymph nodes (popliteal) were harvested for cellular therapy 11 to 16 d later. Each mouse that had been injected IV 3 days previously with 5×10^5 MCA 105 tumor cells was given IV 1.5×10^8 spleen cells or 6×10^7 lymph node cells.
[b] Lungs were harvested and metastases counted on days 14 to 16.
[c] Significantly different from groups without treatment (Wilcoxon rank-sum test).

The principles and methodology established from the animal experimentation have been extrapolated to a clinical trial where patients with metastatic melanoma or renal cell carcinoma were vaccinated with autologous tumor cells admixed with the bacterial adjuvant, BCG. LN draining the vaccination site were resected for IVS culture, and the resulting cells were infused back to the patients. We were able to demonstrate that the majority of the patients (7/9) developed delayed hypersensitivity skin reactions to the autologous tumor cells after cell transfer.[30] However, tumor responses were limited probably due to insufficient numbers of cells transferred to the patients.

ANTI-CD3 ACTIVATION OF TUMOR-DRAINING LYMPH NODE CELLS FOR ADOPTIVE IMMUNOTHERAPY

The generation of immune effector cells by the IVS method for adoptive immunotherapy requires a large number of viable autologous tumor cells to provide specific antigen stimulation.[29] In the clinical setting, this requirement becomes a serious impediment because of the high variability in yield of viable tumor cells between patients. Antigenic stimulation of T cells involves the signal transduction through the T cell antigen receptor (TCR)/CD3 complex. In the absence of antigen, mAb reactive to CD3 molecules have been shown to induce T cell proliferation and lymphokine production.[31] We therefore examined the feasibility of using anti-CD3 as a universal stimulus for the activation of pre-effector cells in the draining LN.

In a series of experiments, we identified a two-step method of T cell activation by anti-CD3 and IL-2 which would allow the greatest cell expansion.[32,33] This procedure involved the stimulation of tumor-draining LN cells with an mAb against the CD3ε chain of the murine TCR/CD3 complex (145-2C11, ref. 34) for 2 days followed by culture in low concentrations of IL-2 (e.g. 10U/ml) for 3 days.[32] With the use of soluble mAb, this procedure induced a cell expansion up to 5-fold in 5 days. Recently, increased cell growth was observed if LN cells were stimulated with anti-CD3 immobilized on plastic surface of the culture vehicle. Although, freshly obtained LN contain approximately 35% T cells, by 5 days, the activated cells were virtually all T cells with ~75% CD8 and 25% CD4 cells.

The in vivo anti-tumor reactivity of the anti-CD3/IL-2 activated tumor-draining LN cells was assessed first in the adoptive immunotherapy of 3-day established pulmonary MCA 106 metastases. In repeated experi-

Table 1.2. Adoptive immunotherapy of established pulmonary MCA 105 metastases with in vitro sensitized lymphoid cells from mice bearing progressively growing tumors

		Adoptive immunotherapy	
		Mean no. metastases (SEM)[c]	
Donor and source of lymphoid cells for IVS[a]	In vivo IL-2[b]	Exp. 1	Exp. 2
–	–	156 (40)	200 (36)
–	+	171 (51)	250
Normal spleen	+	91 (46)	115 (45)
MCA 105 immune spleens	+	1 (1)[d]	11 (8)[d]
14 to 16 day tumor-bearing lymph nodes	+	2 (1)[d]	10 (7)[d]

[a] C57BL/6 mice were inoculated with 5 x 10^5 MCA 105 tumor cells into the footpad. Spleens and lymph nodes (popliteal) were harvested 14 to 16 days later. These cells were cultured by the IVS procedure for 9 days and were given IV 2 x 10^7 to each recipient mouse that had been injected IV 3 days previously with 5 x 10^5 MCA 105 tumor cells.

[b] Recombinant IL-2 (7,500 U) diluted in 0.5 ml of HBSS was given IP twice a day for 4 d after cell transfer.

[c] Lungs were harvested and metastases counted on days 14 to 16.

[d] Significantly different from groups without treatment or treated with IL-2 alone (Wilcoxon rank-sum test).

ments, the IV transfer of 2 x 10^7 activated cells alone could mediate potent anti-tumor effects. As few as 6 x 10^6 cells were found to be highly effective if exogenous IL-2 was also administered to the tumor-bearing animals.[33] To further evaluate the therapeutic efficacy of the anti-CD3/IL-2 activated cells, adoptive immunotherapy was initiated 10 days after tumor inoculation when pulmonary metastases were clearly visible. Mice received no treatment or treated with IL-2 (15000 U, twice/day for 5 days) only succumbed to the growing tumors with median survival time of 30-31 days (Fig. 1.1). Mice treated with 8 x 10^7 activated cells in conjunction with IL-2 treatment demonstrated a prolonged survival (median survival time of 50 days) and 7 of 20 treated animals were cured.[32]

Anti-CD3 has been known to induce T cell activation irrespective of the antigenic specificity. However, the activated LN cells were immunologically specific, against the tumor that stimulated the pre-effector cells in vivo. In a criss-cross experiment, cells from LN draining the MCA 106 or MCA 205 tumors were tested against pulmonary metastases established from the two tumors. The results clearly demonstrated immunologic specificity (Table 1.3) and are consistent with the notion that anti-CD3/IL-2 activation represented a secondary immune activation in vitro.[32,33]

In addition to the MCA 106 and MCA 205 tumors, we have demonstrated the therapeutic efficacy of the activated cells for the treatment of three additional antigenically distinct MCA sarcomas including MCA 105, MCA 203 and MCA 207 (Table 1.4). Also included in Table 1.4 are two poorly immunogenic murine tumors, MCA 102 and B16/BL6 melanoma. These two tumors failed to elicit systemic immunity in syngeneic mice by a variety of immunization procedures, and there was no evidence that pre-effector cells were sensitized during progressive tumor growth. How-

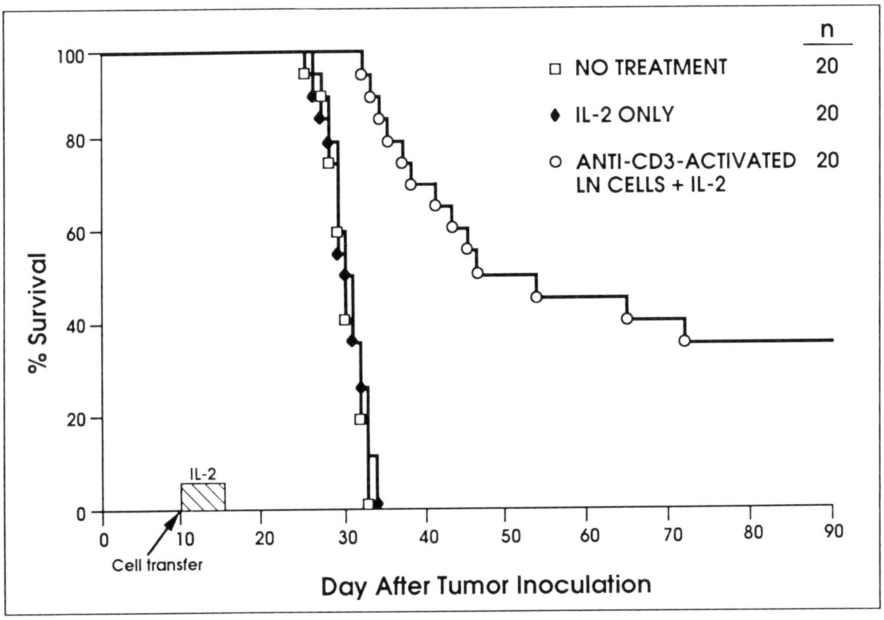

Fig. 1.1. Adoptive immunotherapy of mice with advanced pulmonary MCA 106 metastases. This figure summarizes the combined results of two independent but identically designed experiments. Pulmonary metastases were induced by the IV injection of 10^5 MCA 106 tumor cells. Ten days later, when metastatic nodules were clearly visible, therapy was instituted by IV infusion of 8 x 10^7 anti-CD3/IL-2 activated tumor-draining LN cells. The dose of IL-2 was 15,000 U given ip twice daily, for 5 days. Treatment with activated LN cells and IL-2 resulted in a significant prolongation of survival ($P < 0.05$, Wilcoxon rank sum test).

Table 1.3. Specificity of adoptive immunotherapy mediated by anti-CD3/IL-2-activated tumor-draining LN cells

Source of cells for anti-CD3/IL-2 activation	Adoptive Immunotherapy[b]		
		Mean no. pulmonary metastases (SEM)[c]	
	IL-2	MCA 106	MCA 205
	–	250	250
	+	250	250
LN draining MCA 106[a]	+	0[d]	226 (10)
LN draining MCA 205[a]	+	250	53 (15)[d]

[a] Cells from LN draining intrafootpad MCA 106 or s.c. MCA 205 tumors for 14 days were activated by the anti-CD3/IL-2 culture method.
[b] B6 mice were injected IV with 10^6 MCA 106 or 3 x 10^5 MCA 205 tumor cells to initiate pulmonary metastases. On day 3, activated LN cells (2 x 10^7) were given IV to each mouse. Mice were also treated with IL-2 (15,000) IP twice a day for 4 days.
[c] Lungs were harvested and metastases counted 24 days after tumor inoculation.
[d] Significantly different from groups with no treatment or treated with IL-2 only.

Table 1.4. Therapeutic effect of anti-CD3/IL-2 activated cells in the treatment of immunogenic and nonimmunogenic murine tumors

	Mean no. pulmonary metastases (SEM)[a]				
		Immunogenic		Nonimmunogenic	
Treatment	MCA 105	MCA 203	MCA 207	MCA 102	B16/BL6
None	224 (14)	250	238 (11)	209 (23)	250
IL-2	250	240 (9)	239 (11)	243 (6)	209 (36)
Cells + IL-2	1 (1)	1 (1)	43 (13)	34 (9)	1 (1)

[a] Mice with 3-day established pulmonary metastases were treated by IV transfer of anti-CD3/IL-2 activated lymph node cells draining immunogenic tumors or draining inoculations of nonimmunogenic tumor cells plus *C. parvum* for 9-14 days. IL-2 (15,000 U) was given IP twice daily for 4 days. Two to 5 x 107 cells were given IV to each mouse.

ever, a pre-effector cell response could be artificially induced by inoculating mice with a mixture of tumor cells and the bacterial adjuvant, *C. parvum*. The process of utilizing anti-CD3 for activating T cells has been adapted to modify the previous IVS cell clinical protocol. Some preliminary results of this study are discussed elsewhere in this monograph.

SELECTIVE ACTIVATION OF ANTI-TUMOR T CELLS WITH MICROBIAL SUPERANTIGENS OR mAb

The development of the anti-CD3/IL-2 method for activation of anti-tumor effector T cells has expanded the utility of adoptive immunotherapy for the clinical treatment of cancer. Although the anti-CD3/IL-2 cells displayed exquisite specificity, the polyclonal nature of anti-CD3 interactions must have also predisposed the culture system to the generation of a significant proportion of T cells with irrelevant specificity. A theoretically more practical approach would be the use of reagents capable of selectively activating the subsets of T cells responsible for mediating the desired immune response. In the absence of chemically defined tumor-specific rejection antigens, specific T cell activation was not feasible. However, recent investigations have uncovered a family of potent T cell activating molecules, denoted as superantigens.[35] In contrast to mitogens or conventional antigens, superantigens bind to MHC class II molecules to form ligands that interact with TCR of distinct variable regions of β chain (Vβ). Among the best studied superantigens are toxins produced by gram positive bacteria such as staphylococci and streptococci. We have recently examined several enterotoxins produced by *Staphylococcus aureus* for their ability to stimulate tumor-draining LN cells. MCA 205 draining LN cells stimulated with staphylococcal enterotoxins A (SEA), B (SEB) and C2 (SEC2) resulted in selective expansion of Vβ3 and 11, Vβ3 and 8.1-3, and Vβ8.2 T cells, respectively.[36,37] In adoptive immunotherapy experiments, both SEB and SEC2 activated cells were found to mediate potent anti-tumor effects whereas SEA activated cells were not therapeutically effective (Table 1.5).

The differences in anti-tumor reactivities between T cells activated by different superantigens may reflect the distinct T cell subsets responding to these superantigens. Since multiple Vβ T cells were generated in response to SEB stimulation, we have analyzed the relative contributions of different Vβ T cells by depletion with immunomagnetic beads.[37] In repeated experiments, the elimination of Vβ3 cells resulted in enhancement of therapeutic efficacy while depletion of Vβ8 T cells resulted in a decrease of anti-tumor reactivity. These results suggest that T cells bearing the Vβ8 element constitute the majority of the anti-tumor reactivity and the absence of Vβ8 T cells in SEA stimulated cultures might have contributed to their poor anti-tumor effects. However, since depletion of Vβ8 T cells did not eliminate the entire anti-tumor reactivity and since there was a significant proportion of cells which were non-Vβ3, non-Vβ8, other T cells might have also been involved in the response to growing tumor.

To further delineate whether there are preferential TCR usages in the immune response to malignant tumors, we explored the possibility of activating tumor-draining LN with Vβ specific mAb. Seven mAb specific for TCR Vβ3, 5, 7, 8.1-3, 8.1-2, and 8.2 were analyzed. Tumor-draining LN cells to the murine MCA 205 sarcoma were stimulated with immobilized mAb for 2 days followed by culture in a low concentration (4 U/ml) of recombinant IL-2 for 3 days. Following this 5-day activation, flow cytometric analyses of T cells revealed that each mAb stimulated the proliferation of its corresponding T cells, resulting in ≥ 58% of T cells bearing the Vβ elements. In adoptive immunotherapy of 3-day established pulmonary MCA 205 metastases, significant differences in therapeutic effects among different cells were observed. Cells stimulated with Vβ8.1-2 (MR5.2; Ref. 38) and Vβ 8.1-3 (F23.1; ref. 39) mediated the

Table 1.5. Therapeutic effects of bacterial superantigen-activated tumor-draining lymph node cells

Treatment		Mean no. pulmonary MCA 205 metastases (SEM)[a] Superantigen use for cell activation[b]		
Cells	Interleukin-2	SEA	SEB	SEC2
0	–	250	250	250
0	+	250	250	213 (38)
12 x 10^6	+	242 (7)	3 (2)	1 (1)
6 x 10^6	+	250	19 (10)	103 (29)

[a]Pulmonary metastases were initiated by IV injection of C57BL/6 mice with 3 x 10^5 MCA 205 tumor cells. Three days later, activated cells were given IV and interleukin-2 (15,000 U twice/day) was administered IP for 4 days. Lungs were harvested and counted 21 days after tumor inoculation.
[b]Lymph node cells draining progressive MCA 205 for 12 days were activated

greatest (>90%) reduction in numbers of lung metastases, Vβ8.2 (F23.2; ref. 39) and Vβ5 (MR9.4; ref. 40) ≥ 50%, while Vβ3 (KJ25; ref. 41) and Vβ7 (TR310; ref. 42) activated LN T cells did not have significant therapeutic effects. These results indicate that stimulation of tumor-draining LN cells with some mAb is sufficient to activate immune effector cells. In this study, however, different Vβ mAb displayed different mitogenic activities for LN T cells and the in vivo anti-tumor effects of the activated cells seemed to reflect the mitogenic potency of the antibody used. Nevertheless, our studies clearly demonstrated that the selection of T cells in response to a growing tumor was not reflected in any simple predominance of Vβ usage. To support this notion, we have recently isolated and analyzed 33 T cell clones derived from the MCA 106 tumor-draining LN.[43] Of these 33 clones, 19 expressed Vβ13; 6 expressed Vβ11; and 6 expressed Vβ5. There were two clones whose Vβ phenotypes could not be identified by the available mAb. Virtually, all the clones were capable of mediating the regression of established MCA 106 tumor metastases when adoptively transferred. Despite this demonstration of multiple usage of Vβ elements in response to a single tumor, we have not seen the expression of Vβ2, 3, 6, 7,9 and 14 on anti-tumor effector T cells. The complexity of TCR usage in the anti-tumor immune response may result from the involvement of multiple α and β chain regions of the TCR in response to a single antigenic epitope, or may reflect multiple antigenic determinants expressed on a single tumor. A more definitive answer to this question may only be sought when chemically and molecularly defined tumor antigens become available.

SUMMATION AND FUTURE PERSPECTIVES

Adoptive immunotherapy is an approach to cancer treatment in which tumor-bearing hosts are infused with tumor-sensitized immune T lymphocytes. Principles and insights for the development of adoptive immunotherapy for the treatment of human malignancy have mainly been defined in studies using animal models. In this chapter, we have chronologically reviewed key experimental findings mostly from our own laboratory on the development of adoptive immunotherapy procedures that may be applicable to the treatment of human patients. Based on methodology developed in animal models, two clinical trials have been initiated. Preliminary clinical data on these trials is presented separately in chapter 12.

The use of tumor-draining LN cells as a source of anti-tumor effector cells has enabled successful adoptive immunotherapy in several tumor models. However, the potential anti-tumor reactivity of the draining LN fluctuates depending on the duration of tumor growth.[28] Moreover, the sensitization of draining LN is weak and often insufficient during the normal growth of poorly immunogenic tumors, but can be enhanced with the use of bacterial adjuvants such as *C. parvum*.[44,45] Because of these considerations, the source of lymphocytes in our clinical trials has been from LN draining a vaccination consisting of autologous tumor cells and BCG. Therefore, one of the major goals of future development with regard to T cell therapy is the design of vaccines with increased ability to stimulate the regional LN immune response. One approach, which is already being pursued, is to modify the immunogenicity of tumor cells by the introduction of genes encoding for proteins having immunoregulatory functions. Tumor cells genetically modified to secrete a variety of lymphokines and cytokines have been intensively studied over the past several years. In many experimental systems, the introduction of cytokine genes into tumor cells results in decreased tumorigenicity with concomitant increase in immunogenicity.[46] However, few examples exist indicating that such genetically modified tumor cells can be used successfully as a "tumor vaccine" to treat established parental tumors. The ability of cytokine gene modified tumor cells to stimulate the sensitization of the pre-effector cells has not been thoroughly examined. This approach may prove to be more effective than the current use of BCG in our protocols.

Additional work is also required to improve the techniques for in vitro sensitization of the pre-effector cells. We have developed several methods for this purpose, but each of them has its own drawbacks or shortcomings. One major obstacle is the lack of molecularly defined tumor-specific antigens. Recent work by several groups has demonstrated that peptides and proteins encoded by normal nonmutated cellular genes such as MAGE in melanoma[47] and mucin core protein in pancreatic and breast carcinoma[48] can elicit cytotoxic lymphocyte responses in patients. The use of these defined proteins or peptides will surely provide a means to specifically stimulate the maturation of pre-effector cells in vitro. These are a few examples with which the efficacy of adoptive immunotherapy may be improved. The continued application of advances in cellular and molecular biology to the field of adoptive T cell immunotherapy of tumors should enhance our ability to generate potent immune effector T cells with anti-tumor reactivity. The approach of adoptive immunotherapy is only beginning to be explored and continues to hold promise for further effectiveness.

Acknowledgment

We wish to acknowledge Cetus Corporation, Emeryville, California for the generous gift of recombinant IL-2; Dr. Jeffrey A. Bluestone, University of Chicago, for providing the hybridoma (145-2C11) producing the anti-CD3 mAb; and Drs. O. Kanagawa, P. Marrack, D. H. Raulet and R.J. Hodes for gifts of Vβ mAb producing hybridomas. We also thank Dr. Raoul F. Reiser of the Toxin Technology, Inc., Sarasota, Florida, for preparations of SEA and SEB, and Ms. Debbie Birdsall for skillful secretarial assistance.

This work was supported by grants CA49231, CA58927 and CA64687 from the National Cancer Institute.

References

1. Foley EJ. Antigenic properties of methylcholanthrene-induced tumors in mice of the strain of origin. Cancer Res 13:835-837, 1953.
2. Prehn RT, Main JM. Immunity to methylcholanthrene-induced sarcomas. J Natl Cancer Inst 18:769-778, 1957.
3. Old LJ, Boyse EA. Antigens of tumors and leukemias induced by viruses. Fed Proc 24:1009-1016, 1965.
4. Klein E, Holtermann OA, Papermaster B et al. Immunologic approaches to various types of cancer with the use of BCG and purified protein derivatives. Natl Cancer Inst Monogr. 39:229-239, 1973.
5. McBride WH, Chiang CS, Dubinett SM, Economou JS, Thacher JD, Dougherly GD. Cytokine gene-mediated effects on tumorigenicity and tumor immunogenicity. Proc Annu Meet Am Assoc Cancer Res 34:A2765, 1993.
6. Dillman RO. Monoclonal antibodies for treating cancer. Ann Intern Med 111:592-603, 1989.
7. Rosenberg SA, Terry W. Passive immunotherapy of cancer in animals and man. Adv Cancer Res 25:323-388, 1977.
8. Fefer A, Einstein AB, Cheever MA, Berenson JR. Models for syngeneic adoptive chemoimmunotherapy of murine leukemias. Ann NY Acad Sci 276:573-583, 1976.
9. North RJ. Downregulation of the anti-tumor immune response. Adv Cancer Res 45:1-43, 1985.
10. Awwad, M, North RJ. Cyclophosphamide-induced immunologically mediated regression of a cyclophosphamide-resistant murine tumor: a consequence of eliminating precursor L3T4+ suppressor T cells. Cancer Res 49:1649-1654, 1989.
11. Awwad, M, North RJ. Radiosensitive barrier to T cell-mediated adoptive immunotherapy of established tumors. Cancer Res 50:2228-2233, 1990.
12. Shu, S, Rosenberg SA. Adoptive immunotherapy of newly induced murine sarcomas. Cancer Res 45:1657-1662, 1985.
13. Chang AE, Shu S, Chou T, Lafreniere R, Rosenberg SA. Difference in the effects of host suppression n the adoptive immuno-

therapy of subcutaneous and visceral tumors. Cancer Res 46:3426-3430, 1986.

14. Mosemann TR, Coffman RL. Th1 and Th2 cells: different patterns of lymphokine secretion lead to different functional properties. Ann Rev Immunol 7:145-173, 1989.
15. Shu S, Hunter JT, Rapp HJ, Fonseca LS. Mechanisms of immunologic eradication of a syngeneic guinea pig tumor. I. Quantitative analysis of adoptive immunity. J Natl Cancer Inst 68:673-680, 1982.
16. Morgan DA, Ruscetti FW, Gallop RC. Selective in vitro growth of T lymphocytes from normal human bone marrows. Science 193:1007-1008, 1976.
17. Cheever MA, Greenberg PD, Fefer A. Specific adoptive therapy of established leukemia with syngeneic lymphocytes sequentially sensitized in vivo and in vitro and nonspecifically expanded by culture with interleukin-2. J Immunol 126:1318-1322, 1981.
18. Eberlein TJ, Rosenstein, M, Rosenberg SA. Regression of a disseminated syngeneic solid tumor by systemic transfer of lymphoid cells expanded in interleukin-2. J Exp Med 156:385-397, 1982.
19. Rosenberg SA, Lotze MT. Cancer immunotherapy using interleukin-2 and interleukin-2 activated lymphocytes. Annu Rev Immunol 4:681-709, 1986.
20. Rosenberg SA, Spiess, P, Lafreniere R. A new approach to the adoptive immunotherapy of cancer with tumor-infiltrating lymphocytes. Science 233:1318-1321, 1986.
21. Spiess PJ, Yang JC, Rosenberg SA. In vivo anti-tumor activity of tumor-infiltrating lymphocytes expanded in recombinant interleukin-2. J Natl Cancer Inst 79:1067-1075, 1987.
22. Topalian SL, Solomon, D, Rosenberg SA. Tumor-specific cytolysis by lymphocytes infiltrating human melanomas. J Immunol 142:3714-3725, 1989.
23. Rosenberg SA, Packard BS, Aebersold PM, et al. Use of tumor infiltrating lymphocytes and interleukin-2 in the immunotherapy of patients with metastatic melanoma. A preliminary report. NEJM 319:1676-1680, 1988.
24. Turk JL. Delayed hypersensitivity. North-Holland Publishing Company, Amsterdam, 1967.
25. Shu S, Fonseca LS, Hunter JT, Rapp HJ. Mechanisms of immunologic eradication of a syngeneic guinea pig tumor. II. Effect of methotrexate treatment and T cell depletion of the recipient on adoptive immunity. Transpl 35:56-61, 1983.
26. Stephenson KR, Perry-Lalley DM, Shu, S, Chang AE. The role of regional lymph nodes (RLN) in the development of tumor immunity. Surg Forum 38:438-440, 1987.
27. Shu S, Chou, T, Rosenberg SA. In vitro sensitization and expansion with viable tumor cells and interleukin-2 in the generation of specific therapeutic effector cells. J Immunol 136:3891-3898, 1986.
28. Shu S, Chou, T, Rosenberg SA. Generation from tumor-bearing mice of lymphocytes with in vivo therapeutic efficacy. J Immunol 139:295-304, 1987.
29. Chou T, Chang AE, Shu S. Generation of therapeutic T lymphocytes from tumor-bearing mice by in vitro sensitization: Culture requirements and characterization of immunologic specificity. J Immunol 140:2453-2461, 1988.
30. Chang AE, Yoshizawa H, Sakai K, Cameron MJ, Sondak VK, Shu S. Clinical observations on adoptive immunotherapy with vaccine-primed T lymphocytes secondarily sensitized to tumor in vitro. Cancer Res 53:1043-1050, 1993.
31. Meuer SC, Hussey RE, Cantrell DA, Hodgdon JC, Schlossman SF, Smith KA. and Reinherz EL. Triggering of the T3-Ti antigen receptor complex results in clonal T cell proliferation through an interleukin 2 dependent autocrine pathway. Proc Natl Acad Sci USA 81:1509-1513, 1984.
32. Yoshizawa H, Sakai K, Chang AE, Shu S. Activation by anti-CD3 of tumor-draining lymph node cells for specific adoptive immunotherapy. Cell Immunol 134:473-479, 1991.
33. Yoshizawa H, Chang AE, Shu S. Specific adoptive immunotherapy mediated by tumor-draining lymph node cells sequentially activated with anti-CD3 and IL-2. J Immunol 147:729-737, 1991.
34. Leo O, Foo M, Sachs DH, Samelson LE,

Bluestone JA. Identification of a monoclonal antibody specific for murine T3 polypeptide. Proc Natl Acad Sci USA 84:1374-1378, 1987.

35. Marrack, P, Kappler J. The staphylococcal enterotoxins and their relatives. Science 248:705-711, 1990.
36. Shu S, Sussman JJ, Chang AE. In vivo antitumor efficacy of tumor-draining lymph node cells activated with nonspecific T cell reagents. J Immunother 14:279-285, 1993.
37. Shu S, Krinock RA, Matsumura T, Sussman JJ, Fox BA, Chang AE, Terman DS. Stimulation of tumor-draining lymph node cells with superantigenic staphylococcal toxins lead to the generation of tumor-specific effector cells. J Immunol 152:1277-1287, 1994.
38. Kanagawa O. Antibody mediated activation of T cell clones as a method for screening hybridomas producing Ab to the T cell receptor. J Immunol Meth 110:169-178, 1988.
39. Staerz U, Rammansee H, Benedetto, J, Bevan M. Characterization of a murine monoclonal antibody specific for an allotype determinant on T cell antigen receptor. J Immunol 134:3994-4000, 1985.
40. Reich EP, Sherwin RS, Kanagawa, O, Janeway CA, Jr. An explanation for the protective effect of MHC class II I-E molecule in murine diabetes. Nature 341:326-328, 1989.
41. Pullen AM, Marrack, P, Kappler JW. The T cell repertoire is heavily influenced by tolerance to polymorphic self-antigens. Nature 335:796-801, 1988.
42. Okada CY, Holzmann B, Guidos C, Palmer, E, Weissman EI. Characterization of a rat monoclonal antibody specific for a determinant encoded by the Vβ7 gene segment. J Immunol 144:3473-3477, 1990.
43. Matsumura T, Sussman JJ, Krinock RA, Chang AE, Shu S. Characteristics and in vivo homing of long-term T cell lines and clones derived from tumor-draining lymph nodes. Cancer Res 54:2744-2750, 1994.
44. Shu S, Chou, T, Sakai K. Lymphocytes generated by in vivo priming and in vitro sensitization demonstrate therapeutic efficacy against a murine tumor that lacks apparent immunogenicity. J Immunol 143:740-748, 1989.
45. Geiger JD, Wagner PD, Cameron MJ, Shu, S, Chang AE. Generation of T cells reactive to the poorly immunogenic B16-BL6 melanoma with efficacy in the treatment of spontaneous metastases. J Immunother 13:153-165, 1993.
46. Mulé JJ. Gene therapy for cancer: experimental studies of the gene-modification of tumor cells. Proc Annu Meet Am Assoc Cancer Res 34:581, 1993.
47. Van de Bruggen P, Traversari C, Chomez P, et al. A gene encoding an antigen recognized by cytolytic T lymphocytes on a human melanoma. Science 254:1643-1647, 1991.
48. Jerome KR, Barnd DL, Bendt KM, et al. Cytotoxic T lymphocytes derived from patients with breast adenocarcinoma recognize an epitope present on the protein core of a mucin molecule preferentially expressed by malignant cells. Cancer Res 51:2908-2916, 1991.

CHAPTER 2

CD3 Activation of Tumor-Infiltrating Lymphocytes

Timothy J. Eberlein, George E. Peoples, Ichiro Yoshino
Ulrike L. Burger, Kyung Lee, Hong Li
Linda M. Douville, Peter S. Goedegebuure

INTRODUCTION

At the beginning of this century, the first groundwork was laid for what is now known as biologic cancer therapy. Ehrlich proposed in 1909 that cells which are antigenically sufficiently distinct from normal cells are recognized by elements of the immune system and subsequently eliminated.[1] This theory, known as the immune surveillance theory, was later substantiated by others.[2,3] Failure of the host to mount an appropriate immune response allows the antigenically distinct cells to expand. Biologic cancer therapy is an attempt to boost the host's immune system and correct the imbalance between the immune system and the "foreign invaders". In the case of cancer, transformed normal cells often fail to induce an efficient anti-tumor response. A major goal of tumor immunology has been to document the existence of a host immune response to tumor with the expectation that certain elements of the immune response could be exploited therapeutically. Preclinical studies conducted over the past 10 years have confirmed that for some tumors, T cell immune responses are routinely provoked in the tumor-bearing host.[4-6] Melanoma, renal cell carcinoma (RCC) and ovarian carcinoma are recognized as examples of tumors that provoke T cell responses.[7-9] Our current biologic cancer therapy program attempts to treat cancer patients with T lymphocytes that have reacted to tumor in vivo (adoptive immunotherapy).

At the present time, human tumor-specific cytotoxic T lymphocytes (CTL) can be directly isolated from tumor (tumor-infiltrating lymphocytes

Immunotherapy of Cancer with Sensitized T Lymphocytes, edited by Alfred E. Chang and Suyu Shu.

(TIL))[10,11] or draining lymph nodes.[12] While clinical trials using TIL at some institutions have provided encouraging results, the experience at other institutions has been disappointing. There are several reasons that account for the poor results. First, patients are treated with T cell populations only if a sufficient number of cells have grown (usually >10^{10}). Since each culture possesses different numbers of $CD4^+$ and $CD8^+$ T cells, each patient receives a form of therapy that is based on the growth characteristics of the patients T cell culture rather than the functional traits of T cells required for tumor eradication. Second, most clinical protocols use high-dose IL-2 (≥ 1000 IU/ml) to grow the therapeutic T cells. As documented in several published articles, this method of T cell culture produces oligoclonal populations of T cells as judged by T cell receptor (TCR) variable (V) gene analysis.[9,13] The adoptive transfer of oligoclonal T cell populations would not be expected to eradicate disease unless, by chance, tumor-specific CTL expanded preferentially. Third, we have obtained evidence that the immune response provoked by tumor may include T helper populations incapable of providing T cell help that is required for the induction and maintenance of a strong CTL response.[14] Circumstantial evidence suggests that the same T helper populations *may* have some of the characteristics of suppressor T cells. Alternatively, others have documented the presence of suppressor macrophages in solid tumors.[15] This is clinically relevant because elimination of these cell populations before cellular immunotherapy with CTL and interleukin-2 (IL-2) would be expected to improve response rates. Fourth, we have recently studied a consecutive series of patients with ovarian cancer and have demonstrated that the host immune response to ascites-derived tumor does not include T cells capable of mounting tumoricidal activity against solid tumor obtained from the ovary or omentum.[7]

Since the first two problems are a direct consequence of the in vitro culture conditions (high dose IL-2), we sought an alternative approach to reproducibly expand TIL (1) to therapeutic numbers and (2) with similar functional traits. Our strategy has been to use solid-phase anti-CD3 monoclonal antibody (mAb) activation of TIL for 48 hours and subsequent expansion in low dose IL-2 (<100 IU/ml). As was initially shown by Van Wauwe et al mature T lymphocytes can be activated with anti-CD3 Ab that mimick the antigen-TCR interaction.[16] A requirement for positive activation is the immobilization of the antibody. The underlying thought is that solid-phase anti-CD3 induces a local accumulation of TCR/CD3 complexes that in turn will induce signal transduction via the CD3 molecule.[17] This activation signal is so strong that various T cell functions can be simultaneously observed to include (1) induction of cytolytic activity, (2) induction of cytokine production, (3) induction of proliferation, and, most importantly, (4) suppression of tumor growth in vitro and in vivo. This chapter describes the use of solid-phase anti-CD3 mAb activation in our clinical and preclinical biologic cancer therapy program.

TUMOR-INFILTRATING LYMPHOCYTES

Beginning in the mid 1980s, Rosenberg and others popularized immunotherapy trials utilizing high doses of interleukin-2 (IL-2) with or without activated cellular therapy.[18,19] These studies, however, were criticized because of their extreme toxicity, expense and their relatively low rates of efficacy. Our laboratory initiated cellular immunotherapy trials in 1986 to reduce the life-threatening toxicities associated with systemic IL-2 administration. We used low dose IL-2 (30,000 IU/kg) in conjunction with lymphokine-activated killer cells (LAK) cells. The reduced systemic dosage of IL-2 was compensated by prolonged administration of systemic IL-2 for four days following the final infusion of LAK cells. The laboratory and clinical protocols, as well as the clinical results of the first 18 patients were reported. This trial continued until 40 patients were accumulated.

Overall, the response rate, consisting of both partial and complete responses, was 40 percent. In addition, this trial demonstrated that low dose systemic IL-2 therapy entirely eliminated the life-threatening toxicities that characterized other trials.[20] Furthermore, low dose IL-2 therapy when combined with ibuprofen further reduced the number of minor toxicities but did not alter the response rate to immunotherapy.[21] We also examined the immunomodulatory effects of low dose systemic IL-2 therapy and found similar changes in the immune status to those reported in the high-dose protocols.[22] However, in this and other trials, the mechanism of tumor regression remained unclear. The observation that LAK cells do not "home" to metastatic tumor deposits made it clear that improved rates of response using this form of cellular therapy would be an illusive goal.[23]

A possible solution to this problem was the utilization of (TIL) since adoptively transferred TIL were capable of migrating to tumor, and animal studies showed TIL to be 50 to 200 times as potent on a per cell basis as LAK cells.[23,24] Our experience with TIL cultures indicated that the clinical application of this therapeutic approach was handicapped by the inability to generate therapeutic numbers of T cells from the majority of cancers sampled when high doses of IL-2 were utilized in culture. This limitation prompted the development of an entirely new approach for isolating and expanding TIL for therapeutic application and could be used for virtually any tumor sample. Accordingly, antigen activation signals were provided by exposing the freshly isolated T cell/tumor mixture to flasks coated with a mAb to the CD3 complex (solid-phase anti-CD3) present on all T cells. In addition, low doses of IL-2 (less than 100 IU/ml) were utilized, and this system has improved the expansion of T cells for therapeutic application (Fig. 2.1). Additionally, T cells activated under solid-phase anti-CD3 conditions did not exhibit nonspecific LAK-like patterns of cytotoxicity that are observed when high dose IL-2 is used to culture the cells. Instead, preferential killing of autologous tumor was seen (Fig. 2.2).[25]

STUDIES OF MURINE TIL

Our laboratory was the first to report the use of solid-phase anti-CD3 to isolate and expand murine TIL as well as to show that T cells deliberately activated under these conditions could mediate tumoricidal activity in vitro and demonstrate potent tumor-eradicating properties when adoptively

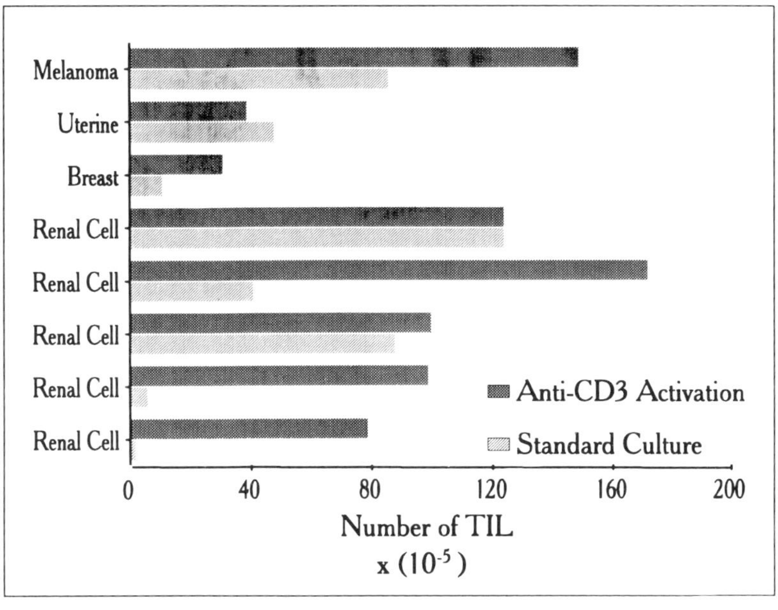

Fig. 2.1. Four million cells from tumor cell suspensions were cultured in 1000 U/ml rIL-2 (Standard culture) or plated on to anti-CD3 mAb coated T-25 flasks. After 48 hours cells were transferred to uncoated flasks with 50 U/ml rIL-2. All cells were harvested after 7 days and incubated with fresh medium. Cells were counted after 14 days and the total number of TIL harvested is reported.

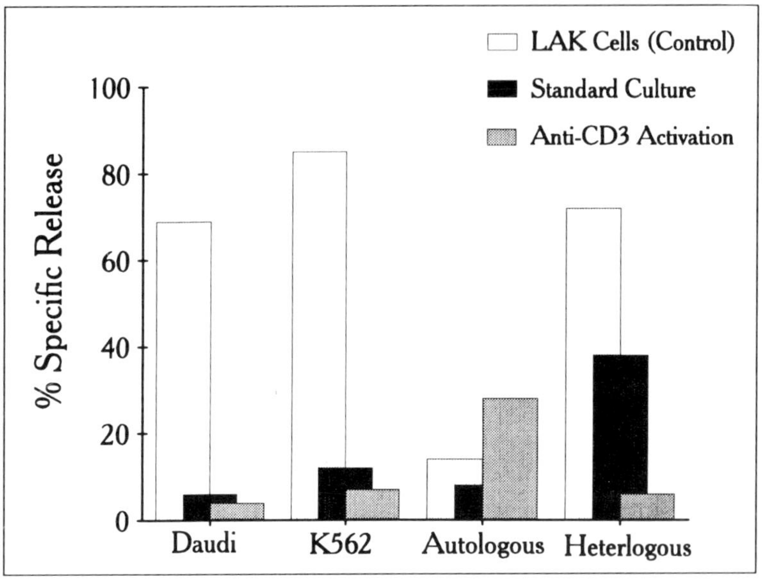

Fig. 2.2. Comparison of cytotoxicity following activation with 1000U/ml rIL-2 or solid-phase anti-CD3. TILs from a patient with ovarian carcinoma were cultured as indicated (Fig. 2.1) and tested for cytotoxicity against fresh autologous tumor cells, histologically matched heterologous tumor cells and the K562 and Daudi cell lines. Effector to target cell ratio was 20:1.

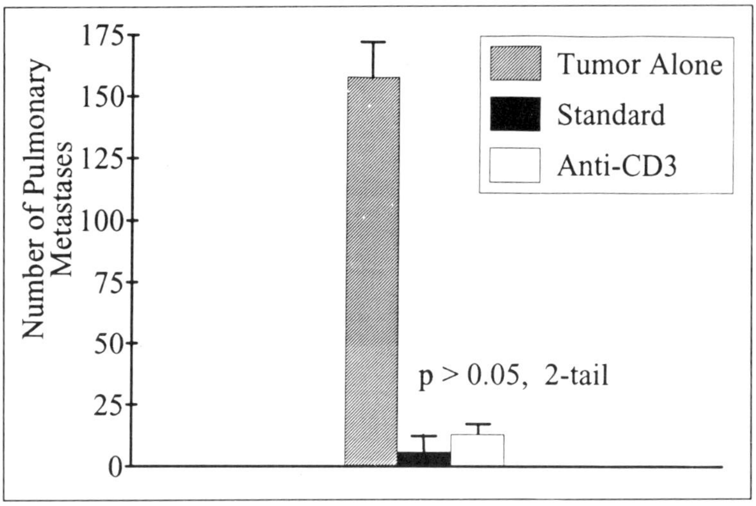

Fig. 2.3. (A) Standard condition (rIL-2 alone) and anti-CD3-stimulated TIL mediated reduction of MC-38 3-day pulmonary micrometastases. No difference in the in vivo activity was noted between the two TIL bulk culture populations ($P > 0.05$). Groups receiving adoptively transferred cells also received rIL-2 (50,000 units/ml, days 3-8, 3 times per day). Each experimental group consisted of 7 to 11 mice.

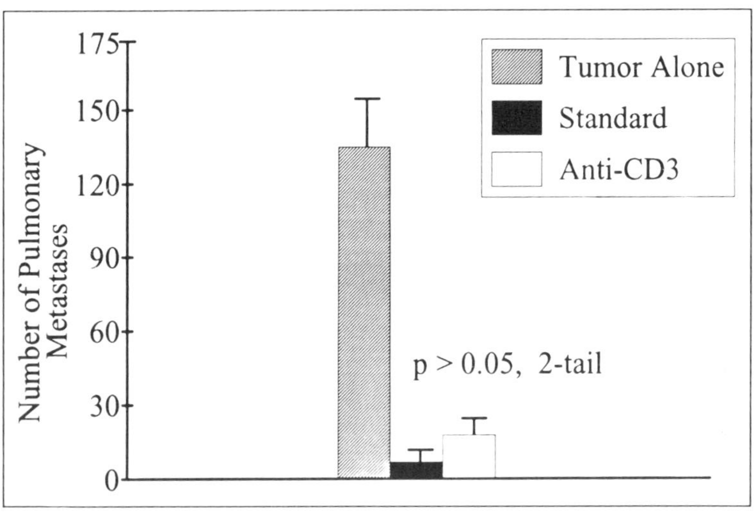

Fig. 2.3. (B) Standard condition and anti-CD-3-stimulated TIL mediated reduction of MCA 105 3-day pulmonary metastases. As with MC-38 tumor, no difference is noted in the ability of the two different culture methods to mediate tumor regression. Both TIL groups experienced significant reduction of tumor as compared to controls ($P < 0.05$).

transferred to tumor-bearing mice[26] (Fig. 2.3). While we could clearly show a tremendous increase in proliferation utilizing solid-phase anti-CD3 in the murine model, there was a discrepancy between the in vivo therapeutic effect of these activated TIL and their in vitro cytotoxicity. Utilizing a restimulation approach, we could demonstrate that TIL restimulated with solid-phase anti-CD3 activation were particularly effective if adoptively transferred within 72 hours of reactivation. Although there was an increase in proliferation and a modest nonspecific increase in cytotoxicity, the effectiveness of the restimulated adoptively transferred cells appeared to be related to the ability of the restimulated cells to produce cytokines, in particular, IL-6, GM-CSF, and IFN-γ (Fig. 2.4)[27] potentially accounting for the discrepancy in in vitro cytoxicity.

The real importance of cytokine production following activation of TIL utilizing solid-phase anti-CD3 is underscored by recent work from our laboratory utilizing a murine pulmonary metastases model.[28,29] Treatment of the host with an anti-CD8 mAb completely abrogated the effectiveness of adoptively transferred TIL plus IL-2. Similar treatment of the host with an anti-CD4 mAb had no effect on the success of the adoptively transferred TIL when exogenous IL-2 was given. This suggested the necessity of recruitment of $CD8^+$ lymphocytes from the host for effective tumor eradication. This recruitment is most likely mediated by the cascade of cytokines produced by the solid-phase anti-CD3 activated TIL. Indeed, when CD8-depleted hosts are given TIL plus IL-2 therapy and, additionally, given normal uneducated syngeneic splenocytes, the effectiveness of the CD3-activated TIL is restored (Fig. 2.5). However, if the uneducated splenocyte population is itself depleted of $CD8^+$ cells and given to a CD8-depleted host, the effectiveness of the CD3-activated TIL immunotherapy is abolished.

CLINICAL STUDIES OF HUMAN TIL

An additional characteristic of solid-phase anti-CD3 activation is that long-term

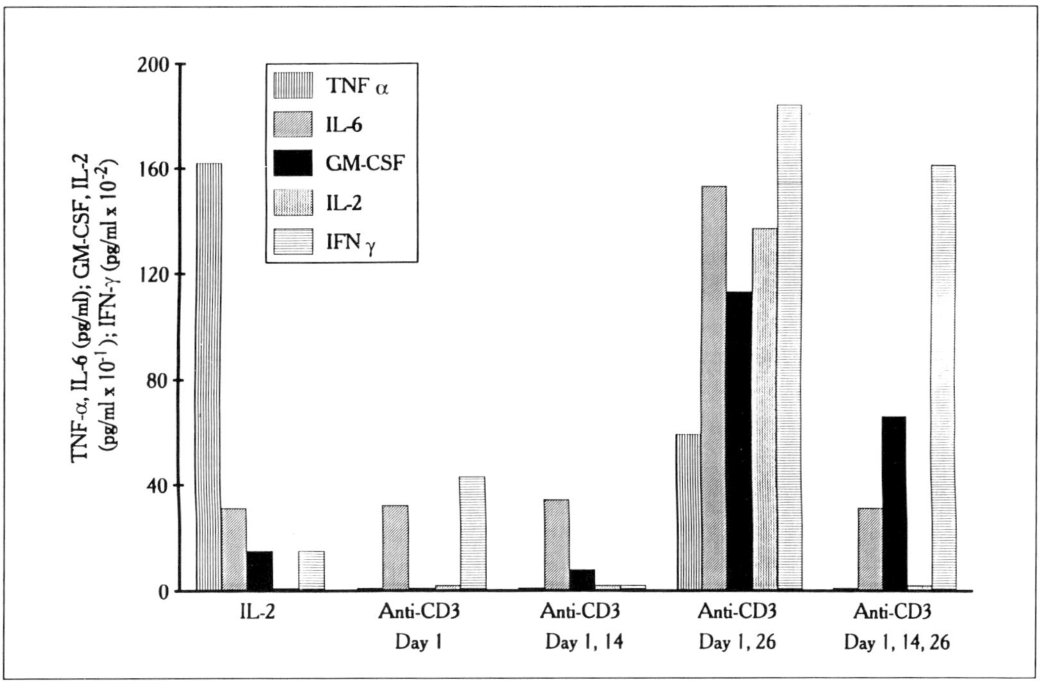

Fig. 2.4. Cytokine production by MCA 105 TIL cultures (re)activated with anti-CD3 or IL-2. Note that the concentrations of GM-CSF and IL-2 are x 10^{-1} and IFN-γ x 10^{-2}.

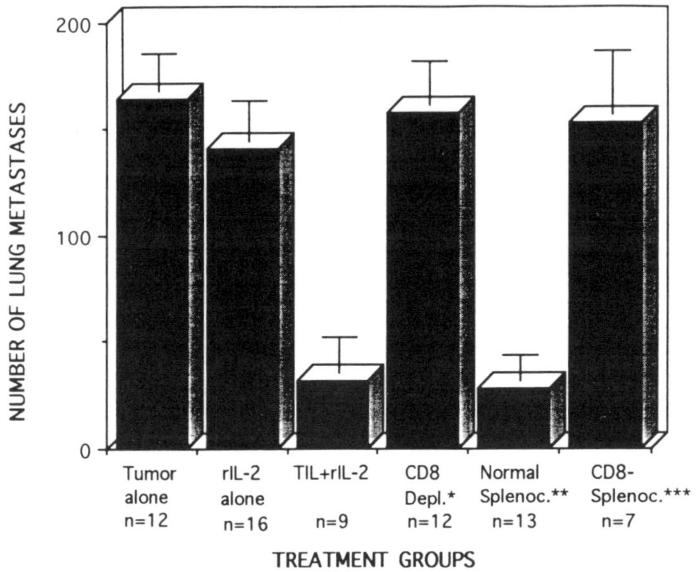

*Fig. 2.5. Splenocyte recruitment experiments. All animal groups were injected IV with MCA 105 tumor cells on day 0 of the protocol. *In this group the host was depleted of its CD8⁺ T cells 24 hours after tumor injection and 48 hours prior to TIL + rIL-2 therapy. **This group represents a CD8-depleted host which received 1 x 10⁸ normal uneducated splenocytes 2 hours after TIL transfer. rIL-2 was administered from day 3-7. ***This group represents a CD8 depleted host which received 1x10⁸ CD8-depleted splenocytes in addition to TIL + rIL-2 treatment on protocol day 3.*

T cell lines are polyclonal in contrast to the oligoclonal T cell cultures which result from culture in high dose IL-2.[9,13] The adoptive transfer of oligoclonal populations may be a disadvantage if they do not possess sufficient anti-tumor activity. Thus, utilizing solid-phase anti-CD3 activation of TIL in conjunction with low dose systemic IL-2, we have conducted clinical trials for melanoma and RCC. To illustrate the in vivo response of tumor to immunotherapy with polyclonal CTL plus low dose IL-2, a patient with extensive metastatic melanoma including a large unresectable perirenal mass was treated. Two months post therapy, the size of the renal mass had significantly diminished (Fig. 2.6). Pathologic examination of the remaining tumor mass adjacent to the right kidney revealed no viable tumor. Almost two years later, the patient is still with no evidence of disease. While we are able to show very dramatic responses, as above, and have approximately a 30% response rate in patients with metastatic melanoma, we still fall short of having solid-phase CD3-activated TILs eradicate tumor in the majority of patients. We, therefore, embarked on a long group of studies to identify the mechanism of how solid-phase anti-CD3 activated TIL recognize tumor with the expectation that we would be able to improve adoptive immunotherapy trials. Anti-CD3 stimulation has allowed us to grow and, therefore, study TIL from a number of different tumors to include RCC, malignant melanoma, and ovarian carcinoma.

THE HOST IMMUNE RESPONSE TO RENAL CELL CARCINOMA

It is interesting that tumor-specific CTL are easily observed in patients with melanoma but only rarely in patients with RCC in spite of a relatively large T cell infiltrate.[30,31] Thus, a program of study was instituted to functionally characterize the T cell subpopulations that infiltrate RCC. T cell clones were established from 20 consecutive patients with RCC. Tumors were disassociated, and T cells were activated for 48 hours on solid-phase anti-CD3 and then subsequently cloned. This approach was intended to maximize the clonal diversity of the T cell clones obtained from each sample. A total of 211 T cell clones were obtained (Fig. 2.7). The vast majority of the clones were $CD4^+$ with only 22% $CD8^+$. To study the tumoricidal characteristics of both $CD8^+$ and $CD4^+$ T cell clones, antibody-redirected lysis (ARL)

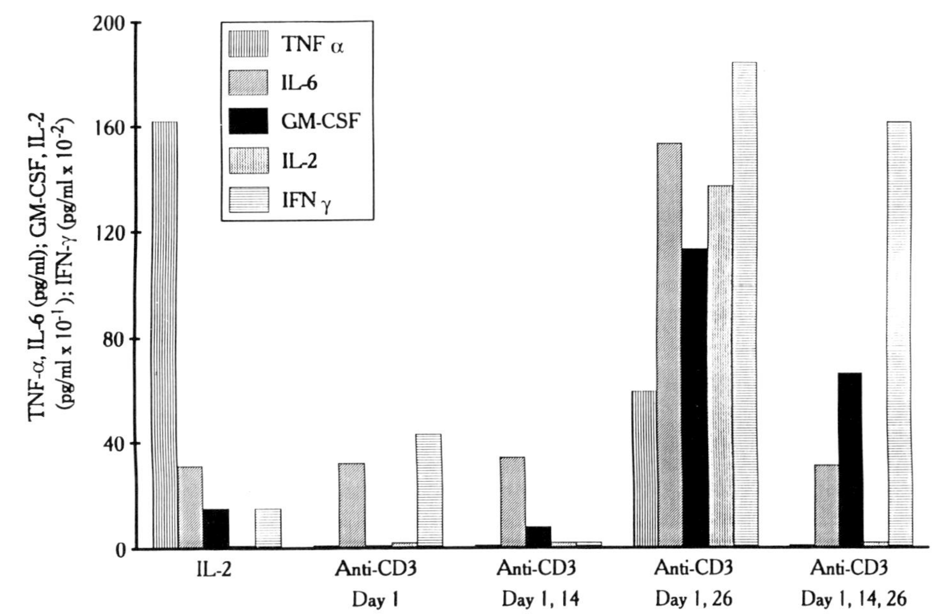

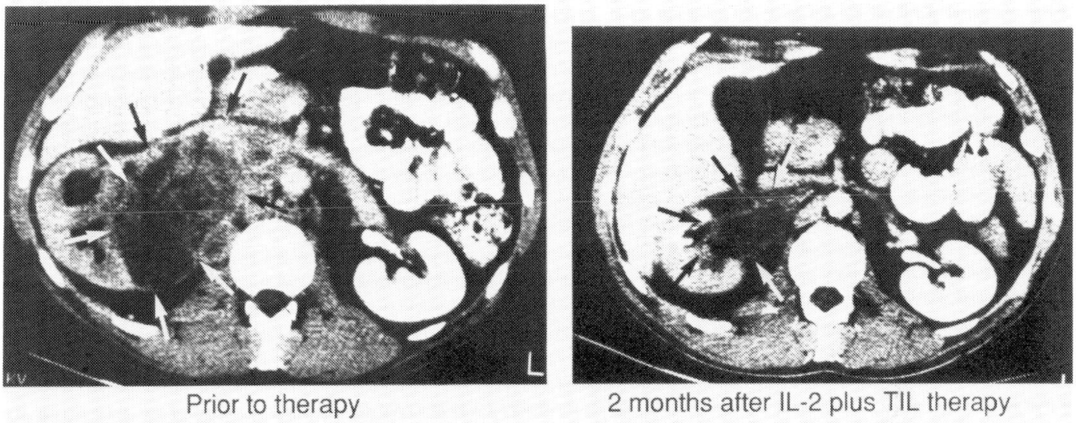

Fig. 2.6. This patient had extensive metastatic disease including progressive unresectable disease in the right kidney as indicated by the arrows (left). The patient received a total of 1 x 10^{10} TIL plus low-dose systemic IL-2. Two months after completing the protocol, the tumor was substantially smaller as indicated by the arrows (right), with normal contour of the diseased kidney returning. The mass was resected as a source for additional TIL therapy, however, microscopic examination of the tissue revealed no viable tumor and all other disease completely resolved.

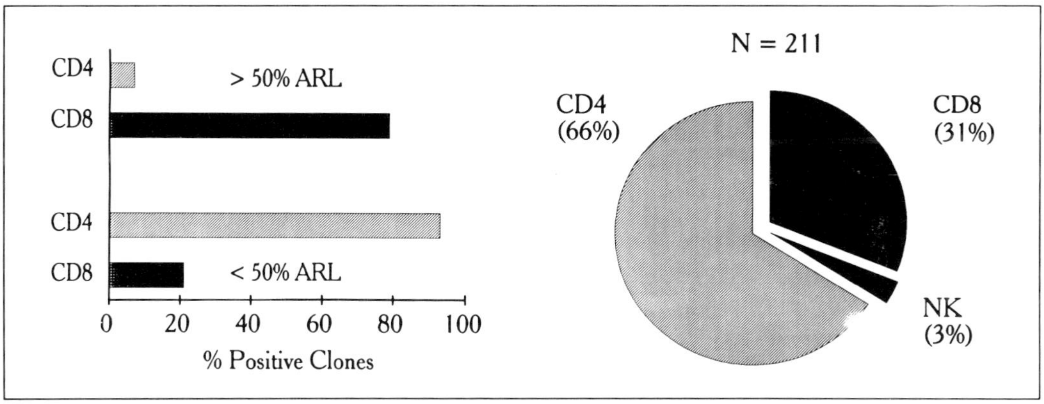

Fig. 2.7. T cell clones (n = 211) were phenotyped and tested for anti-tumor cytotoxicity by ARL against Daudi targets. Cells that killed greater than 50% were arbitrarily classified as strong killers (CD4 = 12/164; CD8 = 37/47), and those that killed less than 50% were classified as poor (CD4 = 152/164; CD8 = 10/47).

with an anti-TCR mAb was utilized to nonspecifically induce cytotoxic T cell function against chromium-labeled Daudi targets. As might be anticipated, 80% of the $CD8^+$ TIL clones possessed strong ARL (defined as greater than 50% specific lysis). In contrast, fewer than 10% of the $CD4^+$ TIL clones possessed strong ARL. With one exception, CTL activity against autologous tumor by ARL^+, $CD4^+$ or $CD8^+$ clones was not observed. Thus, although $CD8^+$ T cell clones can kill tumor if triggered by a strong signal (i.e. anti-TCR mAb), autologous tumor does not appear to trigger CTL responses by $CD8^+$ TIL clones. Therefore, these results indicate that the physiologic response of the immune system to RCC consists primarily of T cells that do not demonstrate anti-tumor cytotoxic function.

These studies were further extended by assessing cytokine production following activation by solid-phase anti-CD3 of 32 $CD4^+$ TIL clones derived from 7 patients. The $CD4^+$ clones could be divided into 2 categories based on the production or nonproduction of IL-2. Twenty-seven out of 32 $CD4^+$ clones failed to produce detectable levels of IL-2 and produced very low amounts of IFN-γ (Fig. 2.8). In addition, the production of IL-4, IL-6, TNF-α and GM-CSF was strong. In contrast, 5/32 CD4+ clones produced high levels of IL-2, IFN-γ; IL-4, IL-6, TNF-α and GM-CSF. Production of cytokines by the IL-2 producing clones was comparable to levels produced by IL-2 non-producers.

These patterns of cytokine production are analogous to the patterns of cytokine production that define subsets of murine CD4+ T cells. Murine Th0 cells are characterized by production of IL-2, IL-4 and IFN-γ. Murine Th1 cells produce IL-2 and IFN-γ but no IL-4. Murine Th2 cells produce IL-4 but no IL-2 or IFN-γ. Examination of these results in the context of IL-2 production indicates that the majority of the cloned CD4+ T cells (greater than 80%) possess the functional traits of murine Th2 cells. Only a minority of these clones possess traits similar to murine Th0 cells. CD4+ clones with the profile of Th1 were not detected in RCC.[14]

These results may have important biological and clinical implications for cancer patients treated with immunotherapy. First, only 5/32 clones produced IL-2. This supports the concept that renal cell tumors in general fail to provoke helper cells capable of providing T cell "help" (IL-2 production) sufficient to support a CTL response (only 47/211 T cell clones from 20 patients were CD8+). Second, studies have shown that the induction of LAK cells is inhibited if exogenous IL-4 is present during the induction phase.[32] Similarly, allogeneic DTH responses are suppressed if IL-4 is present *at the beginning* of culture.[33] IL-4 has also been shown to suppress both the proliferative and tumoricidal responses of human TIL to autologous tumor.[34] Moreover, murine Th2 cells have been recently recognized to be associated with progressive disease in 2 murine models, cutaneous leishmaniasis and experimental systemic yeast infection. In both models, therapy with anti-IL-4 heals the skin lesions in leishmaniasis and protects recipients from

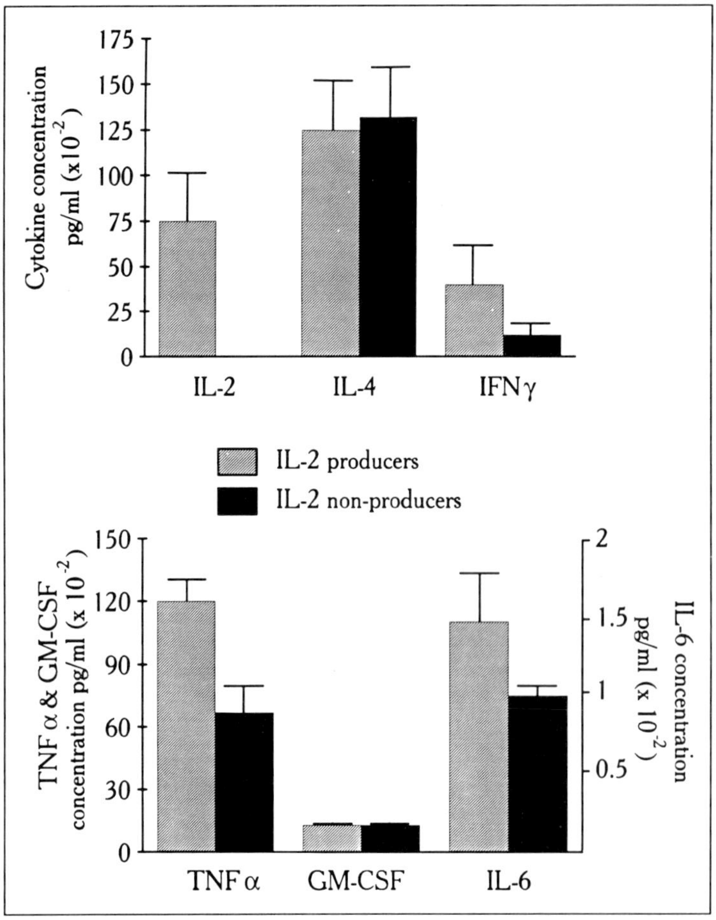

Fig. 2.8. Thirty-two CD4+ TIL clones were activated on solid-phase anti-CD3 for 48 hours. The supernatants were assessed for cytokines by ELISA. Clones were categorized as IL-2 producers or IL-2 non-producers. More than 80% of the clones were IL-2 non-producers. In addition, supernatants from the IL-2 non-producers had very little IFN-γ, but IL-4 was produced. IL-2 producers produced significant quantities of IL-4, IFN-γ as well as TNF-α and IL-6.

fatal yeast infection.[35,36] With anti-IL-4 mAb therapy the levels of Th2 cells decline concomitantly as cells with Th1 phenotype increases. These animal studies along with our findings in RCC suggest that Th2 cells may be associated with progressive disease and suggest methods to eliminate these potentially suppressive cells.

THE HOST IMMUNE RESPONSE TO MALIGNANT MELANOMA

We have recently embarked upon the analysis of cloned $CD4^+$ helper cells isolated for malignant melanoma (ref. 37 submitted). Using an identical experimental approach as detailed for RCC, we have shown that 66% of the $CD4^+$ clones existed as Th0-like cells producing IL-2, IL-4 and IFN-γ. Fifteen percent of the $CD4^+$ clones existed as Th1, producing IL-2 and IFN-γ. Nineteen percent existed as Th2, producing IL-4 but no IL-2 or IFN-γ. Compared to the proportions of Th0, Th1, and Th2 clones isolated from RCC (above), these data demonstrate that our culture conditions did not select for the outgrowth of a particular Th subset, and the presence of better T cell helpers (Th0, Th1) may also help to explain the improved rate of response to T cell immunotherapy for melanoma when compared to RCC.

THE HOST IMMUNE RESPONSE TO OVARIAN CARCINOMA

T Cell Recognition of Ovarian Cancer

In order to further dissect the immune response to tumor, we selected ovarian carcinoma as a model due to its potential immunogenicity as well as the availability of large amounts of tissue, both ascites and solid tumor, from primary debulking surgery. Using anti-CD3 activation, we were able to expand both tumor-associated lymphocytes (TAL) isolated from the ascites and TIL in all patients from 10^7 T cells initiated in culture to greater than 10^{10} lymphocytes in approximately 5 weeks. If T cells from both sources were utilized, an average of 1.5×10^8 lymphocytes would be available to initiate therapeutic cultures and, therefore, shorten the culture time even further.

To grow ovarian TIL, we utilized solid-phase anti-CD3 stimulation for 48 hours, maintenance in low dose IL-2 (50 IU/ml) and repeated stimulation with irradiated autologous tumor every ten to fourteen days.[7] This resulted in the emergence of $CD8^+$ T cell lines in 67% of all cultures. This is in contrast to the work reported by other laboratories using high dose IL-2 (≥ 1,000 IU/ml) which resulted in oligoclonal, predominantly $CD4^+$ cultures,[38,39] or high dose IL-2 and autologous tumor stimulation which resulted in fewer than 30% $CD8^+$ cultures.[40] Interestingly, if we cultured T cells in low dose IL-2 and repeatedly stimulated them with autologous tumor, the cultures became greater than 90% $CD4^+$ thus demonstrating the importance of anti-CD3 activation. These studies, therefore, indicate that $CD4^+$ and $CD8^+$ T cell lines can be established using the appropriate culture conditions in human ovarian carcinoma.

One of the most desirable functional traits of T cells used in cellular therapy is CTL activity. We, therefore, sought to document this activity in ovarian cancer. $CD8^+$ ovarian T cell lines grown with the above-mentioned culture conditions were found to be highly cytotoxic. The cytolytic activity of these T cell lines increased with time and peaked at 7 to 8 weeks in culture (Fig. 2.9). By ten weeks, tumoricidal activity fell dramatically but could be restored with repeated exposure to solid-phase anti-CD3. The specificity of both TAL and TIL cultures was also examined at 7 to 8 weeks of age against autologous tumors, several allogeneic ovarian tumors, and the NK-sensitive K562 cell line. TAL were tested against the ascites tumors, and TIL against solid tumors. Significantly higher CTL activity was observed against autologous tumor when compared with the other targets for both TAL and TIL (Fig. 2.9). These results imply that T cells adoptively transferred at this time would possess strong, specific anti-tumor activity.[7]

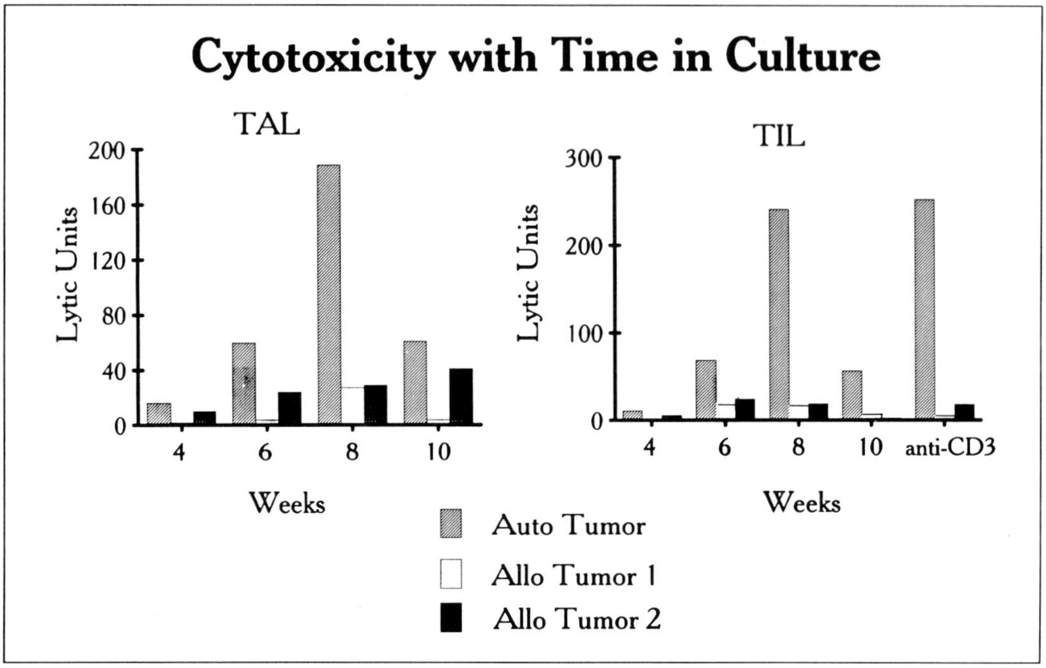

Fig. 2.9. TAL and TIL cultures from the same ovarian cancer patient were tested over time for cytolytic activity against autologous ascites tumor or autologous solid tumor, respectively. In addition, TAL and TIL were tested against two different allogeneic ovarian tumors. TIL were reactivated on solid-phase anti-CD3 after 9 weeks. Results are expressed as $LU_{20}/10^7$ cells.

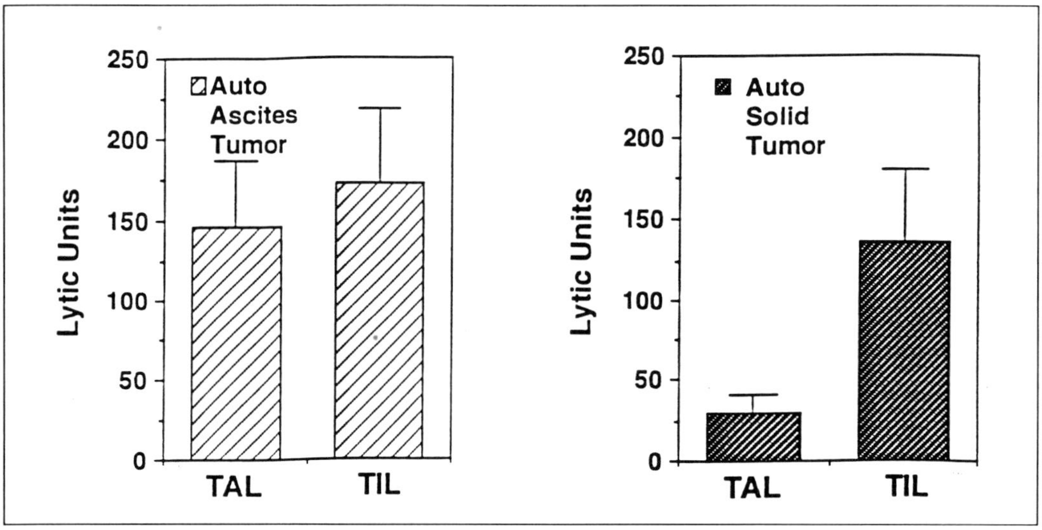

Fig. 2.10. TAL and TIL from the same patient were tested against autologous ascitic tumor and autologous solid tumor in the same experiment. Multiple experiments (3-4) were performed for each of the 6 patients at 5-7 weeks of culture. Results are expressed as lytic units ($LU_{20}/10^7$). Pooled results are presented ± SEM.

An important biologic issue stemming from the two forms of the disease (i.e. ascites and solid) is whether TAL can recognize solid tumor and if TIL can recognize ascites tumor. Aged-matched TAL and TIL were tested against autologous ascites tumor in standard cytotoxicity assays, and cytotoxicity mediated by TAL was not significantly different from TIL. We performed the reciprocal experiments by testing TAL and TIL against autologous solid tumor. In marked contrast, we found that TAL mediated significantly less cytotoxicity against autologous solid tumor as compared to TIL (Fig. 2.10). These data imply that cellular therapy with TAL would not clear the solid disease. Furthermore, these results underscore the need for functional analysis of matched lymphocyte samples in tumor samples of ovarian cancer.[37]

HLA A2 Presents Tumor-Derived Antigens Recognized by Ovarian Tumor Specific CTL

Both TAL and TIL possess functional traits of CTL. Studies performed in our laboratory showed that T cell-mediated killing of tumor could be blocked with mAb to the TCR or CD3 complex. In addition, cytotoxicity could also be inhibited by a mAb to the HLA class I molecule (Table 2.1). In contrast, mAb to HLA class II never blocked killing. These studies are consistent with the suggestion that ovarian tumor cells express antigens in the context of HLA class I molecules which are recognized by the T cell through the TCR. Since the HLA-A2 antigen is present in approximately 45% of the North American population and is known to play a role in the presentation of viral antigens and melanoma antigens, HLA-A2 was tested as a restriction element in ovarian cancer. HLA-A2$^+$ CTL from both ascites and solid tumor promoted significantly higher lytic activity against HLA-A2$^+$ tumors when compared to allogeneic HLA-A2$^-$ tumors. CTL activity mediated by effectors was specific for HLA-A2$^+$ ovarian tumors but not HLA-A2$^+$ melanoma targets indicating that the HLA-A2 molecule itself is not the target of recognition (Fig. 2.11). Finally, the recognition of autologous and allogeneic HLA-A2$^+$ targets by HLA-A2$^+$ CTL was also significantly blocked by pretreating the tumor with the anti-HLA-A2 mAb BB7.2 (Fig. 2.12).[41] The observation that tumor-specific CTL are capable of killing allogeneic ovarian tumors that are matched at the HLA-A2 locus provides evidence that at least one ovarian tumor antigen is shared by different individuals with ovarian cancer. Furthermore, HLA-A2 is confirmed as a major restriction element in ovarian cancer.

To study the possible sources of such TAA, we utilized the drug Brefeldin A (BFA). BFA inhibits the translocation of

Table 2.1. CTL activity inhibited by an anti-HLA Class I antibody and Brefeldin A

Patient No.	Tumor Source	Control	Anti-Class I	Brefeldin A
1	Solid	205	71	119
2	Ascites	243	33	71
3	Ascites	107	13	18
4	Solid	19	0	0
5	Solid	241	46	55
6	Ascites	463	263	233

Results are expressed as lytic units$_{20}$/10^7 cells. The lytic activity of cultures treated with anti-class I antibody were significantly inhibited compared to controls, $p < 0.05$, 2-sided). Lytic activity of cultures treated with Brefeldin A were also significantly inhibited, $p < .05$, 2-sided).

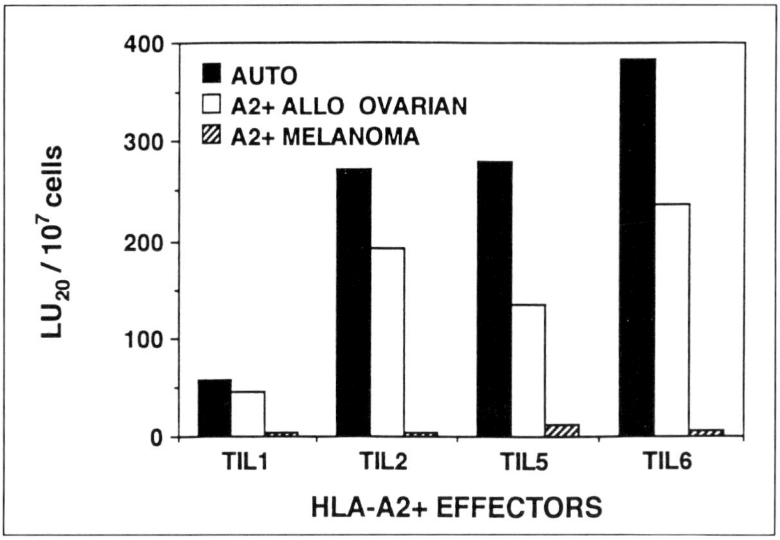

Fig. 2.11. Specific lysis of allogeneic HLA-A2+ ovarian tumor but not HLA-A2+ melanoma by HLA-A2+. CTL from each of the 4 HLA-A2+ patients were tested against autologous tumor, allogeneic HLA-A2+ ovarian tumor, and CTL HLA-A2+ melanoma. Results are expressed as lytic units ($LU_{20}/10^7$). No significant recognition of the A-2+ melanoma was observed; therefore, the HLA-A2 molecule itself is not the target of CTL.

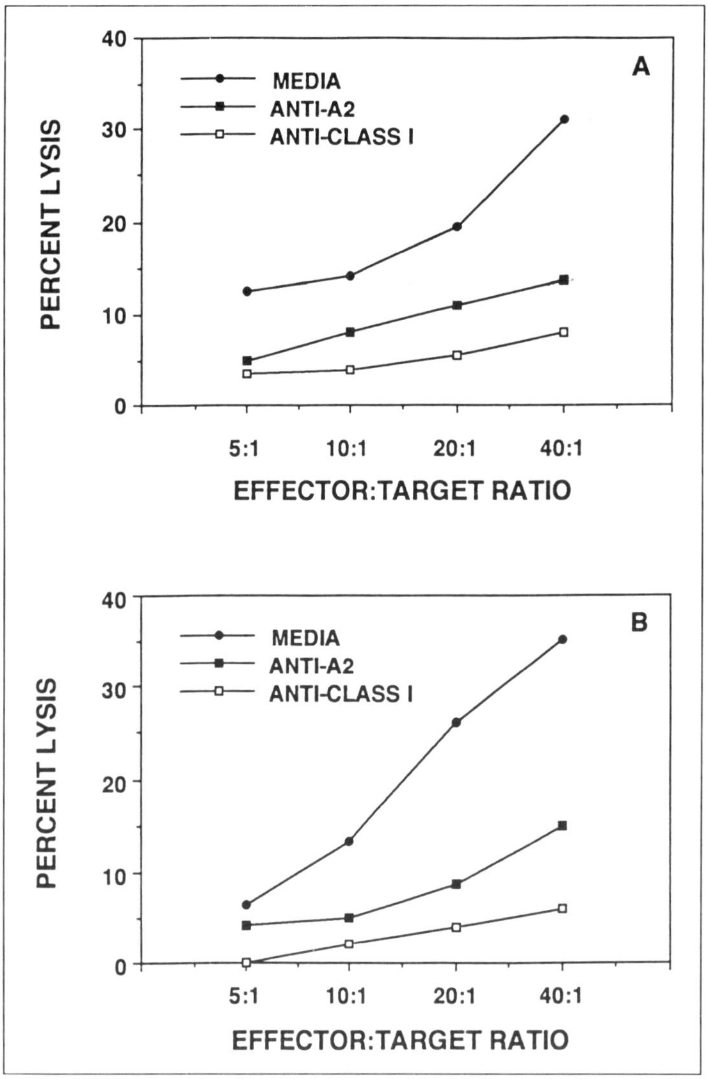

Fig. 2.12. HLA-A2+ effectors blocked by anti-HLA-A2 mAb (BB7.2). Ovarian tumor targets were pretreated with BB7.2 or W6/32 prior to cytotoxicity assays. Representative results are presented from patient 5 (A) and patient 2 (B). Results are expressed in percent lysis for the given E:T ratios.

transport vesicles from the ER to the Golgi apparatus.[42] Since antigenic peptides are known to associate with newly synthesized HLA class I while in the ER, we used BFA to block the association of HLA class I with putative tumor antigen and, therefore, the transport of tumor antigen/HLA class I complex to the cell surface. Treatment of tumor targets with BFA blocked CTL killing of tumor (Table 2.1). However, LAK effector cells killed BFA-treated or untreated targets equally well. Chloroquine (CLQ), which was used to block class II antigen processing pathways, had no inhibitory effect on ovarian CTL killing. This data suggests that ovarian tumor cells are competent to present TAA to CTL and that these antigens are derived from endogenous proteins.

Association between Proto Oncogene Expression and Sensitivity to Ovarian Tumor Specific CTL

Previous studies[43,44] have documented the over-expression of HER2/neu (erbB2) in ovarian tumor. In situ hybridization studies in this laboratory have also confirmed the presence of HER2/neu in our short term tumor cell lines. We, therefore, hypothesized that this oncogene product could serve as a source for tumor antigen. We began our studies by first observing the effect of IFN-γ treatment of the tumor and HER2/neu expression. Our initial observation was that IFN-γ treatment increased HLA class I expression (Fig. 2.13). Instead of increasing cytotoxicity with increasing IFN-γ exposure as one might expect (due to increased HLA class I ex-

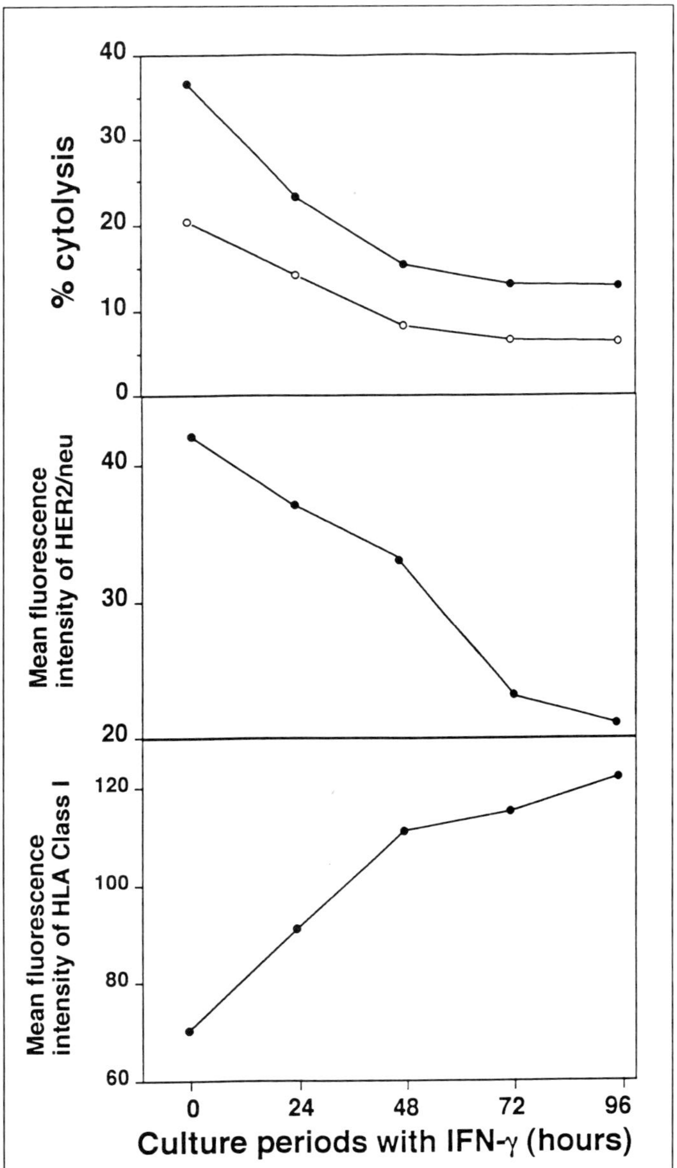

Fig. 2.13. The degree of cell surface expression of HER2/neu was positively correlated with the sensitivity to CTL in OvS1. OvS1 were seeded in 5 separate dishes 5 days before analysis, and 1000 U/ml of IFN-γ was added into each culture at 96, 72, 48 and 24 hours before analysis. Sensitivity of IFN-γ treated cells to autologous CTL was examined at /T ratio of 40:1 (closed circles) and 20:1 (open circles) (shown in the upper square). At the same time, cell surface expression of HER2/neu and HLA Class I was analyzed by flow cytometry (shown in the middle and lower square, respectively). Similar results were obtained in three independent experiments.

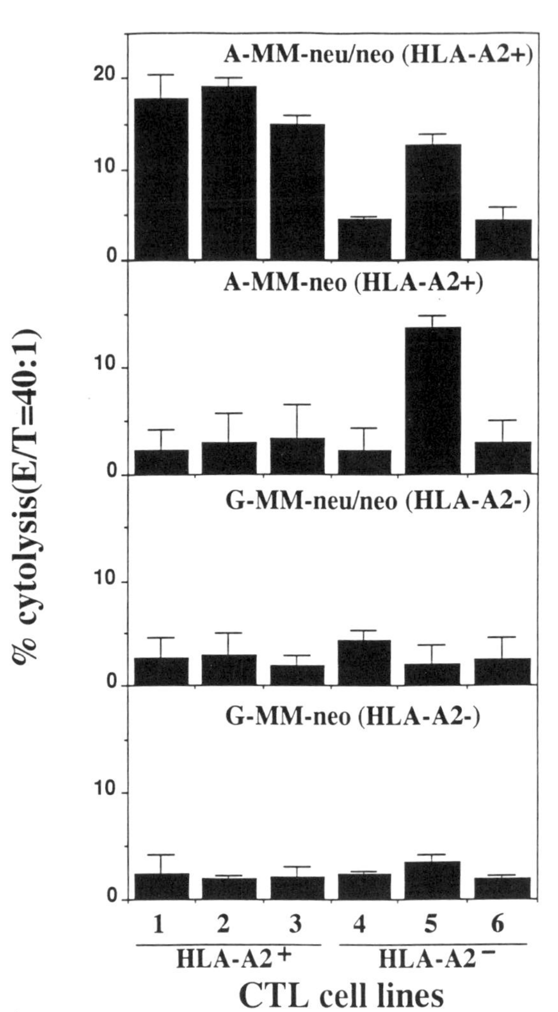

A

pression), we observed a decrease in cytotoxicity. This correlated exactly with a decrease in HER2/neu expression. This simple correlation led us to examine the possible role of HER2/neu in CTL-specific recognition of ovarian cancer. An HLA-A2$^+$ melanoma cell line and an HLA-A2$^-$ melanoma cell line were transfected with the plasmids pSVerbB2 and pMoNeo by lipofection.[45] The pSVerbB2 plasmid contains the 185 Kd Her2/neu gene, and the pMoNeo plasmid contains a neomycin-resistance gene. In addition, the A2$^+$ and A2$^-$ melanoma cells were transfected with pMoNeo alone. Both parental melanoma cell lines were not sensitive to ovarian CTL. As expected, cells transfected with pMoNeo alone did not express HER2/neu and were not sensitive to ovarian cancer-specific CTL (Fig. 2.14A). However, the HLA-A2$^+$ melanoma cells transfected with pSVerbB2 and pMoNeo did express HER2/neu (assessed by flow cytometry) and were sensitive to three ovarian-specific HLA-A2$^+$ CTL lines (Fig. 2.14A). This reactivity could be inhibited with an anti-HLA-A2 mAb (Fig. 2.14B). The HLA-A2$^-$ melanoma transfectant with the pSVerbB2 and pMoNeo was not killed by the same HLA-A2$^+$ ovarian CTL. Finally, both

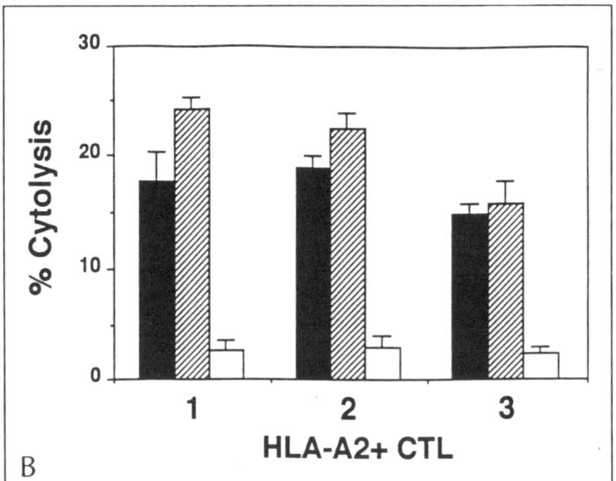

B

Fig. 2.14. Sensitivity of HER2/neu transfectants to a series of ovarian tumor-specific CTL. (A) The sensitivity of the transfectants (A-MM-neu/neo, A-MM-neo, G-MM-neu/neo and G-MM-neo) to six ovarian tumor-specific CTL from six patients was tested in standard four hour ^{51}Cr-release assay. The representative data from four separate experiments are shown. (B) The effect of anti-HLA-A2 mAb on the sensitivity of A-MM-neu/neo to ovarian tumor-specific CTL was examined. Closed bar, without the anti-HLA-A2 mAb; hatched bar, with the anti-HLA-DR mAb; and open bar, with the anti-HLA-A2 mAb. The mean value ± standard error from two separate experiments is shown.

the A2$^+$ and A2$^-$ HER2/neu transfected melanoma cell lines failed to trigger three independent HLA-A2$^-$ ovarian CTL lines. These results suggest that the HER2/neu gene product may contain peptides presented by HLA-A2 and recognized by tumor-specific ovarian CTL. In addition, since HLA-A2$^+$ CTL from three different ovarian cancer patients killed the A2$^+$ transfectant but not the A2$^-$, this data also provides the strongest evidence to date for the existence of shared TAA expressed by individuals with ovarian cancer and HLA-A2 restriction. While it is possible that HER2/neu may regulate the expression of some other protein that is in turn recognized as a target of CTL, we have preliminary data suggesting that at least one synthetic peptide derived from the HER2/neu sequence and containing A2 binding sites is recognized by ovarian tumor-specific CTL.

TCR V Gene Analysis of Ovarian TIL

With the target of T cells more elucidated, our next goal was to determine if a restricted repertoire of TCR is utilized in the recognition of ovarian cancer. The usage of TCR Vβ genes was studied with 22 primers recognizing 20 TCR Vβ families, amplified by PCR, and quantitated by HPLC. In fresh TIL from six consecutive ovarian tumors, six Vβ families were present in increased percentages and shared between patients and included Vβ2, Vβ3, Vβ6, Vβ7, Vβ8 and Vβ13.1. PCR analysis of 7 week tumor-specific TIL cultures revealed an increasingly biased population of T cells as compared to fresh TIL. Vβ2, Vβ3, Vβ6 and Vβ7 were shared between patients and accounted for approximately 50% of the total T cells present at 7 weeks. Comparing the 7 week tumor-specific cultures with the fresh TIL, Vβ2 was augmented by 108% and Vβ6 increased by 61% while no significant increase was seen in Vβ7, Vβ8 or Vβ13.1 (Fig. 2.15). Vβ3 was only marginally increased. No significant difference was seen in the controlled non-tumor stimulated group when comparing fresh with 7 week cultured TIL. Therefore, the change in Vβ repertoire in the tumor stimulated TIL was not just a function of time and culture conditions but related to anti-tumor induced growth. To prove that the increase in Vβ2, Vβ3 and Vβ6 correlated with the increase in cytotoxicity observed over time, anti-TCR Vβ mAb were used to block tumor lysis. Anti-Vβ2 mAb blocked cytotoxicity by 20 ± .3% which is consistent with the 19.1 ± 5.2% average representation of Vβ2 in the 7 week cul-

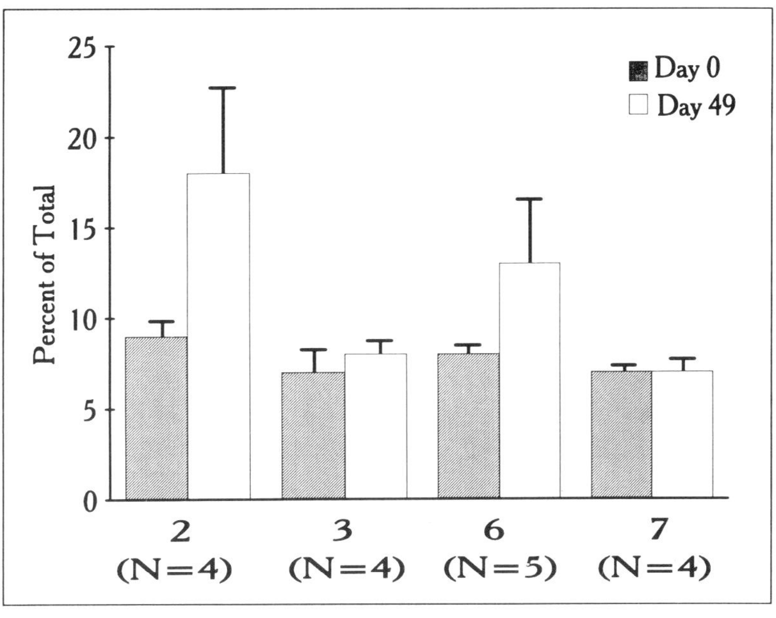

Fig. 2.15. TCR Vβ augmentation with repeated autologous tumor stimulation. A comparison between fresh TIL and tumor-specific 7 week cultured TIL in regards to the level of representation of the TcR Vβ genes found to be important in the latter, revealed that Vβ3 and Vβ6 were significantly augmented by 108% and 61%, respectively ($p < 0.05$).

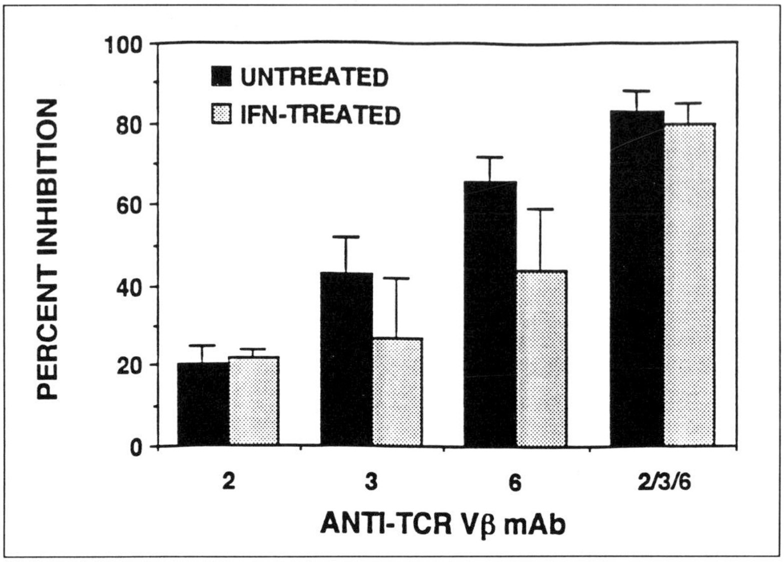

Fig. 2.16. Anti-TCR Vβ mAb blocking of the cytotoxicity against IFN-γ-treated ovarian tumor. IFN-γ-treated (1000 U/ml for 48 hours) OvS1 and untreated OvS1 were used in mAb blocking studies with TIL1. Vβ3 and Vβ6 contributed less to the killing of the HER-2/neu-reduced, IFN-γ-treated target than the untreated control. There was no difference in the level of inhibition by anti-Vβ2. Three separate experiments are pooled and presented as % inhibition ± SEM. Media, anti-TAC, and anti-Vβ12 mAbs were used as controls.

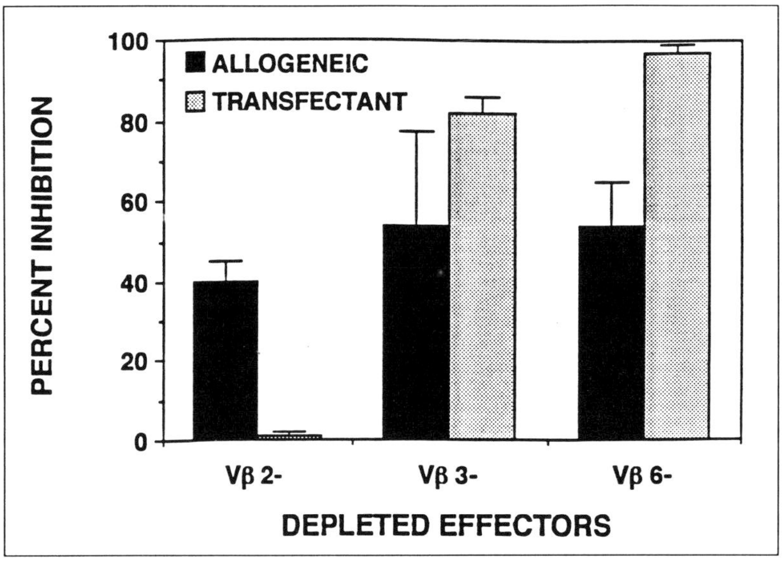

Fig. 2.17. Cytotoxicity against a HER2/neu-transfected melanoma by specific TCR Vβ-depleted CTL. TIL5 was specifically depleted of individual Vβ families by FACS-sorting and tested against the HER2/neu-transfectant in standard cytotoxicity assays. Undepleted TIL5 was used as control. Vβ3⁻ and Vβ6⁻ cultures lost the ability to recognize the HER2/neu-transfectant while Vβ2-depletion had no effect on the cytotoxicity ($p < 0.05$). All depleted populations demonstrated a reduced cytotoxicity for a common HLA-A2⁺ allogeneic ovarian target ($p < 0.05$) confirming the mAb blocking data. Results are pooled from 3 separate experiments and are expressed as % inhibition ±SEM (calculated from LU with E/T ratios of 20, 10, 5:1).

tured TIL tested. Anti-Vβ3 mAb blocked approximately 40% of the cytolytic activity. However, the anti-Vβ6 mAb blocked 48 ± 3.7% of tumor lysis which is well out of proportion to the 13.5 ± 3.5 % average representation of this Vβ family in the 7 week TIL tested. When the mAbs were combined, 63 ± 8.2% of the cytotoxicity could be inhibited in those cultures expressing increasing proportions of both families. Therefore, this data suggests that Vβ2$^+$ and Vβ6$^+$ CTL appear to mediate the majority of anti-tumor activity in ovarian cancer, and Vβ6 may play the predominant role (Ref. 46).

In order to correlate these Vβs with their targets, we utilized mAb blocking and FACS-depleted populations recognizing the stable HER2/neu transfected cells. When the stable transfected tumor was treated with INF-γ (recalling IFN-γ decreased HER2/neu expression and therefore cytotoxicity), the percentage inhibition by anti-Vβ2 mAb was not affected. Anti-Vβ3 and anti-Vβ6 mAb blocking however was markedly decreased after INF-γ treatment (Fig. 2.16). In performing FACS sorting experiments we found that Vβ2 was important in recognition of HLA-A2$^+$ ovarian cancer cells, but played no role in recognizing the stable HER2/neu transfected tumor, whereas Vβ3 and Vβ6 were both important not only in A2-restricted allogeneic recognition but mediated the recognition of the HER2/neu transfected melanoma (Fig. 2.17). We, therefore, concluded that Vβ2 recognizes an A2-restricted, non-HER2/neu- related antigen system. On the other hand, Vβ3 and Vβ6 recognizes an A2-restricted, HER2/neu-related antigen system.[47]

CONCLUSION

In summary, utilizing solid-phase anti-CD3 activation of human TIL, we have been able to improve proliferation and CD8$^+$ TIL augmented cytotoxicity without sacrifice of specificity. Additionally, these solid-phase anti-CD3 activated TILs can be very effective in tumor eradication. In the human, this effect is not uniform, and therefore, mechanisms of tumor identification have been examined. Utilizing solid-phase anti-CD3 activated TIL, we have defined helper cell function in RCC and melanoma and defined lymphocyte-tumor interactions in ovarian cancer. Furthermore, we have utilized this approach to define the specific antigen(s) being recognized in ovarian carcinoma. By thoroughly understanding and dissecting the mechanisms of these lymphocyte-tumor interactions, we will be able to utilize this knowledge for the design of more efficacious and specific immunotherapy and vaccine trials in the future.

REFERENCES

1. Ehrlich P. Uber den Jetzigen Stand der Karzinomforschung. Dutch Journal for Medicine 1:273, 1909.
2. Thomas L. In: HS Lawrence, ed. Cellular and humoral aspects of the hypersensitive states. New York: Hoeber-Harper 1959:529-533.
3. Burnet FM. The concept of immunological surveillance. Prog Exp Tumor Res 13:1, 1970.
4. Parmiani G, Anichini A, Fossati G. Cellular immune response against autologous human malignant melanoma: Are in vitro studies providing a framework for a more effective immunotherapy? J Natl Cancer Inst 82 (5):361-370, 1990.
5. Bookman MA, Bast, Jr. RC. The immunobiology and immunotherapy of ovarian cancer. Seminars in Oncology 18 (3):270-291, 1991.
6. Finke JH, Tubbs R, Connely B, et al. In: J. Battisto T. Plate and G. Shearer, eds. Cytotoxic T cells: Biology and relevance to disease. New York: NY Acad Sci 1988:327-394.
7. Peoples GE, Schoof DD, Andrews J. VR, Goedegebuure PS, Eberlein TJ. T cell recognition of ovarian cancer. Surgery 114 (2):227-234, 1993.
8. Mitchell MS, Harel W, Kempf RA, Hu E, Kan-Mitchell J, Boswell WD, Dean G, Stevenson L. Active-specific immunotherapy for melanoma. J Clin Oncol 8 (5):856-869, 1990.
9. Fishleder AJ, Finke JH, Tubbs R, Bukowski

RM. Induction by interleukin-2 of oligoclonal expansion of cultured tumor-infiltrating lymphocytes. J Natl Cancer Inst 82:124-128, 1990.

10. Rosenberg SA, Spiess P, Lafreniere R. A new approach to the adoptive immunotherapy of cancer with tumor-infiltrating lymphocytes. Science 233:1318-1321, 1986.
11. Rosenberg SA, Packard BS, Aebersold PM, et al. Use of tumor-infiltrating lymphocytes and interleukin-2 in the immunotherapy of patients with metastatic melanoma. N Engl J Med 25:1676-1680, 1988.
12. Yoshizawa H, Chang AE, Shu S. Specific adoptive immunotherapy mediated by tumor-draining lymph node cells sequentially activated with anti-CD3 and IL-2. J Immunol 147 (2):729-737, 1991.
13. Morita T, Salmeron MA, Moser RP, Ross MI, Itoh K. Oligoclonal expansion of Vβ8+ cells in interleukin-2-activated T cells residing in subcutaneous metastatic melanoma. Clin Exp Metastases 10 (1):69-76, 1992.
14. Schoof DD, Terashima Y, Peoples GP, Goedegebuure PS, Andrews J. VR, Richie JP, Eberlein TJ. CD4+ T cell clones isolated from human renal cell carcinoma possess the functional characteristics of Th2 helper cells. Cell Immunol 150:114-123, 1993.
15. Hengst JC, Kan-Mitchell J, Kempf RA, Strumpf IJ, Sharma OP, Kortes VL, Mitchell MS. Correlation between cytotoxic and suppressor activities of human pulmonary alveolar macrophages. Cancer Res 45 (1):459-63, 1985.
16. Van Wauwe JP, Goossens JG. OKT3: a monoclonal anti-human T lymphocyte antibody with potent mitogenic properties. J Immunol 124:2708-2713, 1980.
17. Perez P, Hoffman RW, Shaw S, Bluestone JA, Segal DM. Specific targeting of cytotoxic T cells by anti-T3 linked to anti-target cell antibody. Nature 316:354-356, 1985.
18. Rosenberg SA, Packard BS, Aebersold PM, Solomon D, Topalian SL, Toy ST, Simon P, Lotze MT, Yang JD, Seipp, CAY, et al. Use of tumor-infiltrating lymphocytes and interleukin-2 in the immunotherapy of patients with metastatic melanoma: A preliminary report. N Engl J Med 9:125-127, 1988.
19. Rosenberg SA, Lotze MT, Yang JC, Aebersold PM, Linehan WM, Seipp C. AY, White DE. Experience with the use of high-dose interleukin-2 in the treatment of 652 cancer patients. Ann Surg 210:474-485, 1989.
20. Schoof DD, Gramolini BA, Davidson DL, Massaro AF, Wilson RE, Eberlein TJ. Adoptive immunotherapy of human cancer using low-dose recombinant interleukin-2 and lymphokine-activated killer cells. Cancer Res 48:5007-5010, 1988.
21. Eberlein TJ, Schoof DD, Michie HR, Massaro AF, Burger U, Wilmore DW, Wilson RE. Ibuprofen causes reduced toxicity of IL-2 administration in patients with metastatic cancer. Arch Surg 124:542-547, 1989.
22. Eberlein TJ, Rodrick ML, Massaro AF, Jung SE, Mannick JA, Schoof DD. Immunomodulatory effects of systemic low-dose recombinant interleukin-2 and lymphokine-activated killer cells in humans. Cancer Immunol Immunother 30:145-150, 1989.
23. Griffith KD, Read EJ, Carrasquillo JA, Carter CS, Yank JC, Fisher B, Aebersold P, Packard BS, Yu MY, Rosenberg S.A. In vivo distribution of adoptively transferred indium-111-labeled tumor-infiltrating lymphocytes and peripheral blood lymphocytes in patients with metastatic melanoma. J Natl Cancer Inst 81:1709-1717, 1989.
24. Rosenberg SA, Spiess P, Lafreniere R. A new approach to the adoptive immunotherapy of cancer with tumor-infiltrating lymphocytes. Sience 233:1318-1321, 1986.
25. Schoof DD, Selleck C, Massaro AF, Jung SE, Eberlein TJ. Activation of human tumor-infiltrating lymphocytes by monoclonal antibodies directed to the CD3 complex. Cancer Res 50:1138-1143, 1990.
26. Massaro AF, Schoof DD, Rubinstein A, Jung SE, Wilson RE, Eberlein TJ. Solid-phase anti-CD3 antibody activation of murine tumor-infiltrating lymphocytes. Cancer Res 50:2587-2592, 1990.
27. Goedegebuure PS, Zuber M, Leonard-Vidal DL, Burger UL, Cusack Jr. JC, Chang MP,

Douville LM, Eberlein TJ. Reactivation of murine tumor-infiltrating lymphocytes with solid phase anti-CD3 antibody: in vitro cytokine production is associated with in vivo efficacy. J Surgical Oncol 3: 79-89, 1994.

28. Burger UL, Chang MP, Goedegebuure PS, Eberlein TJ. Tumor eradication with tumor-infiltrating lymphocytes and rIL-2 requires the recruitment of host CD8+ T cells. Surgery, In press.
29. Burger UL, Chang MP, Adams SL, Schoof DD, Eberlein TJ. The role of CD4+ and CD8+ T cells during TIL+ rIL-2 treatment in cancer immunotherapy. Surg Forum 44:467-469, 1993.
30. Finke JH, Rayman P, Alexander J, Edinger M, Tubbs RR, Connelly R, Pontes E, Bukowski R. Characterization of the cytolytic activity of CD4+ and CD8+ tumor-infiltrating lymphocytes in human renal cell carcinoma. Cancer Res 50:2363-2370, 1990.
31. Kim TY, Von Eschenbach AC, Filaccio MD, Hayakawa K, Parkinson DR, Balch CM, Itoh K. Clonal analysis of lymphocytes from tumor peripheral blood and non-tumorous kidney in primary renal cell carcinoma. Cancer Res 50:5263-5268, 1990.
32. Nishioka Y, Sone S, Okubo A, Ogura T. Suppression by interleukin-4 of activation of human blood monocytes to the tumoricidal state. Jpn J Cancer Res 81:936-941, 1990.
33. Yamahsita U, Tanaka Y. Suppressive activity of interleukin-4 on the induction of antigen-specific cytotoxic T. Cells in humans. Jpn J Cancer Res 82:585-592, 1991.
34. Yamada T, Holmes EC, Golub SH. Differential regulation by interleukin-4 and interferon-γ of an autologous melanoma-specific cytotoxic T cell clone and tumor-infiltrating lymphocytes from which it was established. Cancer Comm 2:113-121, 1990.
35. Sadick M, Heinzel FP, Holaday F, Pu RT, Dawkins RS, Locksley RM. Cure of murine leishmaniasis with anti-interleukin-4 monoclonal antibody: Evidence for a T cell-dependent, interferon–γ independent mechanism. J Exp Med 171:115-127, 1990.
36. Romani L, Mencacci A, Grohmann U, Mocci S, Mosci P, Puccetti P, Bistoni, F Neutralizing antibody to interleukin-4 induces systemic protection and T helper type 1-associated immunity in murine candidiasis. J Exp Med 176:19-25, 1992.
37. Goedegebuure PS, Lee KY, Matory YL, Andrews JVR, Richie JP, Schoof DD, Eberlein T.J. CD4+ Th2 cells dominate the immune response to renal cell cancer. Surg Forum 44:783-785, 1993.
38. Belldegrun A, Kasid A, Uppenkamp M, Topalian SL, Rosenberg S.A. Human tumor-infiltrating lymphocytes: An analysis of lymphokine mRNA expression and relevance to cancer immunotherapy. J Immunol 142:4520-4526, 1989.
39. Bennett WT, Pandolfi F, Grove BH, Hawes GE, Boyle LA, Kradin RL, Kurnick JT. Dominant rearrangements among human tumor-infiltrating lymphocytes. Analysis of T cells derived from 32 patients with melanoma, lung, and renal cell carcinoma. Cancer 69:2379-2384, 1992.
40. Lotzova E, Savary CA, Freedman RS, Edwards CL, Morris M. Comparison of recombinant interleukin-2-activated peripheral blood and tumor-infiltrating lymphocytes of patients with epithelial ovarian carcinoma: Cytotoxicity, growth kinetics and phenotype. Cancer Immunol. Immunother 31:169-175, 1990.
41. Peoples GE, Goedegebuure PS, Andrews JVR, Schoof DD, Eberlein T.J. HLA-A2 presents shared tumor-associated antigens derived from endogenous proteins in ovarian cancer. J. Immunol 151:5481-5491, 1993.
42. Yewdell JW, Bennink JR. Bredfeldin A specifically inhibits presentation of protein antigens to cytotoxic T lymphocytes. Science, 244:1072-1075, 1989.
43. Heo DS, Whiteside T.L, Kanbour A, Herberman RB. Lymphocytes infiltrating human ovarian tumors. I. Role of Leu-19 (NKH-1)-positive recombinant IL-2-activated cultures of lymphocytes infiltrating human ovarian tumors. J Immunol 140:4042-4049, 1988.
44. Ioannides CG, Freedman RS, Ioannides MG, Fisk B, O'Brian CA. CTL clones isolated from ovarian tumor-infiltrating lymphocytes can recognize peptides with sequences cor-

responding to the HER2/neu gene product. FASEB J 6:A1404(2711), 1992.

45. Yoshino I, Peoples GE, Goedegebuure PS, Maziarz R, Eberlein TJ. Association of HER2/neu expression with sensitivity to tumor-specific CTL in human ovarian cancer. J Immunol. J Immunol 152: 2393, 1993.
46. Peoples GE, Davey MP, Goedegebuure PS, Schoof DD, Eberlein TJ. T cell receptor Vβ2 and Vβ6 mediate tumor-specific cytotoxicity by tumor-infiltrating lymphocytes in ovarian cancer. J Immunol 151:5472-5480, 1993.
47. Peoples GE, Yoshino I, Douville CC, Andrews JVR, Goedegebuure PS, Eberlein, TJ. T cell receptor $V\beta3^+$ and $V\beta6^+$ cytotoxic T lymphocytes recognize tumor-associated antigens related to HER2/neu expression in HLA-$A2^+$ ovarian cancers. J Immunol 152: 4993, 1994.

CHAPTER 3

Adoptive Immunotherapy with Pharmacologically Activated T Lymphocytes

Harry D. Bear, Todd M. Tuttle

Adoptive immunotherapy is the transfer of immunologically competent cells with anti-tumor activity into tumor-bearing hosts (TBH), with the objective of inducing tumor regression in the adoptive host. Although the initial goal of research in this area was focused on activation and growth of T lymphocytes with antigen-specific responses, the first clinical trials which showed that immunocompetent cells could mediate tumor regression were carried out with nonspecific lymphokine activated killer (LAK) cells.[1,2] Generated in high concentrations of the T cell growth factor interleukin 2 (IL-2), these cells were essentially a laboratory artifact found in the process of trying to grow T cells in vitro. Although LAK cells could mediate regression of tumors in a minority of patients with melanoma and renal cell cancer, their activity required very high and toxic doses of IL-2 given concomitantly.[1,3] Nevertheless, these trials did establish the feasibility of treating human cancer with adoptive transfer of autologous lymphocytes activated in vitro.

More recently, tumor-infiltrating lymphocytes (TILs) and lymphocytes from tumor-draining lymph nodes (DLN) from animals and humans with progressively growing tumors have been shown to have potent anti-tumor activity when stimulated in vitro with tumor cells and cultured with lower doses of IL-2.[4-11] The T cells obtained using these protocols have been shown to be 50-100 times more effective on a per cell basis than LAK cells and can induce tumor regression with much lower and non-toxic doses of IL-2 given concomitantly.[4,9] Optimal therapeutic activity requires large numbers of cells and optimal growth of T cells using the in vitro sensitization (IVS) protocol requires large numbers of autologous tumor cells for serial stimulation.[7,11,12] Unfortunately,

---

Immunotherapy of Cancer with Sensitized T Lymphocytes, edited by Alfred E. Chang and Suyu Shu.

for many patients sufficient tumor is not available for this to be accomplished.[13] Moreover, tumor cells may be very poor stimulators of T cell activation, because of weak expression of tumor or MHC antigens[14-17] or because of release of immunosuppressive factors.[18-21]

A number of possible solutions to this problem have been tested, including the use of allogeneic tumor cells or cell lines,[22-24] monoclonal antibodies to the T cell antigen receptor (TCR)/CD3 complex and pharmacologic doses of IL-2.[4,25-28] Allogeneic cells may not be adequate, since classical T cell recognition of target antigens occurs in the context of syngeneic MHC class I or class II.[29,30] Moreover, the use of allogeneic tumor cells is predicated on the assumption that cancers of similar histologic type from different individuals will share relevant antigens.

Recently, several groups have used antibodies to the TCR/CD3 complex to mimic antigen ligand and activate tumor-specific T cells from TBH mice.[25,27,28,31] These cells appear to have similar anti-tumor activity as T cells activated with autologous tumor antigen in classical IVS regimens. However, the growth of these cells is usually quite limited, and the optimal concentration of antibody is extremely critical. In fact, the antibody concentration that produces the best growth in terms of cell numbers may actually yield cells without therapeutic activity.[28,32] Moreover, optimal T cell activation with anti-CD3 monoclonal antibodies (mAb) occurs only in the presence of accessory cells, or the antibody must cross-linked by a secondary antibody or by binding to a solid substrate.[25,33-35] The ability of anti-CD3 to activate frozen-thawed cells may also be limited, since such cells generally have limited accessory cell function. In light of data indicating that T cells from TBH with visceral metastases cannot be activated to become therapeutically effective,[36] this limitation is particularly important. Ideally, T cells obtained from patients as early as possible in their clinical course would be stored until later use, either at the time of recurrence or after other treatment. For this to be possible, frozen-thawed cells must be able to be activated and expanded with retention of in vivo efficacy. With current regimens, which may require many weeks to months to obtain sufficient numbers of lymphocytes, cancer progression in prospective recipients often makes treatment impractical. By accelerating the growth of therapeutically active cells, this problem may be avoided.

Antigen binding to the TCR triggers a bifurcated pathway initiated by the activation of phospholipase C. This enzyme then cleaves phosphotidylinositol biphosphate into inositol triphosphate (IP3) and diacylglycerol (DG). IP3 induces an increase in the concentration of intracellular Ca^{2+}, an effect that can also be produced by calcium ionophores, such as ionomycin or anti-CD3 antibody.[37-40] DG causes activation and translocation of protein kinase C (PKC), which can also be achieved by exposure to phorbol esters. In combination, phorbol esters and ionophores can activate T cells for IL-2 responsiveness and growth in vitro, even in the absence of accessory cells.[41,42] Based on our knowledge of these events, we set out to test the hypothesis that T cells derived from the draining lymph nodes (DLN) of tumor-bearing mice could be expanded for adoptive immunotherapy by using pharmacologic activation of this signal transduction pathway followed by culture in low concentrations of IL-2.

ADOPTIVE IMMUNOTHERAPY WITH PDBu/Io-ACTIVATED DLN

Initially, we showed that T cells from the lymph nodes draining progressive murine tumors could be activated and expanded to large numbers using phorbol dibutyrate (PDBu) and ionomycin (Io). PDBu was chosen because previous studies from our institution had demonstrated that, unlike phorbol myristate acetate, PDBu could be removed from cells by washing in warm medium, allowing for a well-defined and limited period of protein kinase C (PKC) stimulation.[43] PDBu/Io activation was therefore compared with antigen stimulation using a tumor model originally described by Shu et al.[44] Briefly, naive C57Bl/6 mice were inoculated with MCA 105 sarcoma cells in the hind footpad. Ten days later, the popliteal draining lymph nodes (DLN) were harvested, and DLN cells were either stimulated with irradiated autologous tumor cells every 7 days (the standard IVS protocol) or stimulated with PDBu/Io for 18 hours on Days 0 and 14 of culture. All DLN cells were cultured in IL-2 (20 IU/ml) for 21 days. Under these conditions, PDBu/Io-activated lymphocytes grew up to 500-fold (9 to 16-fold more than antigen-stimulated cells). When the therapeutic efficacy of PDBu/Io-activated lymphocytes was assessed, these cells could induce regression of established sarcoma lung metastases in vivo.[45] Despite the non-specific stimulus used to activate these cells, the anti-tumor effects were tumor-specific (Table 3.1).

USE OF BRYOSTATIN 1 TO ACTIVATE TUMOR-SPECIFIC T CELLS

Even using a phorbol ester that could be washed out of the cells, however, there would remain a theoretical concern about treating patients with cells that had been exposed to a tumor-promoting agent. Bryostatin 1 (Bryo), a macrocyclic lactone derived from a marine invertebrate (*Bugula neritina*) also activates lymphocyte PKC, and has been shown to stimulate human lymphocyte proliferation and cytokine production in combination with a calcium ionophore and/or exogenous IL-2.[46,47] Unlike the phorbol esters, Bryo has no tumor-promoting activity.[48] In fact, it actually inhibits tumor promotion by phorbol esters and has direct anti-tumor activity itself.[49-52] The reasons for this difference are not entirely clear, and are being actively investigated in several labs. Recent studies have shown that Bryo has anti-tumor activity against a variety of tumors in vivo, but this activity was not felt to be immunologically mediated—based mainly on the fact that Bryo inhibited LAK generation in vitro.[51]

Before testing Bryo for activation of tumor-reactive T cells, an optimal dose combination of Bryo and Io for T cell growth was first established using normal cells. In the protocol selected, lymphocytes are incubated for 18 hr. in 5 nM Bryo plus 1 μM Io. Bryo/Io activation was then compared with antigen stimulation using the MCA 105 sarcoma model as described above. Again, DLN were either stimulated with irradiated autologous tumor cells every 7 days or stimulated with Bryo/Io on Days 0 and 14, and cells were cultured in 20 IU/ml of IL-2. DLN cells stimulated every 7 days with MCA 105 tumor cells expanded an average 15-fold, while DLN cells stimulated with Bryo/Io expanded an average 131-fold during 3 weeks in culture. With IL-2 alone, cell numbers gradually declined until none remained by 3 weeks. DLN lymphocytes stimulated only

Table 3.1. Therapeutic efficacy and specificity of DLN cells activated with PDBu/Ionomycin

Cells transferred[a]	IL-2[b]	Metastases (s.d.)[c]	
		MCA 105	MCA 203
None	–	250 (0)	250 (0)
PDBu/I-DLN (MCA 105)	+	7 (8)[d]	250 (0)

[a]After activation with PDBu/Io and culture in IL-2, 5 x 10^6 DLN cells obtained from MCA 105-bearing mice were given IV 3 days after IV tumor injection.
[b]IL-2 given as 7500 U IP twice a day for three days starting on day of adoptive transfer. Treatment with IL-2 alone had no effect on the number of lung metastases (data not shown).
[c]Fourteen days after tumor injection, mice were sacrificed and pulmonary metastases counted. Each value represents the mean for at least 5 animals per group. Standard deviations are shown in parentheses.
[d]Significantly different from untreated groups ($P < 0.05$, two-sided values; Wilcoxon rank-sum test).

with autologous tumor were all Thy1+, CD8+, and CD4−. DLN cells activated with Bryo/Io were also all Thy1+, but contained a mixed population of CD8+ and CD4+ T cells (approximately 80% and 20%, respectively).[53]

The therapeutic efficacy of Bryo/Io-activated lymphocytes was assessed in the sarcoma IV lung metastasis model. Untreated mice or mice treated with exogenous IL-2 alone had greater than 250 MCA 105 pulmonary nodules 14 days after tumor injection. However, the adoptive transfer of Bryo/Io-activated DLN cells plus IL-2 treatment three days after tumor injection completely eradicated pulmonary metastases. In contrast, freshly harvested DLN cells, not activated with Bryo/Io and cultured in IL-2, were ineffective (Table 3.2). Moreover, although lymph node cells from normal mice and non-draining lymph node cells from tumor-bearing mice could be expanded just as well as tumor-draining lymph node cells using Bryo/Io, they did not reduce pulmonary metastases (Table 3.2).[53] In other words, the anti-tumor activity of these cells depended upon prior in vivo sensitization with tumor cells. This also showed that the therapeutic effect cannot be attributed to IL-2 alone nor to some nonspecific LAK-like activity.

THE EFFECTS OF BRYO/Io-ACTIVATED T CELLS ARE ANTIGEN SPECIFIC DESPITE NONSPECIFIC STIMULATION

Despite the use of a nonspecific method of T cell activation in vitro, the therapeutic effect of Bryo/Io activated cells was tumor-specific. Adoptive transfer of DLN cells obtained from MCA 105 TBH significantly reduced MCA 105 pulmonary metastases after expansion with Bryo/Io, but these same cells had no effect on MCA 203 metastases (Table 3.3). Conversely, Bryo/Io-expanded DLN cells obtained from MCA 203 TBH eliminated MCA 203, but not MCA 105, lung metastases. These data suggest that the in vivo sensitization of DLN T cells provides an enriched population of tumor-specific pre-effector cells that can be expanded in vitro without the necessity for further antigen stimulation. Recently, using limiting dilution methodology to analyze allo-specific T cell precursor frequency, we have also found that Bryo/Io selectively activates previously sensitized T cells, resulting in a 10-fold increased frequency of these cells. This, along with a high fraction of tumor-specific T cell clones in the DLN probably accounts for the activity of these T cells in vivo despite the use of a nonspecific stimulus.

Table 3.2. Tumor draining lymph nodes contain pre-effector cells which require in vitro activation with Bryo/Io

Cells transferred[a]	IL-2[b]	Lung metastases (s.d.)[c]
none	+	250 (0)
Fresh DLN	+	250 (0)
TBH Mes LN + B/I	+	250 (0)
NLN + B/I	+	250 (0)
DLN + B/I	+	10 (10)[d]

[a]Fresh DLN: Freshly harvested DLN cells from day 10 MCA 105 tumor-bearing mice (without B/I activation).
TBH Mes LN + B/I: Mesenteric lymph nodes from mice with 10-day footpad tumors expanded with B/I.
NLN + B/I: Axillary lymph nodes from normal mice expanded with B/I. DLN + B/I: DLN cells activated with B/I and cultured in IL-2
[b]IL-2 given as 7500 U IP twice a day for three days starting on day of adoptive transfer.
[c]Fourteen days after tumor injection, mice were sacrificed and pulmonary metastases counted. Each value represents the mean for at least 5 animals per group. Standard deviations are shown in parentheses.
[d]significantly different from untreated groups ($P < 0.05$, two-sided values; Wilcoxon rank-sum test).

Table 3.3. Specificity of in vivo anti-tumor activity of Bryo/Io-expanded DLN cells

Lung Metastases (SD)[c] Transferred Cells	IL-2[b]	MCA 105	MCA203
none	–	250 (0)	250 (0)
MCA 105 DLN + B/I	+	23 (20)[d]	250 (0)
MCA 203 DLN + B/I	+	250 (0)	0 (0)[d]

[a] DLN cells obtained from either MCA105 or MCA203 TBH were activated with B/I and cultured in IL-2.
[b] IL-2 given as 7500 U IP twice a day for three days starting on day of adoptive transfer.
[c] Fourteen days after tumor injection, mice were sacrificed and pulmonary metastases counted. Each value represents the mean for at least 5 animals per group. Standard deviations are shown in parentheses.
[d] significantly different from untreated groups ($P < 0.05$, two-sided values; Wilcoxon rank-sum test).

BRYO/Io-ACTIVATED DLN CAN TRAFFIC TO TUMOR IN SITES OTHER THAN LUNG

Previous studies have shown that cultured T cells traffic abnormally in vivo after adoptive transfer.[54,55] To exclude the possibility that tumor regression induced by Bryo/Io-activated cells is dependent upon nonspecific trapping of lymphocytes in the lung, the activity of these cells against tumors at other sites was tested.[56] To establish MCA 105 liver metastases, sarcoma cells were injected into the spleens of anesthetized mice and the spleens were removed. Three days later, activated DLN cells were given IV with exogenous IL-2. A single IV injection of Bryo/Io-stimulated lymphocytes + IL-2, but not IL-2 alone induced complete regression of MCA 105 liver metastases (Table 3.4). Bryo/Io-activated DLN cells also mediated tumor-specific P815 mastocytoma metastatic to the liver.[57] Additional experiments showed that activated DLN cells given IV could also induce regression of intradermal sarcomas. Again, tumor regression was immunologically specific (Fig. 3.1); adoptive transfer of Bryo/Io-activated lymphocytes from MCA 105 tumor-bearing animals induced the regression of MCA 105 i.d. tumors, but had no anti-tumor activity against MCA 203 sarcomas. After regression of intradermal tumors, mice remained tumor-free for at least 3 months. In collaboration with the Neurosurgery group at our institution, we have also shown in a rat glioblastoma model that Bryo/Io-activated T cells from DLN draining a site of vaccination could induce regression of intracerebral tumors when administered IV[58] This has important implications, not only for the treatment of primary brain tumors, but also for cellular therapy of other cancers, since there has been concern that metastatic foci of tumor in the central nervous system might not be reached by T cells after intravenous adoptive transfer.

BRYO/Io-DLN T CELLS CONFER IMMUNOLOGIC MEMORY ON THE ADOPTIVE HOST

One of the major theoretical advantages to the use of antigen-specific T cells over LAK cells or other nonspecific effector cells is that T cells may provide long-term immunologic memory and resistance to tumor challenge or re-growth. To determine whether Bryo/Io-activated T cells could fulfill this objective, DLN cells obtained from MCA 105 tumor-bearing hosts were activated with Bryo and Io, grown in low-dose IL-2 and transferred to sublethally irradiated hosts. This treatment conferred resistance to subsequent IV tumor challenge up to 23 weeks later (Table 3.5), and like the therapeutic effect described above, this resistance was immunologically specific (data not shown, ref. 59). In contrast to Bryo/Io-activated DLN cells, the adoptive transfer of fresh noncultured DLN cells did *not* protect the hosts from subsequent IV tumor challenge.[59] Exogenous IL-2 was not given to these mice at any time in these experiments. The resulting immunity after transfer of Bryo/Io-activated DLN cells also appears to be systemic; mice challenged by footpad injections of MCA 105 tumor cells were also protected (Fig. 3.2). All mice given B/I-DLN cells remained tumor-free at least three months after footpad tumor challenge. Other investigators have found that antigen-stimulated cultured CD4⁺ and CD8⁺ T cells survived 120 days after adoptive immunotherapy,[60] and we found that in vivo elimination of either CD4⁺ or CD8⁺ T cell subsets with mAb abrogated the immunologic protection conferred by Bryo/Io-activated DLN T cells.[59] These results, implicate the participation of both CD4⁺ and CD8⁺ T cells in establishing long-term tumor immunity. The transfer of CD4⁺ helper cells may provide lymphokines, such as IL-2, that are essential for in vivo proliferation and survival of effector cells. Administration of exogenous IL-2 either at the time of adoptive transfer

Table 3.4. Adoptive transfer of DLN induces regression of liver metastases

Cells transferred[a]	IL-2[b]	MCA 105 Liver Metastases[c]	
		Exp 1.	Exp 2.
None	–	174 (76)	250 (0)
DLN + B/I	+	0 (0)[d]	0 (0)[d]

[a] After activation with B/I and culture in IL-2, 2 x 10^7 DLN cells/mouse were given IV 3 days after intrasplenic tumor injection.
[b] IL-2 given as 7500 U IP twice a day for three days starting on day of adoptive transfer.
[c] Fourteen days after tumor injection, mice were sacrificed and liver metastases counted. Each value represents the mean for at least 5 animals per group. Standard deviations are shown in parentheses.
[d] significantly different from untreated groups ($P < 0.05$, two-sided values; Wilcoxon rank-sum test).

Table 3.5. Adoptive transfer of B/I-stimulated DLN cells protects the host from IV metastases for 15 to 23 weeks

	MCA 105 Pulmonary Metastases[a]	
	Cells transferred[b]	
Week of Tumor Challenge	None[c]	B/I-DLN
Experiment 1		
1	250 (0)	0 (0)[d]
2	243 (16)	0 (0)[d]
3	250 (0)	0 (0)[d]
5	208 (24)	0 (0)[d]
7	250 (0)	0 (0)[d]
10	232 (23)	4 (5)[d]
15	250 (0)	29 (66)[d]
Experiment 2		
5	229 (34)	0 (0)[d]
15	250 (0)	132 (92)[d]
23	250 (0)	46 (54)[d]

[a] Irradiated (500 rad) C57Bl/6 mice received 1 x 10^7 B/I-DLN cells IV and were then challenged with tumor cells IV at various times thereafter. Two weeks after tumor injection, mice were sacrificed and lung metastases counted.
[b] B/I-DLN: Lymphocytes were obtained from the popliteal lymph nodes draining an MCA 105 footpad tumor, stimulated with 5 nM bryostatin 1 and 1 μM ionomycin, and then cultured for 7 days with 20 U/ml IL-2 (B/I-DLN).
[c] Each value represents the mean of at least 5 animals per group. Standard deviations are shown in parentheses.
[d] Significantly different from untreated groups ($p < 0.05$, Wilcoxon rank-sum test).

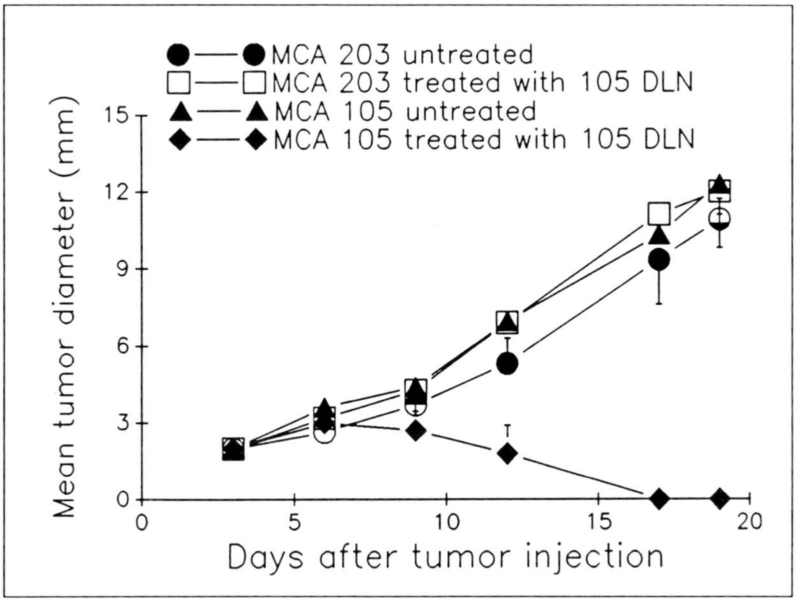

Fig. 3.1. Regression of intradermal tumors is immunologically specific. Irradiated (500 R) mice were injected intradermally with 2 x 10^5 MCA 105 or MCA 203 tumor cells. Three days later, 4 x 10^7 B/I-stimulated cells obtained from lymph nodes draining MCA 105 sarcomas were given in the tail vein. IL-2 was given as 15,000 U IP twice a day for 5 days starting on the day of adoptive transfer. Values shown represent the means and standard deviations of the average of two perpendicular tumor diameters for each tumor. Values in parentheses indicate the number of tumor-free mice at 3 months as a fraction of total number of animals injected with tumor.

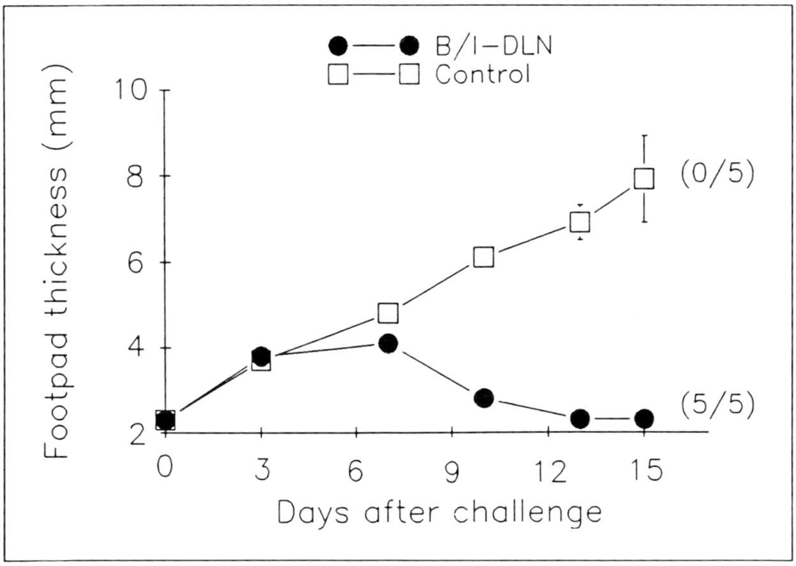

Fig. 3.2. Footpad tumor challenge 5 weeks after IV injection of B/I-DLN cells into naive irradiated mice. Normal mice were used as controls. Values shown represent the means and standard deviations of footpad thickness. Values in parentheses indicate the number of tumor-free mice at 3 months after tumor challenge as a fraction of total number of animals injected with tumor.

or at the time of tumor challenge might overcome the need for CD4⁺ helper cells.

MECHANISMS OF ACTION OF BRYO/Io-ACTIVATED T CELLS

Tumor-draining lymph node cells activated with Bryo/Io and cultured in IL-2 were a mixed population of $CD8^+$ and $CD4^+$ T cells. Using both in vitro and in vivo depletion methods, we found that $CD8^+$ cells retained only a modest in vivo effect, but these lymphocytes no longer completely eliminated experimental metastases (Table 3.6). Conversely, depleting $CD4^+$ cells did not alter the therapeutic effect at all. In vivo subset depletion gave similar results (data not shown, ref. 53). Thus, $CD8^+$ cells appear to be the predominant mediators of this in vivo effect. Furthermore, using Thy-1 congenic strains of C57Bl/6 mice, we showed that only the adoptively transferred T cells are required; the recipient hosts' T cells do not appear to play role.[61]

When the need for exogenous IL-2 to induce regression of lung metastases was evaluated, we found that Bryo/Io-activated DLN cells had potent in vivo anti-tumor activity even when IL-2 was not given.[56] At borderline cell numbers (e.g., 2.5×10^6 per mouse), IL-2 did seem to improve the therapeutic effect, but no exogenous cytokine was required if ≥ 5 million lymphocytes were given. Although $CD8^+$ cells appear to mediate in vivo tumor regression, the adoptive transfer of $CD4^+$ helper cells may provide lymphokines such as IL-2 which induce in vivo growth of effector cells and therefore, may bypass the requirement for exogenous IL-2 administration.

In some model systems, the in vivo anti-tumor activity of transferred lymphocytes correlates with in vitro cytotoxicity and is apparently mediated by direct cytolysis,[62-65] but others have found that noncytolytic $CD4^+$ and $CD8^+$ T cells can also mediate regression of certain tumors.[66-68] At all effector:target ratios tested, Bryo/Io-activated DLN cells did not lyse autologous tumor cells which were, however, susceptible to lysis by lymphokine activated killer (LAK) cells (Fig. 3.3). Recent experiments in our lab demonstrate that this lack of cytotoxicity is *not* the result of ineffective triggering mechanisms or cytolytic effector function resulting from exposure to Bryo/Io. Bryo/Io-activated DLN *can* mediate antibody-redirected cytotoxicity, even with anti-TCR antibodies, which require intact PKC to trigger cytolysis (data not shown).[69]

Since Bryo/Io-activated DLN cells have potent in vivo anti-tumor activity despite minimal in vitro cytotoxicity, we postulated that cytokine release might play a key role in tumor regression. For example, interferon-γ (IFN-γ) and tumor necrosis factor-α (TNF-α) were found to be important me-

Table 3.6. Effect of in vitro depletion of $CD4^+$ and $CD8^+$ cells prior to adoptive immunotherapy

Cells transferred[a]	In vitro treatment[b]	Lung Metastases (s.d.)[c]
none	-	144 (44)
DLN + B/I	C	0 (0)[d]
DLN + B/I	anti-CD4 + C	1 (1)[d]
DLN + B/I	anti-CD8 + C	62 (20)[d,e]

[a] DLN + B/I = DLN cells from MCA 105-bearing mice expanded with B/I. IL-2 was given as 7500 U twice a day for 3 days starting on the day of adoptive transfer.
[b] After expansion with B/I, DLN cell cultures were treated with monoclonal antibody plus complement prior to adoptive immunotherapy.
[c] Means and standard deviations () of at least 5 animals/group.
[d] significantly different from untreated group ($P < 0.05$, two-sided values; Wilcoxon rank-sum test).
[e] significantly different from C' alone group ($P < 0.05$, two-sided values; Wilcoxon rank-sum test).

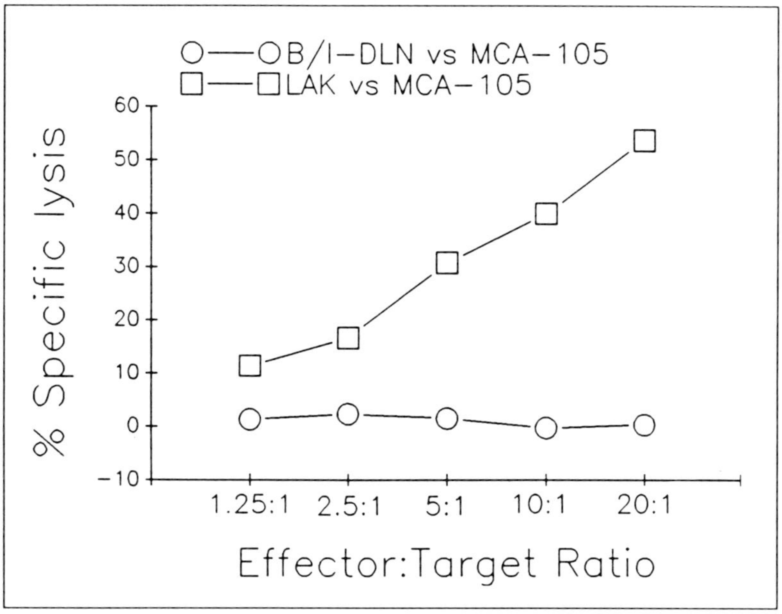

Fig. 3.3. Activated tumor-draining lymph node cells lack in vitro cytotoxicity. Popliteal lymph node cells draining MCA 105 footpad sarcomas were activated with bryostatin 1 plus ionomycin and cultured in 20 U/ml IL-2 for 7 days. LAK cells were generated by culturing normal C57Bl/6 splenocytes with 1000 U/ml IL-2 for 3 days. The cytolytic activity of the effector cells against MCA 105 was determined in a 4 hour ^{51}Cr-release assay.

diators of the anti-tumor effect of murine TIL from sarcomas.[70] To test the role of INF-γ in our system, mice with established lung metastases were pretreated with 0.25 mg of monoclonal rat anti-mouse IFN-γ or control rat IgG 24 hr before adoptive immunotherapy with Bryo/Io-activated DLN cells. The neutralizing antibody against IFN-γ significantly inhibited the in vivo activity of activated DLN cells in three independent experiments (Fig. 3.4). Anti-TNF-α antibody, however, had a much less significant effect. Moreover, DLN cells obtained from MCA 105 tumor-bearing hosts and expanded in IL-2 after activation with Bryo/Io, secreted high concentrations of IFN-γ in response to specific tumor cells, but little or none in response to irrelevant tumor cells (Table 3.7). Fresh DLN cells *not* activated with Bryo/Io and cultured in IL-2 did not secrete IFN-γ when stimulated with the appropriate tumor cells (Table 3.8). In contrast, Bryo/Io-activated DLN cells did *not* secrete TNF-α in response to specific tumor cells.[61] IFN-γ secretion in response to autologous tumor was markedly reduced by removing $CD8^+$ lymphocytes; depletion of $CD4^+$ cells had no significant effect (Fig. 3.5A). Moreover, release of IFN-γ was blocked by addition of anti-CD8, but not anti-CD4, directly to co-cultures (Fig. 3.5B). This suggests a role for CD8 in tumor cell recognition and/or triggering of IFN-γ secretion, as one would expect for a classical MHC Class I-restricted T cell response.

Previous studies have demonstrated that IFN-γ has both direct cytotoxicity and anti-proliferative effects on murine and human tumors.[71-73] Neither high concentrations (1000 U/ml) of recombinant murine IFN-γ nor supernatants from DLN/tumor co-cultures were directly cytotoxic in vitro to MCA 105 (data not shown), but recombinant murine IFN-γ did have a significant anti-proliferative effect against MCA 105 tumor cells (Fig. 3.6). Similarly, supernatants obtained from DLN/autologous

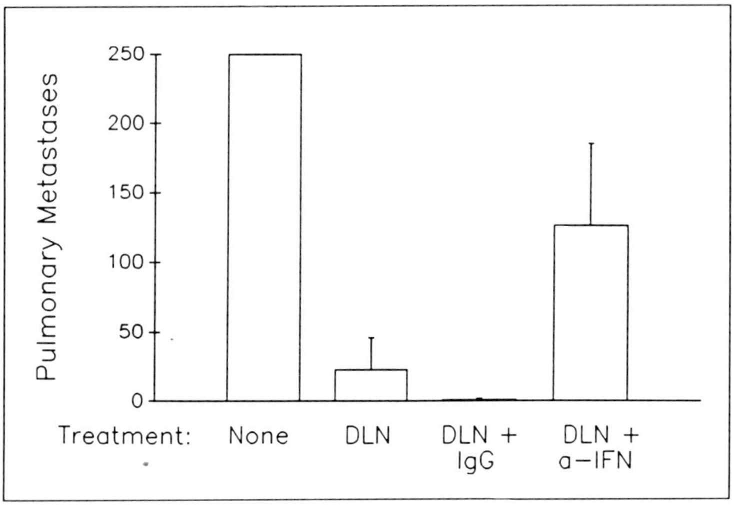

Fig. 3.4. Antibody against IFN-γ partially blocked in vivo effect induced by DLN cells. On day 0, normal C57Bl/6 mice received 4 x 10^5 MCA 105 tumor cells IV Two days later, 250 μg of either anti-IFN-γ or control rat IgG were given IP On day 3, 5 x 10^6 activated DLN cells were injected IV IL-2 was given as 7500 U IP twice/day x 3 days. All groups were significantly different from each other and controls (Wilcoxon-rank sum test, $p < 0.05$).

Table 3.7. Activated tumor-draining lymph node cells secrete interferon-gamma in response to specific tumor

Responder[a]	Stimulator[b]	IFN-γ (U/ml)
DLN	medium	0
DLN	MCA 105	31.3
DLN	MCA 203	11.0
none	MCA 105	0
none	MCA 203	0

[a]Popliteal draining lymph node cells from MCA 105 tumor-bearing mice were stimulated with bryostatin 1 and ionomycin for 18 hr and then cultured for 7 days in 20 U/ml IL-2.
[b]After 7 days in culture, 5 x 10^5 activated draining lymph node cells were incubated with either medium alone or 1 x 10^6 tumor cells in 2 ml of a 24-well plate. Eighteen hours later, the supernatants were collected, and the concentration of IFN-g was determined by ELISA.

Table 3.8. Bryo/Io-activated and expanded but not freshly harvested DLN secrete IFN-γ in response to specific tumor

Responder	Stimulator	IFN U/ml
B/I-activated DLN[a]	medium	0
B/I-activated DLN	MCA 105	61.2
Fresh DLN[b]	medium	0
Fresh DLN	MCA 105	0.2

[a]Popliteal draining lymph node cells from MCA 105 tumor-bearing mice were stimulated with bryostatin 1 and ionomycin for 18 hr and then cultured for 7 days in 20 U/ml IL-2. 5 x 10^5 activated draining lymph node cells were then incubated with either media alone or 1 x 10^6 tumor cells in 2 ml of a 24-well plate. Eighteen hours later, the supernatants were collected, and the concentration of IFN-g was determined by ELISA.
[b]5 x 10^5 freshly harvested popliteal draining lymph node cells from MCA 105 tumor-bearing mice were incubated immediately with either medium alone or 1 x 10^6 tumor cells in 2 ml of a 24-well plate. Eighteen hours later, the supernatants were collected, and the concentration of IFN-g was determined by ELISA.

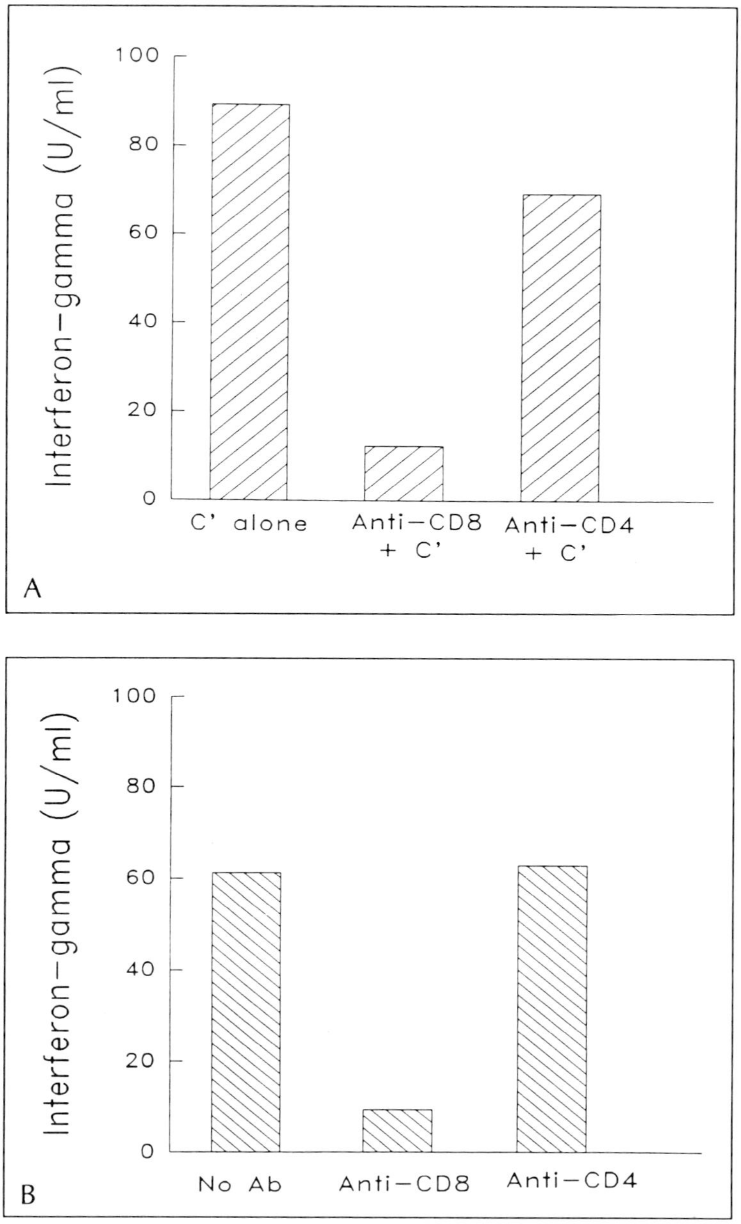

Fig. 3.5. Tumor-stimulated secretion of IFN-γ by B/I-DLN is mediated by CD8⁺ lymphocytes (A) and depends upon CD8 for recognition (B)

A. DLN from C57Bl/6 mice bearing MCA 105 sarcomas were activated with B/I and cultured for 7 days in IL-2 (20 IU/ml). Cells harvested from cultured were treated either with C′ alone, anti-CD8 Ab + C′ or anti-CD4 Ab + C′ and then cultured overnight with irradiated MCA 105 tumor cells. Supernatants were then harvested and assayed for IFN-γ by ELISA. Data shown are means of triplicate assays. B/I-DLN cells incubated with medium only secreted almost no detectable IFN-γ (0-1 U/ml).

B. Experiment was similar to that in panel A, except that B/I-DLN cells harvested from culture were co-cultured with MCA 105 overnight in the presence or absence of anti-CD8 or anti-CD4 antibody (ascites at a final dilution of 1:40). The addition of antibody to supernatants did not affect the IFN-γ ELISA (not shown).

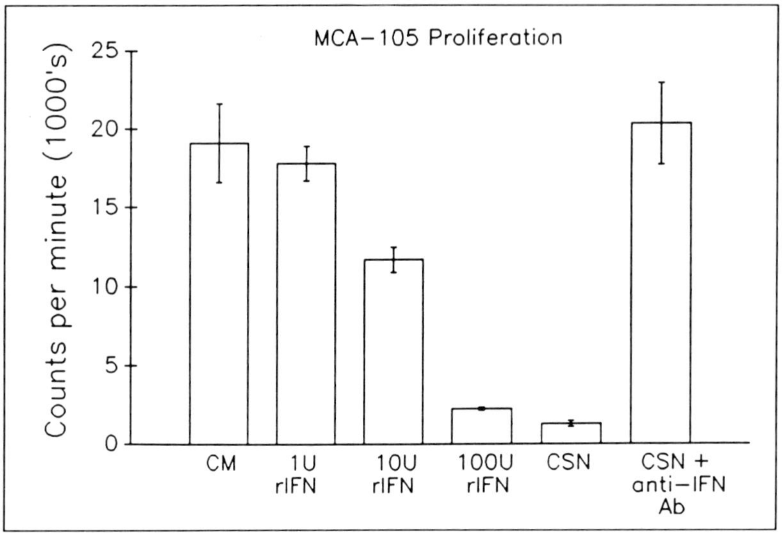

Fig. 3.6. IFN-γ inhibits proliferation of MCA 105 tumor cells. MCA 105 tumor cells were incubated for 3 days in complete medium (CM), various concentrations of recombinant murine IFN-γ, or supernatant (CSN) from cultures of activated DLN cells plus autologous tumor with or without anti-IFN-γ antibody. ^{3}H-thymidine was added 18 hours before harvesting the cells.

tumor co-cultures significantly inhibited MCA 105 proliferation; this anti-proliferative effect was abrogated by the addition of anti-IFN-γ antibody to the cultures.[61] These results suggest that at least part of the anti-tumor effect of Bryo/Io-activated DLN cells may be mediated by the anti-proliferative effect of IFN-γ in this tumor model. Other effects, such as immunomodulation by secreted cytokines or the development of cytolytic activity in vivo may also be involved.

BRYO/Io CAN BE USED TO EXPAND DLN FROM PATIENTS WITH BREAST CANCER

The principles derived from our experiments in mice have been applied to expansion of human T lymphocytes as well. After determining an optimal concentration of Bryo for activation of human T cells (50 nM), axillary draining lymph nodes which had been obtained from patients with breast cancer and stored frozen in liquid nitrogen were thawed and stimulated overnight with Bryo/Io using essentially the same regimen as had been used successfully for murine DLN. For 20 patients' DLN, the average expansion over 17 days of culture in IL-2 (20 IU/ml) was nearly 2,000-fold. The absence or presence of metastases detected histologically in these nodes did not appear to affect the growth response, and in no instance was the expansion less than 250-fold. Starting with 5 to 10 lymph nodes containing on average 8 x 10^7 cells each, obtaining more than 10^{11} cells for most patients should present no difficulty.

As we had seen with murine DLN cells expanded after Bryo/Io activation, the expanded human DLN cells were >90% CD3$^+$ T cells, mostly CD8$^+$ with some CD4$^+$ cells also seen (4 to 30%). These cells were not cytolytic for autologous tumor cells, but in 5 out of 6 patients tested, these T cells released significant amounts of IFN-γ and TNF-α in response to autologous tumor cells but not in response to an irrelevant tumor (a melanoma cell line, see Table 3.9). Thus, it appears that Bryo/Io can be used to activate and then grow large numbers of T cells from human tumor-draining lymph nodes. Moreover, these cells display similar features and functions as those which in the murine models were able to induce regression of metastatic cancers.

FUTURE PLANS

Currently, we are further refining our understanding of the T cells obtained using this regimen and their responses to tumor cells in man. In addition, further refinements are being made in the murine pre-clinical models to increase the logistic practicality and applicability of this approach, especially to patients with micro-

Table 3.9. Cytokine production by Bryo/Io-activated and expanded DLN lymphocytes from patients with breast cancer

	Stimulators[a]		
Source of DLN	**None**	**Autol. Tumor**	**SK-MEL**
IFN-γ (units/10^6 cells)			
BC-1	0	30.1 (4.2)[b]	0
BC-2	0	24.7 (2.3)	0
BC-3	0	29.8 (6.0)	0
BC-4	0	7.0 (1.0)	0
BC-7	0	5.3 (0.1)	0
BC-12	0	0	0
SK-MEL	0	ND	ND
TNF (units/10^6 cells)			
BC-1	0	3.6 (0.5)[b]	0
BC-2	0	17.0 (3.5)	0
BC-3	0	4.4 (0.2)	0
BC-4	0	12.7 (3.5)	0
BC-7	0	54.0 (20.0)	0
BC-12	0	0[c]	0
SK-MEL	0	ND	ND

[a]Bryo/Io-activated DLN cells from 6 different breast cancer patients were incubated with irradiated autologous tumor cells or SK-MEL melanoma cells or no cells for 24 hours. Culture supernatants were then harvested and assayed for IFN-γ or TNF-α by ELISA.
[b]Units/million lymphocytes are shown with standard deviations for duplicate wells. Neither SK-MEL nor any of the breast cancer cells secreted detectable levels of either cytokine when cultured alone (data not shown for breast cancer cells).
[c]DLN cells from BC-12 did secrete TNF when stimulated with anti-CD3 antibody (not shown).

scopic metastatic disease. Soon, clinical trials based on this pharmacologic T cell activation strategy should be underway.

SUMMARY

These studies demonstrate that by using our knowledge of the signal transduction pathway triggered by binding of antigen to the TCR, pharmacologic agents can be substituted for antigen in the activation of T cells from tumor-bearing hosts. Despite the nonspecific stimulus used in vitro, T cells expanded in IL-2 after this treatment mediate potent anti-tumor effects in vivo, and they retain tumor specificity that is determined by the prior sensitization of pre-effector cells in the donors. The phenotypes and activities that account for the anti-tumor effects are similar to TIL and to anti-CD3-activated T cells, with the anti-tumor effect apparently dependent on secretion of IFN-γ. Because this method induces very rapid expansion of T cells from mice or humans in low concentrations of IL-2, it appears to have great potential to increase the practicality of cellular adoptive immunotherapy. Moreover, these agents may be able to be used in ways that minimize or eliminate the need for prolonged cell culture and the resulting expense.

REFERENCES

1. Rosenberg SA, Lotze MT, Muul LM, Chang AE, Avis FP, Leitman S, Linehan WM, Robertson CN, Lee RE, Rubin JT, Seipp CA, Simpson CG, White DE. A progress report on the treatment of 157 patients with advanced cancer using lymphokine-activated killer cells and interleukin-2 or high dose interleukin-2 alone. New Eng J Med 316:889-897, 1987.
2. Rosenberg SA. Cancer therapy with Interleukin-2: Immunologic manipulations can

mediate the regression of cancer in humans. J Clin Onc 6:403-406, 1988.
3. Lotze MT, Matory YL, Rayner AA. Clinical effects and toxicity of interleukin-2 in patients with cancer. Cancer 58:2764-2772, 1986.
4. Rosenberg SA, Spiess P, Lafreniere R. A new approach to the adoptive immunotherapy of cancer with tumor-infiltrating lymphocytes. Science 233:1318-1321, 1986.
5. Itoh K, Tilden AB, Balch CM. Interleukin 2 activation of cytotoxic T-lymphocytes infiltrating into human metastatic melanomas. Cancer Res 46:3011-3017, 1986.
6. Rosenberg SA, Packard BS, Aebersold PM, Solomon D, Topalian SL, Toy ST, Simon P, Lotze MT, Yang JC, Seipp CA, Simpson C, Carter C, Bock S, Schwartzentruber D, Wei JP, White DE. Special Report: Use of tumor-infiltrating lymphocytes and interleukin-2 in the immunotherapy of patients with metastatic melanoma. New Eng J Med 319:1676-1680, 1988.
7. Chou T, Bertera S, Chang AE, Shu S. Adoptive immunotherapy of microscopic and advanced visceral metastases with in vitro sensitized lymphoid cells from mice bearing progressive tumors. J Immunol 141:1775-1781, 1988.
8. Lynch DH, Miller RE. Immunotherapeutic elimination of syngeneic tumors in vivo by cytotoxic T lymphocytes generated in vitro from lymphocytes from the draining lymph nodes of tumor-bearing mice. Eur J Immunol 21:1403-1410, 1991.
9. Stephenson KR, Perry-Lalley D, Griffith KD, Shu S, Chang AE. Development of antitumor reactivity in regional draining lymph nodes from tumor-immunized and tumor-bearing murine hosts. Surgery 105:523-528, 1989.
10. Slingluff CL, Darrow TL, Seigler HF. Human T cells specifically activated against autologous malignant melanoma. Arch Surg 122:1407-1411, 1987.
11. Itoh K, Platsoucas CD, Balch CM. Autologous tumor-specific cytotoxic T lymphocytes in the infiltrate of human metastatic melanomas. Activation by interleukin 2 and autologous tumor cells and involvement of the T cell receptor. J Exp Med 168:1419-1441, 1988.
12. Chou T, Chang AE, Shu S. Generation of therapeutic T lymphocytes from tumor-bearing mice by in vitro sensitization. J Immunol 140:2453-2461, 1988.
13. Chang AE, Yoshizawa H, Sakai K, Cameron MJ, Sondak VK, Shu S. Clinical observations on adoptive immunotherapy with vaccine-primed T-lymphocytes secondarily sensitized to tumor in vitro. Cancer Res 53:1043-1050, 1993.
14. Blieden TM, McAdam AJ, Frelinger JG, Lord EM. Mechanism of cytolytic T lymphocyte killing of a low class I-expressing tumor. J Immunol 147:1433-1438, 1991.
15. Weber JS, Jay G. MHC class I gene expression by tumors: Immunotherapeutic implications. Curr Top Microbiol Immunol 137:140-147, 1988.
16. Weber JS, Rosenberg SA. Modulation of murine tumor major histocompatibility antigens by cytokines in vivo and in vitro. Cancer Res 48:5818-5824, 1988.
17. Momburg F, Ziegler A, Harpprecht J, Möller P, Moldenhauer G, Hämmerling GJ. Selective loss of HLA-A or HLA-B antigen expression in colon carcinoma. J Immunol 142:352-358, 1989.
18. Cornelius JG, Normann SJ. Isolation of a low molecular weight inhibitor of lymphocyte proliferation from tumorous ascites. J Immunol 141:2175-2180, 1988.
19. Kuppner MC, Hamou M-F, Bodmer S, Fontana A, De Tribolet N. The glioblastoma-derived T-cell suppressor factor/transforming growth factor $beta_2$ inhibits the generation of lymphokine-activated killer (LAK) cells. Int J Cancer 42:562-567, 1988.
20. Nelson M, Bremner JAG, Nelson DS. Tumour cell products inhibit both functional and immunoreactive interleukin 2 production by human blood lymphocytes. Br J Cancer 60:161-163, 1989.
21. Sulitzeanu D. Immunosuppressive factors in human cancer. Adv Cancer Res 60:247-267, 1993.
22. Crowley NJ, Slingluff CL,Jr, Darrow TL, Seigler HF. Generation of human autologous melanoma-specific cytotoxic T-cells using HLA-A2-matched allogeneic melanomas. Cancer Res 50:492-498, 1990.

23. Barnd DL, Lan MS, Metzgar RS, Finn OJ. Specific major histocompatibility complex-unrestricted recognition of tumor-associated mucins by human cytotoxic T cells. Proc Natl Acad Sci USA 86:7159-7163, 1989.
24. Jerome KR, Barnd DL, Bendt KM, Boyer CM, Taylor-Papadimitriou J, McKenzie IFC, Bast RC,Jr, Finn OJ. Cytotoxic T-lymphocytes derived from patients with breast adenocarcinoma recognize an epitope present on the protein core of a mucin molecule preferentially expressed on malignant cells. Cancer Res 51:2908-2916, 1991.
25. Schoof DD, Selleck CM, Massaro AF, Jung S-E, Eberlein TJ. Activation of human tumor-infiltrating lymphocytes by monoclonal antibodies directed to the CD3 complex. Cancer Res 50:1138-1143, 1990.
26. Yannelli JR, Crumpacker DB, Good RW, Friddell CD, Poston R, Horton S, Maleckar JR, Oldham RK. Use of anti-CD3 monoclonal antibody in the generation of effector cells from human solid tumors for use in cancer biotherapy. J Immunol Methods 130:91-100, 1990.
27. Nijhuis EWP, Wiel-van Kemenade EVD, Figdor CG, Van Lier RAW. Activation and expansion of tumour-infiltrating lymphocytes by anti-CD3 and anti-CD28 monoclonal antibodies. Cancer Immunol Immunother 32:245-250, 1990.
28. Yoshizawa H, Chang AE, Shu S. Specific adoptive immunotherapy mediated by tumor-draining lymph node cells sequentially activated with anti-CD3 and IL-2. J Immunol 147:729-737, 1991.
29. Townsend A, Bodmer H. Antigen recognition by class I-restricted T lymphocytes. Annu Rev Immunol 7:601-624, 1989.
30. Doyle C, Strominger JL. Interaction between CD4 and class II MHC molecules mediates cell adhesion. Nature(Lond) 330:256-259, 1987.
31. Crossland KD, Lee VK, Chen W, Riddell SR, Greenberg PD, Cheever MA. T cells from tumor-immune mice nonspecifically expanded in vitro with anti-CD3 plus IL-2 retain specific function in vitro and can eradicate disseminated leukemia in vivo. J Immunol 146:4414-4420, 1991.
32. Davis LS, Wacholtz MC, Lipsky PE. The induction of T cell unresponsiveness by rapidly modulating CD3. J Immunol 142:1084-1094, 1989.
33. Dixon JFP, Law JL, Favero JJ. Activation of human T lymphocytes by crosslinking of anti-CD3 monoclonal antibodies. J Leukocyte Biol 46:214-220, 1989.
34. Van Lier RAW, Brouwer M, Rebel VI, Van Noesel CJM, Aarden LA. Immobilized anti-CD3 monoclonal antibodies induce accessory cell-independent lymphokine production proliferation and helper activity in human T lymphocytes. Immunology 68:45-50, 1989.
35. Geppert TD. and Lipsky PE. Immobilized anti-CD3-induced T cell growth: Comparison of the frequency of responding cells within various T cell subsets. Cell Immunol 133:206-218, 1991.
36. Sondak VK, Wagner PD, Shu S, Chang AE. Suppressive effects of visceral tumor on the generation of anti-tumor T cells for adoptive immunotherapy. Arch Surg 126:442-446, 1991.
37. Ullman KS, Northrop JP, Verweij CL, Crabtree GR. Transmission of signals from the T lymphocyte antigen receptor to the genes responsible for cell proliferation and immune function: The missing link. Annu Rev Immunol 8:421-452, 1990.
38. Weiss A, Imboden J, Hardy K, Manger B, Terhorst C, Stobo J. The role of the T3/ Antigen receptor complex in T-cell activation. Ann Rev Immunol 4:593-619, 1990.
39. Hara T, Fu SM. Human T cell activation. I. Monocyte-independent activation and proliferation induced by anti-T3 monoclonal antibodies in the presence of tumor promoter 12-O-tetradecanoyl phorbol-13-acetate. J Exp Med 161:641-656, 1985.
40. Chatila T, Silverman L, Miller R, Geha R. Mechanisms of T cell activation by the calcium ionophore ionomycin. J Immunol 143:1283-1289, 1989.
41. Kumagai N, Benedict SH, Mills GB, Gelfand EW. Induction of competence and progression signals in human T lymphocytes by phorbol esters and calcium ionophores. J Cell Physiol 137:329-336, 1988.
42. Truneh A, Albert F, Golstein P, Schmitt-Verhulst A-M Calcium ionophore

plus phorbol ester can substitute for antigen in the induction of cytolytic T lymphocytes from specifically primed precursors. J Immunol 135:2262-2267, 1985.

43. McCrady CW, Ely CM, Westin E, Carchman RA. Coordination and reversibility of signals for proliferative activation and interleukin-2 mRNA production in resting human T lymphocytes by phorbol ester and calcium ionophore. J Biol Chem 263:18537-18544, 1988.
44. Shu S, Chou T, Rosenberg SA. Generation from tumor-bearing mice of lymphocytes with in vivo therapeutic efficacy. J Immunol 139:295-304, 1987.
45. Tuttle TM, Inge TH, McCrady CM, Bethke KP, Bear HD. Activation of $CD8^+$ murine T cells from tumor-draining lymph nodes by phorbol dibutyrate plus calcium ionophore. J Immunother 12:32-40, 1992.
46. Hess AD, Silanskis MK, Esa AH, Pettit GR, May WS. Activation of human T lymphocytes by bryostatin. J Immunol 141:3263-3269, 1988.
47. Trenn G, Pettit GR, Takayama H, Hu-Li J, Sitkovsky MV. Immunomodulating properties of a novel series of protein kinase C activators. The bryostatins. J Immunol 140:433-439, 1988.
48. Blumberg PM, Pettit GR, Warren BS, Szallasi A, Schuman LD, Sharkey NA, Nakakuma H, Dell'Aquila ML, de Vries DJ. The protein kinase C pathway in tumor promotion. In: Slaga TJ ed. Skin Carcinogenesis: Mechanisms and Human Relevance. New York: Alan R Liss 1989:201-212.
49. Pettit GR, Day JF, Hartwell JL, Wood HB. Antineoplastic components of marine animals. Nature(Lond) 227:962-963, 1970.
50. Hennings H, Blumberg PM, Pettit GR, Herald CL, Shores R, Yuspa S. Bryostatin 1, an activator of protein kinase C inhibits tumor promotion by phorbol esters in Sencar mouse skin. Carcinogenesis 9:1343-1346, 1987.
51. Schuchter LM, Esa AH, May WS, Laulis MK, Pettit GR, Hess AD. Successful treatment of murine melanoma with bryostatin 1. Cancer Res 51:682-687, 1991.
52. Hornung RL, Pearson JW, Beckwith M, Longo DL. Preclinical evaluation of bryostatin as an anticancer agent against several murine tumor cell lines: In vitro versus in vivo activity. Cancer Res 52:101-107, 1992.
53. Tuttle TM, Inge TH, Bethke KP, McCrady CW, Pettit GR, Bear HD. Activation and growth of murine tumor-specific T-cells which have in vivo activity with bryostatin 1. Cancer Res 52:548-553, 1992.
54. Lotze MT, Line BR, Mathisen DJ, Rosenberg SA. The in vivo distribution of autologous human and murine lymphoid cells grown in T cell growth factor (TCGF): implications for the adoptive immunotherapy of tumors. J Immunol 125:1487-1493, 1980.
55. Dailey MO, Falkman CG, Butcher EC, Pillemer E, Weissman I. Abnormal migration of T lymphocyte clones. J Immunol 128:2134-2136, 1982.
56. Tuttle TM, Bethke KP, Inge TH, McCrady CW, Pettit GR, Bear HD. Bryostatin 1-activated T cells can traffic and mediate tumor regression. J Surg Res 52:543-548, 1992.
57. Tuttle TM, Inge TH, Wirt CP, Frank JL, McCrady CM, Bear HD. Bryostatin 1 activates T cells that have anti-tumor activity. J Immunother 12:75-81, 1992.
58. Rice CD, Baldwin NG, Bear HD, Merchant RE. Adoptive immunotherapy of intracranial glioma models with tumor-sensitized lymphocytes. Proc Am Assoc Cancer Res 34:483, 1993 (Abstract).
59. Tuttle TM, Inge TH, Lind DS, Bear HD. Adoptive transfer of bryostatin 1-activated T cells provides long-term protection from tumor metastases. Surg Oncol 1:299-307, 1992.
60. Cheever MA, Thompson DB, Klarnet JP, Greenberg PD. Antigen-driven long term-cultured T cells proliferate in vivo distribute widely mediate specific tumor therapy and persist long-term as functional memory cells. J Exp Med 163:1100-1112, 1986.
61. Tuttle TM, McCrady CW, Inge TH, Salour M, Bear HD. Gamma-interferon plays a key role in T-cell-induced tumor regression. Cancer Res 53:833-839, 1993.
62. Greenberg PD. Therapy of murine leukemia with cyclophosphamide and immune

Lyt-2+ cells: cytolytic T cells can mediate eradication of disseminated leukemia. J Immunol 136:1917-1922, 1986.

63. Rosenstein M, Eberlein TJ, Rosenberg SA. Adoptive immunotherapy of established syngeneic solid tumors: Role of T lymphoid subpopulations. J Immunol 132:2117-2122, 1984.
64. Dye ES, North RJ. Adoptive immunization against an established tumor with cytolytic versus memory T cells. Immediate versus delayed onset of regression. Transplantation 37:600-605, 1984.
65. Fernandez-Cruz E, Halliburton B, Feldman JD. In vivo elimination by specific effector cells of an established syngeneic rat Moloney virus induced sarcoma. J Immunol 123:1772-1777, 1979.
66. Greenberg PD, Cheever MA, Fefer A. Eradication of disseminated murine leukemia by chemoimmunotherapy with cyclophosphamide and adoptively transferred immune syngeneic Lyt-1+2- lymphocytes. J Exp Med 154:952-963, 1981.
67. Fujiwara H, Fukuyawa T, Yoshioka T, Nakajima H, Hamaoka T. The role of tumor specific Lyt-1+2- T cells in eradicating tumor cells in vivo. J Immunol 133:1671-1676, 1984.
68. Kahn M, Sugawara H, McGowan P, Okuno K, Nagoya S, Hellström KE, Hellström I, Greenberg P. CD4+ T cell clones specific for the human p97 melanoma-associated antigen can eradicate pulmonary metastases from a murine tumor expressing the p97 antigen. J Immunol 146:3235-3241, 1991.
69. Hengel H, Wagner H, Heeg K. Triggering of CD8+ cytotoxic T lymphocytes via CD3-ε differs from triggering via α/β T cell receptor: CD3-ε-induced cytotoxicity occurs in the absence of protein kinase C and does not result in exocytosis of serine esterases. J Immunol 147:1115-1120, 1991.
70. Barth RJ,Jr, Mulé JJ, Spiess PJ, Rosenberg SA. Interferon t and tumor necrosis factor have a role in tumor regressions mediated by CD8+ tumor-infiltrating lymphocytes. J Exp Med 173:647-658, 1991.
71. Tyring S, Klimpel GR, Fleischman WR,Jr, Baron S. Direct cytolysis by partially-purified preparations of immune interferon. Int J Cancer 30:59-64, 1982.
72. Ratliff TL, Kadmon D, Shapiro A, Jacobs AJ, Heston WDW. Inhibition of mouse bladder tumor proliferation by murine interferon-gamma and its synergism with interferon-beta. Cancer Res 44:4377-4381, 1984.
73. Sacchi M, Klapan I, Johnson JT, and Whiteside TL. Antiproliferative effects of cytokines on squamous cell carcinoma. Arch Otolaryngol Head Neck Surg 117:321-326, 1991.

CHAPTER 4

CD4+ T Cells in Tumor Rejection: Past Evidence and Current Prospects

Peter A. Cohen

Difficulties maintaining functional CD4+ T cells in culture have historically limited out ability to study their role in tumor rejection. Better understanding of other immune components, such as CD8+ T cells, natural killer (NK) cells, and macrophages has created a strong impetus to define optimal culture conditions for growing anti-tumor CD4+ T cells.

INTRODUCTION

During the past two decades, thanks largely to the discovery and subsequent availability of interleukin-2 (IL-2), it has been possible to propagate antigen specific CD8+ T cells in vitro with considerable ease. This has led to progress in the area of antimicrobial cellular adoptive therapy,[1,2] and has also enabled in depth characterization of CD8+ T cell responses to tumor related antigens. Definitive CD8+ T cell adoptive therapy experiments in murine tumor models led to clinical trials in cancer patients; striking tumor regressions have been noted in many mouse models[3,4] as well as in melanoma patients.[5] Nonetheless, there are apparent well defined limits to what has been achievable with anti-tumor CD8+ therapy in murine tumor models. For example, cultured murine anti-tumor CD8+ T cells, notably effective against three- to ten-day experimental pulmonary metastases, are ineffective when used to treat three to five day established syngeneic subcutaneous sarcomas.[6] This is despite the fact that adoptive transfer of fresh unfractionated immune splenocytes can cure established syngeneic subcutaneous tumors, even without coadministration of exogenous IL-2.[7,8]

To explain such observations some investigators have postulated that prolonged culture may impair the ability of T cells to traffic to certain

Immunotherapy of Cancer with Sensitized T Lymphocytes, edited by Alfred E. Chang and Suyu Shu.

extravascular locations such as the skin. In contrast to mouse studies, however, cultured human tumor infiltrating lymphocytes (TILs) from melanoma patients frequently traffic to and cause striking regressions of subcutaneous melanoma nodules when given as adoptive therapy.[5,9,10] One major feature which distinguishes the treatment of human cancers from that of experimental animal tumors is the presence of a natural host immune response at the time of adoptive therapy. Syngeneic adoptive transfer therapy of animals usually begins between 0 to 14 days after first exposure to tumor cells; in addition, mice are often sublethally irradiated or given cyclophosphamide before tumor challenge to minimize confounding elements of the host immune response.[11,12] In contrast, human cancer patients may have been exposed to tumor antigen for many years prior to adoptive therapy with autologous cells, and elements of a long-term host response may have significant impact on exogenously administered T cells. Subcutaneous human melanoma nodules may be susceptible to cultured T cell adoptive therapy because of host elements already present in the tumor which facilitate homing and activation of the adoptively transferred cells. The absence of such host elements in many murine therapy models may result in altered traffic of cultured T cells.

Even in murine studies it is occasionally possible to develop cultured anti-tumor T cell lines which are highly effective for the treatment of widely disseminated tumors: for example, cultured $CD8^+$ T cell lines raised against the murine lymphoma FBL-3 have been used adoptively to cure sublethally irradiated mice of widespread tumor burdens (intrafootpad, lymph node, bone marrow and hematogenous).[13] One distinguishing feature of these anti-FBL-3 $CD8^+$ cells is that they are IL-2-producing, so-called helper-independent T ("HIT") cells.[14] Because in this model the administration of exogenous IL-2 is still required to achieve a full therapeutic effect,[15] it is likely to be some property other than IL-2 production which renders these cells superior to "helper-dependent" $CD8^+$ T cells. Whatever the critical property, these experiments are further proof that culturing per se is not the only reason why cultured anti-tumor T cells are sometimes ineffective as adoptive therapy.

In response to these observations two basic strategies have widely been contemplated: (1) to grow, or genetically engineer, "helper-independent"-type $CD8^+$ T cells in tumor systems other than FBL-3; (2) to grow anti-tumor $CD4^+$ T cells to guide and facilitate "helper-dependent" $CD8^+$ T cells. The first strategy has been unsuccessful to date. It appears that much of the $CD8^+$ HIT cell repertoire is naturally eliminated during thymic maturation, possibly as protection against autoimmune disease.[16] It has not routinely been possible to demonstrate "helper-independent" $CD8^+$ T cells among the immune responses to other murine or human tumors, and it is likely that the $CD8^+$ "HIT" cell response to the FBL-3 lymphoma is an anomaly related to that tumor's strong viral antigenicity. Efforts to genetically engineer $CD8^+$ HIT cells have also been unsuccessful,[17] and in any case may not be achievable simply by transferring the ability to synthesize interleukin-2. As the limits of current pure $CD8^+$ T cell anti-tumor therapy have become apparent in the mouse, it is of increasing interest to understand the ways in which anti-tumor $CD4^+$ T cells may guide and potentiate anti-tumor $CD8^+$ T cells in vivo, or even function independently of $CD8^+$ T cells. As will be elucidated below, the main constraint on studying anti-tumor $CD4^+$ T cells has been the difficulty growing them with sustained functional characteristics in vitro. Nonetheless, a great deal has been learned about the therapeutic value of $CD4^+$ T cells against tumors, as well as their value in facilitating the therapeutic effects of anti-tumor $CD8^+$ T cells.

$CD4^+$ T CELLS PROVIDE MORE THAN INTERLEUKIN-2 TO $CD8^+$ T CELLS

Non-IL-2-producing $CD8^+$ T cells are dependent upon IL-2-producing cells such as CD4+ T cells to proliferate following antigen exposure. In addition, other studies have indicated that CD8+ T cells may be dependent upon CD4+ T cells for optimal trafficking to extravascular sites, as well as for functional activation at sites of rejection. Thivolet et al demonstrated in a murine model of autoimmune pancreatitis that adoptively transferred, antigen specific CD8+ T cells were unable to generate pancreatitis or accumulate significantly within the recipients' pancreases unless anti-pancreas CD4+ T cells were also administered; in contrast, the anti-pancreas CD4+ T cells were able to accumulate in pancreas when administered alone, but generated only a mild form of pancreatitis.[18] Thus, an absolute symbiosis between CD4+ and CD8+ T cells was demonstrated in this rejection model. In a murine anterior chamber ocular tumor model, Ksander et al demonstrated that presensitized anti-tumor CD8+ T cells were unable to mediate tumor rejection unless reactivated within the tumor site by CD4+ T cells;[19] the requisite activating cytokines or interactions were not identified.

It would be useful to identify such essential relationships between CD4+ and CD8+ T cells in other tumor models, but progress has been slow because of the difficulty growing functional anti-tumor CD4+ T cells in vitro. Most adoptive therapy studies have been restricted to the use of freshly harvested or very short-term cultured immune CD4+ T cells. Alternatively, in vivo CD4/CD8 depletions have been utilized to delineate the relative contribution of each subset to rejection events. As discussed below, these studies have often implied a potent therapeutic role for anti-tumor CD4+ T cells, even though they could not be expanded readily in culture for subsequent characterization.

ADOPTIVE THERAPY STUDIES UTILIZING CD4+ T CELLS

In pioneering studies performed in the late 1970s, Fernandez-Cruz et al analyzed the immunologic rejection of two syngeneic rat sarcoma models, one Moloney virus based, the other chemically induced. Unfractionated splenocytes obtained from rats immunized to either tumor could be briefly cultured, then used in adoptive therapy to cure syngeneic rats with large established subcutaneous tumors.[20,21] Tumor rejection required several weeks to develop fully but cured the rats. In vitro selection of subsets prior to adoptive transfer demonstrated that the essential component of therapy was a W3/25+, W3/13+ T cell of the type currently described as CD4+; this T cell was nonlytic to tumor targets in vitro.[22] At the same time, a W3/25−, W3/13+ subpopulation was present in the immune spleen preparations which was lytic for tumor targets in vitro, but paradoxically enhanced tumor growth when administered adoptively. Unfortunately, at the time of these studies, neither subpopulation could be expanded in long-term culture.

In other pioneering work, Greenberg and coworkers demonstrated that the class II non expressing murine lymphoma FBL-3 could be cured by adoptive transfer of non lytic CD8- anti-tumor T cells (presumed CD4+ T cells; antibodies for positive identification of murine CD4 were unavailable at that time). Congenic Thy-1.1 mice immunized to FBL-3 lymphoma were used as a source of fresh immune T cells; the latter were depleted of CD8+ cells, and administered to thymectomized, irradiated, T-depleted bone marrow-reconstituted five day tumor bearers following cyclophosphamide treatment. Such adoptively treated tumor-bearing mice were cured of their tumors without receiving exogenous recombinant IL-2 (rIL-2), and there was, as expected, no evidence of direct anti-tumor cytolytic activity by the adoptively transferred cells in vitro.[23]

As noted previously, syngeneic mice bearing palpable cubcutaneous MCA sarcomas or the FBL-3 lymphoma can be cured by the adoptive transfer of fresh unfractionated splenocytes harvested from syngeneic mice previously immunized to the tumors, even without coadministration of exogenous rIL-2.[7,8] Efforts in the mid

1980s to identify T cell subsets essential to such rejections were impaired by the unavailability of antibodies to murine CD4.[8,23] It was noted, however, that even brief (five day) culture of fresh immune splenocytes caused them to lose their ability to cure recipient animals unless exogenous IL-2 was also administered to the tumor-bearing mice.[24] As culture techniques subsequently improved to allow expansion of immune splenocytes for many weeks in rIL-2, it was discovered that such cultured cell lines, always exclusively CD8⁺ in murine studies, were consistently ineffective as therapy against established small subcutaneous tumors even with concomitant administration of IL-2.[6] (The notable exception was the anti-FBL-3 CD8⁺ cultured "HIT" cell.[13,15]) Although such cultured CD8⁺ anti-tumor T cell lines lacked the wider efficacy easily demonstrable for fresh immune splenocytes, they could be used with pronounced success to treat experimental established pulmonary and hepatic metastases.[3,4,25]

After monoclonal antibodies (mAb) to both murine CD4 and CD8 were developed it became possible to perform in vitro and in vivo CD4 or CD8 depletions in murine tumor studies.[3] Such studies have demonstrated, for example, that exogenous rIL-2 can fully substitute for CD4⁺ T cells when either fresh immune or cultured anti-tumor CD8⁺ T cells are used to treat experimental pulmonary metastases.[3,26,27] It remained possible, however, that rIL-2 cannot substitute for immune CD4⁺ T cells in the treatment of tumors at other extravascular locations. We have therefore begun to utilize CD4/CD8 depletion techniques to assess the role of anti-tumor CD4⁺ T cells in those circumstances where cultured CD8⁺ T cells plus exogenous rIL-2 are ineffective in the mouse.

In two recent experiments utilizing the weakly immunogenic, non-class II expressing methylcholanthrene (MCA) sarcoma 203 (one study of five day established subcutaneous tumors, one study of three day pulmonary metastases), we demonstrated that adoptive transfer of fresh splenocytes from tumor immune mice yielded highly significant tumor reduction at either location in recipient mice which had been sublethally irradiated prior to tumor challenge; similar results had previously been shown for other MCA sarcomas.[8,12] Portions of these experiments are shown in Tables 1 and 2. Administration of exogenous rIL-2 augmented responses in all subcutaneous tumor treatment groups, possibly due to activation of passenger cells within the fresh tumor digest inoculum. Nonetheless, the therapeutic benefit of adoptive cellular therapy was significantly linked to the transferred immune CD4⁺ component, and, as might be expected for fully functional CD4⁺ T cells, their efficacy was intact whether or not exogenous rIL-2 was co-administered. We are currently repeating and extending these preliminary studies which suggest that fresh immune CD4⁺ T cells can function independently of CD8⁺ T cells to achieve tumor rejections in this non-class II expressing tumor.

Two other recent studies have emphasized that anti-tumor CD4⁺ T cells can have therapeutic impact without apparent involvement of CD8⁺ T cells, even against non-Class II expressing tumors. Nagarkatti et al studied the mechanism by which syngeneic mice were cured of intraperitoneal lymphoma (the non-class II expressing LSA tumor) following BCNU chemotherapy and presented substantial evidence that cure was mediated by tumor specific CD4⁺ T cells.[28] Following BCNU treatment intraperitoneal CD4⁺ T cells increased from 3 to 41% of the infiltrating population, while CD8⁺ T cells increased only from 5 to 9%. The infiltrating CD4⁺ T cells secreted "Th1" rather than "Th2" cytokines (i.e., IL-2 and interferon-γ, but not IL-4 or IL-5[29,30]), and when the CD4⁺ T cell subset was purified and transferred into nude mice it conferred protection against simultaneous tumor challenge as well as demonstrable tumor-specific delayed type hypersensitivity.[28] In other work, Levitsky et al studied the mechanism by which syngeneic mice immunized to a class I deficient variant of B16 melanoma resisted

Table 4.1. Treatment of established subcutaneous murine sarcoma MC 203 with syngeneic splenocytes

Treatment Group		Progressive Tumors Death by Day 81 (% tumor free survivors) A. No IL-2 Given	B. IL-2 x 7 days
1.	5 x 10^7 Non-immune spleen	5/6 (17%)	2/5 (60%)
2.	5 x 10^7 Immune spleen	0/6 (100%)	0/6 (100%)
3.	5 x 10^7 CD4/CD8 depleted	5/6 (17%)	2/6 (67%)
4.	5 x 10^7 CD8 depleted	1/6 (87%)	0/6 (100%)
5.	5 x 10^7 CD4 depleted	4/6 (33%)	2/5 (60%)

Wilcoxin Rank Sum Analysis Comparing Group Survival

2A vs 1A	p2 = 0.005
2A vs 4A	p2 = 0.316
2A vs 3A	p2 = 0.005
2A vs 5A	p2 = 0.019
3A vs 4A	p2 = 0.027
3A vs 5A	p2 = 0.523

Naive C57BL/6 female mice were sublethally irradiated (500R), then inoculated subcutaneously with 5 x 10^5 viable MC 203 tumor cells from a freshly digested, serially passed tumor. Five days later when palpable tumors were evident adoptive therapy was begun. Adoptive splenocytes were obtained either from naive mice or from mice immunized to MC 203 by a *C. parvum* based protocol;[69,70] two days prior to adoptive therapy, certain donor mice were depleted of $CD4^+$ and/or $CD8^+$ T cells by intravenous administration of GK 1.5 or 2.43 antibody respectively. On the day of adoptive therapy, donors splenocytes were harvested, depletions confirmed by FACS, then 5 x 10^7 splenocytes were administered to each tumor-bearing mouse by the tail vein route. Some groups received seven days of exogenous rHIL-2 therapy (50,000 Cetus units IP bid). Mice were randomized; tumor size and survival were recorded in a double blind fashion. Data shows proportion of mice which developed progressive tumors which led to death by day 81. Surviving mice at that time were all tumor free. Two-tailed survival statistics by Wilcoxon rank sum analysis is shown.

Table 4.2. Treatment of three day MC 203 experimental pulmonary metastases with syngeneic splenocytes

Treatment	Number of Macroscopic Lung Metastases per Mouse Day 14
No treatment	> 250 >250 > 250 > 250
Whole naive splenocytes	> 250 160 > 250 240 164
Whole naive splenocytes plus IL-2	150 > 250 > 250 240 164
CD8⁺ depleted naive splenocytes	160 160 236 >250 >250
CD8⁺ depleted immune splenocytes	0 4 0 0 18
CD8⁺ depleted immune splenocytes plus IL-2	16 0 0 8 0

Naive C57BL/6 female mice were sublethally irradiated (500R) then inoculated by the tail vein with 5 x 10^5 viable MC203 tumor cells from a freshly digested serially passed tumor. Three days later adoptive therapy was begun. Adoptive splenocytes were obtained as in Table 4.1; each tumor bearing mouse received 2.5 x 10^7 splenocytes. by the tail vein route. Some groups received rIL-2 therapy as in Table 4.1. 14 days later, mice were sacrificed, and macroscopic pulmonary metastases scored in a double blind fashion. Table shows number of metastases in individual mice of each treatment group.

subsequent tumor challenge. Resistance was not affected by systemic treatment with anti-CD8 antibody, but was blocked by treatment with either anti-CD4 or anti-NK-1.1 antibody, indicating essential roles for the latter two cell types in the rejection of this tumor.[31]

MECHANISM OF CD4⁺ T CELL PARTICIPATION IN TUMOR REJECTION

The above studies indicate that anti-tumor CD4⁺ T cells can mediate rejections of a variety of tumors, most of which do not express detectable levels of MHC class II markers. Such rejections occur in at least some instances without notable participation of CD8⁺ T cells. How can such rejections proceed? This question has two components: (1) how can an anti-tumor CD4⁺ T cell recognize tumor deposits if the tumor cells do not express class II; (2) how can the CD4⁺ T cell mediate tumor rejection if it cannot itself bind to the tumor target (for lack of class II expression)?

Many tumors contain cells which express MHC class II molecules;[32-38] many tumor cell lines also express class II or can be upregulated to do so in vitro by treatment with interferon-γ (IFN-γ) or other cytokines.[39-41] class II expressing tumor cells can process and present endogenous antigen or possibly exogenous tumor debris in a class II context.[42-44] In either case, antigen presentation to CD4⁺ T cells may be ineffective unless the tumor cell also expresses a variety of costimulatory and adhesion molecules, such as B7 and ICAM-1.[44-46] Since tumor cells often do not express all of these molecules simultaneously, class II expressing normal passenger cells within the tumor stroma may be the most reliable presenters of tumor antigen to CD4⁺ T cells within the tumor. Many tumors contain large numbers of such class II expressing passenger cells (unpublished observations), which in theory can process and present exogenous tumor debris. An example is shown in Figure 4.1; double stain FACS analysis of a fresh breast tumor digest revealed the presence of many class II expressing cells; readily identifiable non-tumor passenger cells (B cells, T cells, monocytes) accounted for over 80% of all class II expressing cells within the tumor.

The mechanism by which CD4⁺ T cells mediate tumor rejection is probably similar to that by which CD8⁺ T cells appear to mediate tumor rejection: specific cytokine secretion.[47] The notion that anti-tumor CD8⁺ T cells primarily function in vivo through direct target lysis was recently disproved by Barth et al, who prepared a variety of murine CD8⁺ T cell lines which recognized relevant syngeneic tumor targets as evidenced by specific cytokine secretion;[48,49] only a subset of these CD8⁺ T cell lines also lysed their relevant target in vitro. However, lytic and nonlytic CD8⁺ T cell lines were equally effective when used in adoptive therapy against experimental pulmonary metastases so long as they displayed specific secretion of IFN-γ in vitro.[47] Systemic administration of anti-IFN-γ and/or anti-TNF-α antibody blocked tumor rejections. Such data indicated that release of cytokines by CD8⁺ T cells following exposure to tumor targets in vitro, rather than direct tumor cell killing, correlated most closely to their therapeutic effect.

The importance of T cell cytokine secretion provides a common link to explain how either CD4⁺ or CD8⁺ T cells can mediate tumor rejection. CD8⁺ T cells and the Th1 subset of CD4⁺ T cells both secrete IFN-γ, TNF-α, TNF-β, and GM-CSF; in addition, many CD4⁺ T cells and the rare "HIT" subset of CD8⁺ T cells secrete IL-2.[14,30] The net effect of such cytokine secretion by either CD4⁺ or CD8⁺ T cells appears to be accumulation and activation of accessory cells which are capable of distinguishing and killing tumor cells via non T cell receptor mediated mechanisms.[50-53]

Under the influence of CD4⁺ or CD8⁺ cytokines, NK cells and other precursors are activated to become tumoricidal LAK cells,[50,51] and monocytes are activated to become tumoricidal macrophages (TMφ).[52,53] It is difficult to prove that such activated accessory cells are the final effec-

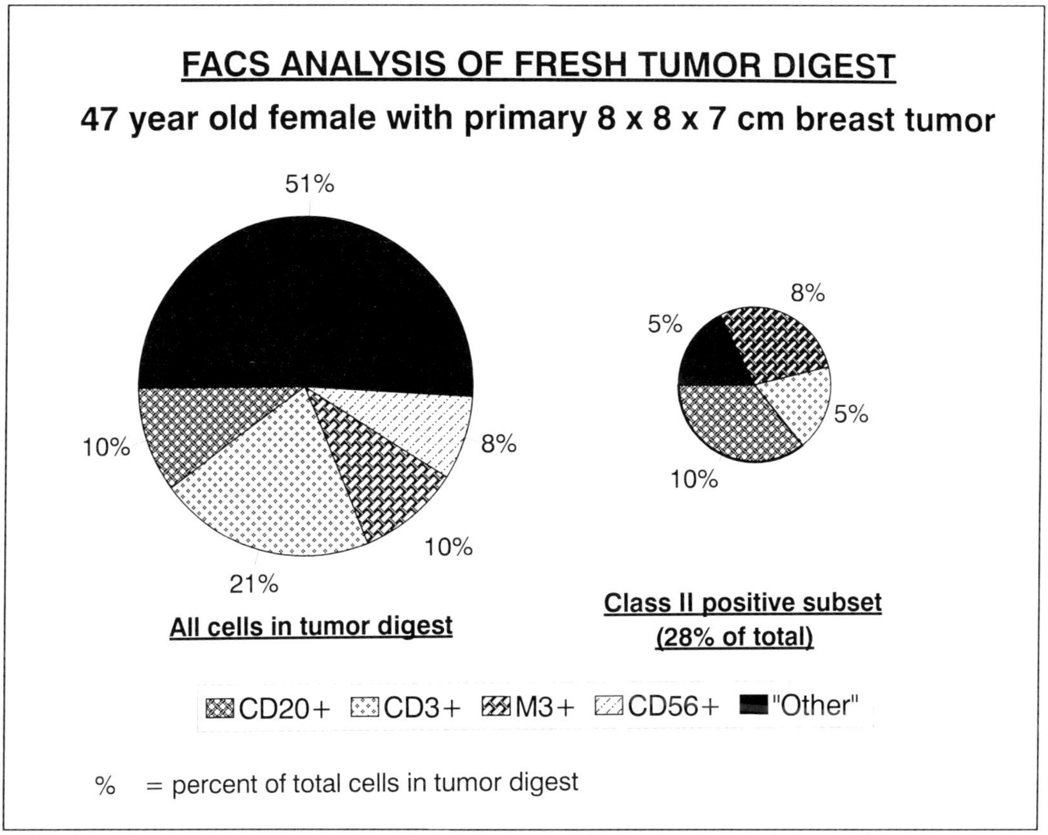

Fig. 4.1. Double stained fluorescent activated cell sorter (FACS) analysis of freshly digested primary breast tumor revealing a large subpopulation of Class II expressing cells. Digest cells were stained with FITC-conjugated anti-Dr and one or a cocktail of the following PE-conjugates: anti-CD3 (T cell), anti-CD20 (B cell and dendritic cell), anti-M3 (monocyte), and/or anti-CD56 (NK cell). Left pie chart shows representation of individual cell groups in the total digest population. Right pie chart shows individual cell subsets comprising the 28% of all cells which expressed Dr (Class II). Only 5% of all digest cells were Dr+ and not identifiable as CD3+, CD20+, M3+ or CD56+.

tors in immunologic tumor rejection, but suggestive evidence for an essential role has been provided by several groups, who have shown that anti-macrophage or anti-NK cell agents can block successful immune tumor rejection in particular murine tumor models.[31,54,55] Such a mechanism of tumor rejection would ideally permit either CD4+ or CD8+ T cells to mediate regressions even when antigen is non uniformally expressed within a tumor: recognition of antigen on even a small subset of tumor or passenger cells could lead to cytokine release and accumulation of LAK and TMφ which recognize and kill all tumor targets regardless of antigen expression.[50-53] This pattern of rejection is probably that which occurs when adjuvants such as *Bacille Calmette Guérin* (BCG) or *Corynebacterium parvum (C. parvum)* are injected directly into tumors.[56-57]

IN VITRO GROWTH OF ANTIGEN-SPECIFIC CD4+ T CELLS

The above studies indicate a therapeutic role for CD4+ T cells in many animal tumor models. Nonetheless, the optimal anti-tumor CD4+ T cell for therapeutic purposes—probably one with pronounced Th1-like characteristics[28]—may not occur in the natural host response to "tumor bearing" or even to standard methods of "tumor immunization". Hence, the true potential of CD4+ adoptive therapy can only be demonstrated when it is possible to grow anti-tumor CD4+ T cells with defined, stable characteristics in culture such as is already often possible for anti-tumor CD8+ T cells. It may also be necessary to convert CD4+ T cells in vitro from one type of behavior to another more suitable for adoptive therapy (e.g., conversion from a Th2 to a Th1 phenotype).

While CD8+ T cells can often be grown in relatively simple, rIL-2-based culture conditions to generate predictable antigen specificities and functional properties, this remains difficult to accomplish with CD4+ T cells. To aggravate the problem, the properties of CD4+ T cells which emerge following cloning attempts are often seemingly random or unpredictable. In efforts to grow and characterize anti-tumor CD4+ T cells in vitro, Matis et al immunized syngeneic mice to the Friend leukemia virus induced, class I expressing, class II non expressing FBL-3 lymphoma, and collected draining lymph node cells for cloning purposes. Specific CD8+ T cell clones were easily derived in vitro when lymph node cells were cultured in the presence of irradiated FBL-3 tumor cells. However, it was only possible to derive specific anti-tumor CD4+ T cell clones in vitro when the lymph node cells were cultured with purified Friend virus in the presence of syngeneic splenocytes as a source of antigen presenting cells (APCs). After establishing the CD4+ T clones, however, the latter proliferated specifically in the presence of splenic APCs pulsed with intact or killed FBL-3 tumor cells.[58] Thus, anti-tumor CD4+ T cell lines could be established in this study, but only when a strong antigen was isolated to drive the culture.

Kahn et al used a similar technique to derive cultured CD4+ anti-tumor T cell lines against a murine melanoma for adoptive therapy experiments. Mice were immunized with a vaccinia construct of the human p97 melanoma antigen, then used as a source of anti-p97 CD4+ T clones. The derived clones were I-A^k or I-E^k class II restricted, and could not directly recognize a non I-A, non-I-E expressing murine melanoma line, K1735, which was transduced to express human p97. Nonetheless, the CD4+ T clones were quite effective when given adoptively to treat two day or six day experimental p97-transduced K1735 pulmonary metastases, even without the administration of exogenous rIL-2. In vitro incubation of CD4+ T clones with p97-pulsed splenocyte APCs resulted in specific release of uncharacterized factors into the supernatant which rendered macrophages tumoricidal.[59]

Purifiable tumor associated antigens such as Friend leukemia virus and melanoma p97 are not available for the vast majority of murine and human cancers; thus, the above techniques are not broadly applicable to growing anti-tumor CD4+ T cells. Furthermore, standard rIL-2 based culture techniques generally give rise only to CD8+ T cell lines in the mouse for reasons not completely understood at this time. Investigators have therefore attempted to identify stimuli which would favor and propagate CD4+ T cells as well. Working with draining lymph node cells from mice bearing syngeneic sarcomas, Shu and coworkers have succeeded in expanding murine anti-tumor T cells which include a 20-40% CD4+ subpopulation by adding either anti-CD3 or staphylococcal-derived superantigens to rIL-2-driven cultures.[60-62] CD4 depletion studies demonstrated that such anti-tumor CD4+ T cells have tumor specific therapeutic value when given adoptively to treat experimental pulmonary or brain metastases, as is discussed elsewhere in this volume. The in vitro characterization of these CD4+ T cells is in progress.

As noted above, rIL-2-based culture of murine lymphocytes usually gives rise to T cell lines which are exclusively CD8+; in contrast, similar culture techniques applied to human lymphocytes frequently give rise to persistent subpopulations of CD4+ T cells, the function of which is under study. CD4+ T cells grown from tumor digests (tumor infiltrating lymphocytes) frequently secrete cytokines when co-cultured with fresh tumor digests or tumor cell lines,[63-66] but the significance of such secretion is unclear because activated CD4+ T cells also secrete cytokines nonspecifically when cocultured with any class II expressing cells.[67] Stringent proof that CD4+ TILs recognize specific tumor antigens requires the use of "third party" antigen-presenting cells such as autologous monocytes or Epstein-Barr transformed B cell lines; such APCs can be pulsed with tumor lysates to present specific peptides to CD4+ T cells, while unpulsed or irrelevantly pulsed APCs provide controls for nonspecific cytokine release.[67] Recent work employing such third party APCs suggests that CD4+ TILs grown from melanoma nodules can recognize either non-shared or shared melanoma antigens, but that such cells may often represent only small subpopulations of the bulk TIL.[68]

Since culture conditions which promote the growth of functional anti-tumor CD8+ T cells may be suboptimal for CD4+ T cells, it is desirable to define those conditions which favor the growth of CD4+ T cells with readily demonstrable anti-tumor specificity and stable physiologic patterns of cytokine release. A first step towards accomplishing this is to incorporate a reliable source of antigen presentation into the culture system. In the case of tumor cells, where specific antigens are usually not known, a "professional" APC could ideally be used to process autologous whole tumor cell lysates, thus permitting presentation of the broadest possible repertoire of both putative and unidentified, both shared and non shared tumor antigens, in a class II context. Alternatively, allogeneic tumor cell lysates could be used as a source of shared tumor antigens when autologous tumor materials are not available; lysates are preferable to irradiated or viable tumor cell materials because killed tumor cells provide a source of tumor antigen without being directly allostimulatory.

In the mouse, we have succeeded in using syngeneic spleen dendritic cells (DC) or Langerhans cells to present the antigen(s) contained in tumor lysates to CD4+ T cells.[69,70] Snap freeze-thawed tumor cells are used to pulse fresh DC overnight; then the latter are cocultured with CD4+ T cells freshly prepared from mice immunized to particular syngeneic MCA sarcomas (using a *C. parvum* adjuvant protocol). Short-term (five-day) ^{3}H-thymidine proliferation assays demonstrated that such immune CD4+ T cells recognize non shared tumor antigen(s) unique to the particular sarcoma used in immunization (Fig. 4.2), similar to CD8+ T cells derived from the same immunized mice.[71] Early experiments suggested that CD4+ T cells from such tumor immune mice recognized shared antigens on other tumors, but this proved to be an artifact of enzymatic tumor digestion: DC pulsed with only the bacterial collagenase used in digestion were also "cross recognized."[70] We are currently investigating whether CD4+ T cells derived from the lymph nodes of tumor-bearing mice recognize true shared antigens as was previously demonstrated for CD8+ T cells from such mice.[71]

Having demonstrated that freshly harvested murine anti-tumor CD4+ T cells can proliferate specifically in short term culture, the next goal is to expand such cells indefinitely in vitro, maintaining their specificity and function. While CD4+ T cells cocultured with syngeneic DC expand in number when either rIL-2 or rIL-7 is added to culture, it is difficult to demonstrate antigen specificity when these CD4+ T cells are restimulated after two to three weeks' expansion. At that time, the cultured CD4+ T cells are highly dysfunctional: they proliferate strongly in the presence of non pulsed syngeneic DC, and even appear to apoptose when cocultured with DC pulsed in the relevant tumor lysate ("specific negative proliferation") (Fig. 4.3).[67] Surprisingly, preliminary experiments demonstrated that such cultured CD4+ T cells remained moderately effective when used in adoptive therapy, though now dependent on administration of exogenous rIL-2 for their therapeutic effect (unpublished observations). This, of course, falls far short of the goal to grow CD4+ T cells with the original properties which

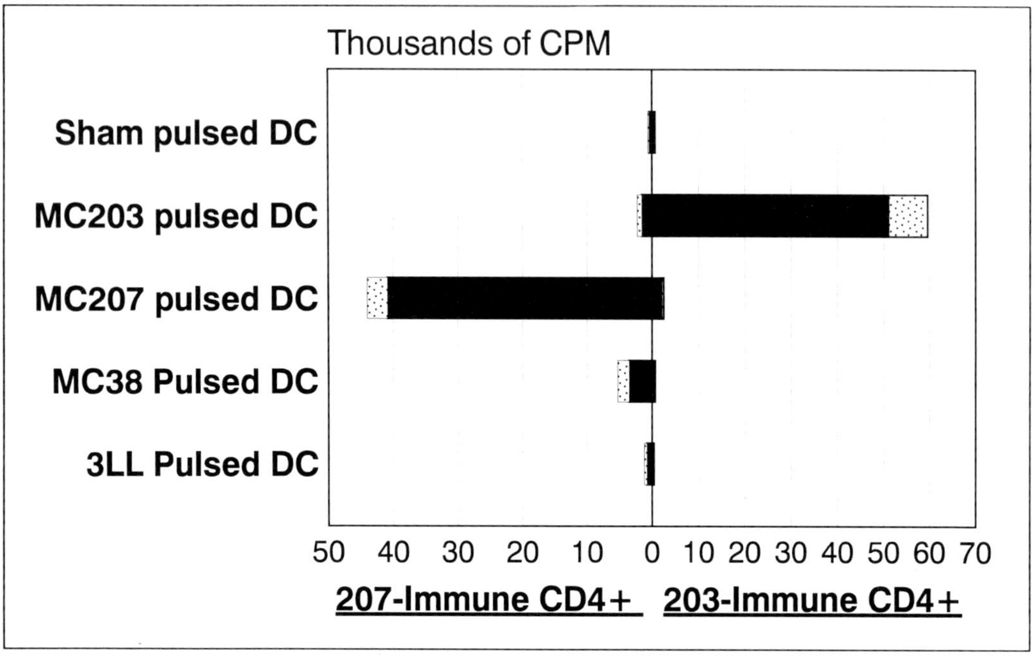

Fig. 4.2. Initial specific proliferative responses of fresh immune murine $CD4^+$ T cells to tumor antigen. $CD4^+$ cells were collected from spleens of mice immunized to 207 (left) or 203 (right) MC sarcomas. DCs were sham-pulsed or pulsed with freeze-thawed tumor lysates. $CD4^+$ T cells were co-cultured with antigen-pulsed DC (20:1 ratio) for five days. DC were irradiated (1000R) just prior to coculture; ^{3}H-thymidine was added 18 hours prior to harvest. (Stippled bar caps indicate ±SEM.) Reprinted with permission of J. Immunotherapy.

enabled them to adoptively cure subcutaneous or pulmonary tumors even without administration of exogenous rIL-2.

To accomplish this last goal, we have found the use of several recombinant cytokines in culture to be helpful or obligatory. The addition of rIFN-γ during both DC preparation and subsequent coculture with $CD4^+$ T cells provides two benefits: it reduces autoreactive "background" in ^{3}H-thymidine proliferation assays, and also promotes expansion of $CD4^+$ T cells which are competent to proliferate specifically upon subsequent reexposure to antigen.[67] We have further determined that addition of rIL6 and/or rIL1 is essential to maintain longterm $CD4^+$ T cell numerical expansion, even though these cytokines are not necessary to maintain demonstrable antigen specificity.[72] We have also been able to demonstrate that bulk (non cloned) cultures of antigen specific $CD4^+$ T cells can be made to develop pronounced "Th1" or "Th2" behavior (i.e., they specifically secrete either IL-2/IFN-γ or IL-4/IL-10[30]); we are currently categorizing the complex combinations of cytokines necessary to maintain such behaviors reliably in long term culture.[72]

The orchestrated use of several recombinant cytokines in addition to (or instead of) rIL-2 has enabled the preparation of cultured $CD4^+$ T cells whose function closely resembles that of fresh (noncultured) immune $CD4^+$ T cells. In vitro expansion of $CD4^+$ T cells which recognize syngeneic sarcoma antigens and manifest "Th1" or "Th2" behavior provides the opportunity to assess which $CD4^+$ T cell properties are critical for successful adoptive therapy, and such experiments are now in progress. The same culture techniques are also being applied to grow anti-tumor $CD4^+$ T cells from the peripheral blood of melanoma patients; elutriated monocytes are utilized to provide processing and presentation of autologous or allogeneic tumor lysates.[67]

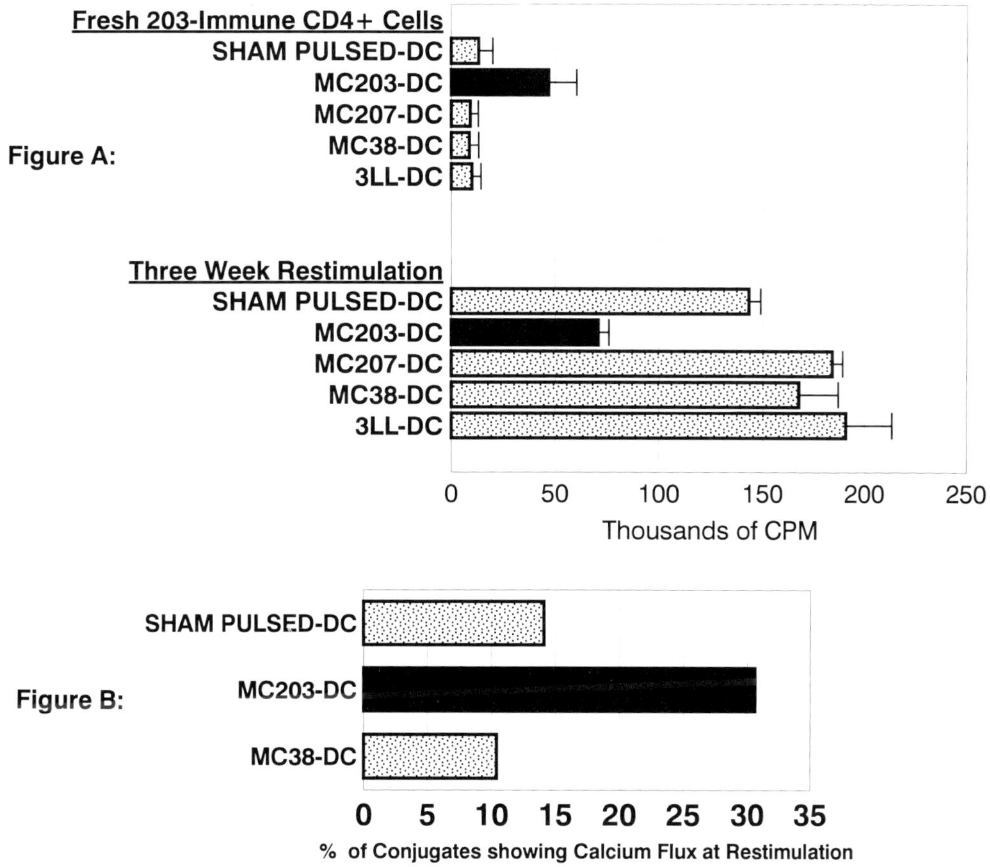

Fig. 4.3. (A) shows representative pre-culture and post-expansion ^{3}H-thymidine proliferation assays of murine anti-tumor CD4$^+$ splenocytes. Low background responses and specific anti-203 responses were initially seen when fresh 203-immune CD4$^+$ cells were cocultured with pulsed DC. However, after three weeks' expansion in the presence of 203-pulsed DC and rhIL-7 (100 ng/ml added day 2), restimulation assay showed elevated background responses and specifically impaired proliferation to 203-pulsed DC. (B) shows a calcium flux assay for expanded 203-immune CD4$^+$ T cells at the time of restimulation; CD4$^+$ cells were loaded with indo-1 and mixed with freshly prepared DC followed by prompt FACS analysis. Graph shows the proportion of CD4$^+$ T cells conjugating with DC with increased intracellular calcium flux. Even though cultured 203-immune CD4$^+$ T cells show impaired proliferation in the presence of 203-pulsed DC, they showed a specifically increased burst of calcium signaling when first cocultured with the same 203-pulsed DC. Reprinted with permission of J. Immunotherapy.

SUMMARY

A sizable body of evidence indicates that anti-tumor CD4$^+$ T cells can play an important role in the rejection of syngeneic tumors. Of particular interest are the findings that CD4$^+$ T cells can function therapeutically against class II non expressing tumors, perhaps utilizing class II expressing passenger cells within the tumors to recognize processed tumor antigen. It is unlikely in the case of either CD4$^+$ or CD8$^+$ T cells that T cells themselves directly kill all tumor cells within a tumor deposit; it is much more likely that accessory cells (LAK, TMφ) activated by either CD4$^+$ or CD8$^+$ T cell cytokines kill the bulk of tumor cells; in addition, T cell cytokines such as TNF can destroy tumor cells indirectly by effects on the microvasculature.[73]

$CD4^+$ T cells can potentiate the therapeutic value of $CD8^+$ T cells by providing IL-2, as well as by chemotactic guidance and activation through mechanisms not yet well characterized. $CD8^+$ T cells may potentiate the therapeutic value of $CD4^+$ T cells by expanding the repertoire of antigen recognition within a tumor, by secreting cytokines such as IFN-γ which lead to further accessory cell activation, and possibly by the direct killing of class I positive tumor targets. The additional possibility exists that $CD4^+$ T cells can function, sometimes of necessity, without support from $CD8^+$ T cells, particularly in the instance of class I non expressing (e.g., β_2-microglobulin-deficient[74,75]) tumors. In fact, anti-tumor $CD4^+$ T cells do appear to function effectively without $CD8^+$ T cell support in several murine tumor models. This is not surprising, since $CD8^+$ T cell lysis of tumor targets does not appear to be an essential component of tumor rejection and Th1-type $CD4^+$ T cells can release the same cytokines as $CD8^+$ T cells, plus the IL-2 seldom secreted by $CD8^+$ T cells.

As it becomes apparent that a very wide range of potential CD4 behaviors exists in the normal host (Th0, Th1, Th2 and many other permutations[30]), it is clear that a new generation of culture techniques will be necessary before an optimally performing anti-tumor $CD4^+$ T cell is available for adoptive therapy studies. It is fortunate that improved availability of recombinant cytokines is enabling progress in this area both in murine and in human studies. Use of appropriate APCs such as dendritic cells in the mouse and elutriated monocytes in the human has enabled processing and presentation of antigens present within tumor lysates even when purified tumor antigens are unknown and/or unavailable in chemically defined forms.

Acknowledgments

I would like to express my deepest gratitude to Steven A. Rosenberg, Suyu Shu, Richard L. White, Daniel J. Fowler, Hyun Kim, and Brian J. Czerniecki for their helpful comments in the preparation of this manuscript.

References

1. Hammond SA, Bollinger RC, Stanhope PE et al. Comparative clonal analysis of human immunodeficiency virus type 1 (HIV-1)-specific $CD4^+$ and $CD8^+$ cytolytic T lymphocytes isolated from seronegative humans immunized with candidate HIV-1 vaccines. J Exp Med 176:1531-42, 1992.
2. Riddell SR, Watanabe KS, Goodrich JM et al. Restoration of viral immunity in immunodeficient humans by the adoptive transfer of T cell clones Science 257:238-41, 1992.
3. Shu S, Chou T, Takaaki C, Rosenberg SA. Generation from tumor-bearing mice of lymphocytes with in vivo therapeutic efficacy. J Immunol 139:295-304, 1987.
4. Rosenberg SA, Spiess P, Lafreniere R: A new approach to the adoptive immunotherapy of cancer with tumor infiltrating lymphocytes, Science 233:1318-21, 1986.
5. Rosenberg SA, Packard BS, Aebersold PM et al. Use of tumor-infiltrating lymphocytes and interleukin-2 in the immunotherapy of patients with metastatic melanoma, special report. N Engl J Med 319:1676-80, 1988.
6. Chou T, Bertera S, Chang AE, Shu S. Adoptive immunotherapy of microscopic and advanced visceral metastases with in vitro sensitized lymphoid cells from mice bearing progressive tumors. J Immunol 141:1775-91, 1988.
7. Rosenstein, M, Eberlein TJ, Rosenberg SA. Adoptive immunotherapy of established syngeneic solid tumors: role of T lymphoid subpopulations. J Immunol 132:2117-22, 1984.
8. Shu S, Rosenberg SA. Adoptive immunotherapy of newly induced murine sarcomas. Cancer Res 45:1657-62, 1985.
9. Fisher B, Packard BS, Read EJ et al. Tumor localization of adoptively transferred indium-111 labeled tumor infiltrating lymphocytes in patients with metastatic melanoma. J Clin Oncol 7:250-261, 1989.
10. Rosenberg SA, Aebersold P, Cornetta K et al. Gene thransfer into humans—Immunotherapy of patients with advanced melanoma, using tumor-infiltrating lymphocytes modified by retroviral gene transduction. N Engl J. Med 323:570-8, 1990.

11. Berendt MJ, North RJ. T-cell-mediated suppression of anti-tumor immunity: an explanation for progressive growth of an immunogenic tumor. J Exp Med 151:67-80, 1980.
12. Chang AE, Shu S, Chou T et al. Differences in the effects of host suppression on the adoptive immunotherapy of subcutaneous and visceral tumors. Cancer Res 46:3526-30, 1986.
13. Rosenstein M, Rosenberg SA. Generation of lytic and proliferative lymphoid clones to syngeneic tumor: in vitro and in vivo studies, J Natl Cancer Inst 72:1161-5, 1984.
14. Klarnet JP, Kern DE, Dower SK et al. Helper-independent CD8$^+$ cytotoxic T lymphocytes express IL-1 receptors and require IL-1 for secretion of IL-2. J Immunol 142:2187-91, 1989.
15. Matis LA, Shu S, Groves ES et al. Adoptive immunotherapy of a syngeneic murine leukemia with a tumor-specific cytotoxic T cell clone and recombinant human interleukin 2: correlation with clonal IL 2 receptor expression. J Immunol 136:3496-501, 1986.
16. Mizuochi T, Singer A. Intrathymic differentiation and tolerance induction of lymphokine-secreting Lyt-2$^+$ T helper cells. J Immunol 140:1421-4, 1988.
17. Greenberg, P Watanabe, K Gilbert M et al. Reconstitution of viral immunity in immunocompromised humans by the adoptive transfer of T cell clones. J Cellular Biochem Suppl 17D:99, 1993.
18. Thivolet C, Bendelac A, Bedossa P et al. CD8$^+$ T cell homing to the pancreases in the nonobese diabetic mouse is CD4$^+$ T cell-dependent. J Immunol 146:85-8, 1991.
19. Ksander PR, Acevedo J, Streilein JW. Local T helper cell signals by lymphocytes infiltration intraocular tumors. J Immunol 148:1955-63, 1992.
20. Fernandez-Cruz E, Feldman JD. In vivo elimination by specific effector cells of an established syngeneic rat moloney virus-induced sarcoma. J Immunol 123:1772-7, 1979.
21. Fernandez-Cruz E, Gilman SC, Feldman JD. Immunotherapy of a chemically-induced sarcoma in rats: characterization of the effector T cell subset and nature of suppression. J Immunol 128:1112-7, 1982.
22. Fernandez-Cruz E, Woda BA, Feldman JD. Elimination of syngeneic sarcomas in rats by a subset of T lymphocytes. J Exp Med 152:823-41, 1980.
23. Greenberg PD, Kern DE, Cheever, MA. Therapy of disseminated murine leukemia with cyclophosphamide and immune Lyt-1$^+$,2$^-$ T Cells: tumor eradication does not require participation of cytotoxic T cells. J Exp Med 161:1122-34, 1985.
24. Shu S, Rosenberg SA. Adoptive immunotherapy of a newly induced sarcoma: immunologic characteristics of effector cells. J Immunol 135:2895-2903, 1985.
25. Spiess PJ, Yang JC, Rosenberg SA. In vivo antitumor activity of tumor-infiltrating lymphocytes expanded in recombinant interleukin-2. J Natl Cancer Inst 79:1067-1075, 1987.
26. Shu S, Chou T, Rosenberg SA. In vitro differentiation of T-cells capable of mediating the regression of established syngeneic tumors in mice. Cancer Res 47:1354-1360, 1987.
27. Ward BA, Shu S, Chou T et al. Cellular basis of immunologic interactions in adoptive T cell therapy of established metastases from a syngeneic murine sarcoma. J Immunol 141:1047-53, 1988.
28. Nagarkatti M, Clary SR, Nagarkatti PS. Characterization of tumor-infiltrating CD4$^+$ T cells as Th1 cells based on lymphokine secretion and functional properties. J Immunol 144:4898-4905, 1990.
29. Mosmann TR, Cherwinski H, Bond MW et al. Two types of murine helper T cell clone: I. Definition according to profiles of lymphokine activities and secreted proteins. J Immunol 136:2348-57, 1986.
30. Street NE, Mosmann TR. Functional diversity of T lymphocytes due to secretion of different cytokine patterns. FASEB J. 5:171-7, 1991.
31. Levitsky HI, Pardoll DM. The effect of tumor class I MHC expression on the generation of two distinct cytolytic anti-tumor responses. J Cellular Biochem 17D: 119, 1993.
32. Rubin JT, Elwood LJ, Rosenberg SA et al, Immunohistochemical correlates of response

to recombinant interleukin-2 based immunotherapy in humans. Cancer Res 49:7086-92, 1989.

33. Horie Y, Chiba M, Iizuka M, Masamune O Class II (HLA-DR, -DP, and -DQ) antigens on intestinal epithelia in ulcerative colitis, Crohn's disease, colorectal cancer and normal small intestine. Gastroenterol Jpn 25(5):575-84, 1990,
34. Concha A, Esteban F, Cabrera T, Ruiz-Cabello F, Garrido F Tumor aggressiveness and MHC class I and II antigens in laryngeal and breast cancer. Semin Cancer Biol 2(1):47-54, 1991.
35. Brunner CA, Gokel JM, Riethmüller, Johnson JP. Expression of HLA-D subloci DR and DQ by breast carcinomas is correlated with distinct parameters of favourable prognosis. Eur J Cancer 27:411-6, 1991.
36. Dammrich J, Buchwald J, Papadopoulos T, Muller-Hermelink HK. Special subtypes of pulmonary adenocarcinomas indicated by different tumor cell HLA-expression and stromal infiltrates. A light, electron microscopic and immunohistologic study. Virchows Arch B Cell Pathol 61:9-18, 1991.
37. Kamma H, Yazawa T, Ogata T et al. Expression of MHC class II antigens in human lung cancer cells. Virchows Arch B Cell Pathol 60:407-12, 1991.
38. Banner BF, Burnham JA, Bahnson RR et al. Immunophenotypic markers in renal cell carcinoma. Mod Pathol 3:129-34, 1990.
39. Hoon DS, Okun E, Banez M et al. Interleukin 4 alone and with gamma-interferon or alpha-tumor necrosis factor inhibits cell growth and modulates cell surface antigens on human renal cell carcinomas. Cancer Res 51:5687-93, 1991.
40. Beniers AJ, Peelen WP, Debruyne FM, Schalken JA. HLA-class-I and -class-II expression on renal tumor xenografts and the relation to sensitivity for alpha-IFN, gamma-IFN and TNF. Int J Cancer 48:709-16, 1991.
41. Leon JA, Mesa-Tejada R, Gutierrez MC et al. Increased surface expression and shedding of tumor associated antigens by human breast carcinoma cells treated with recombinant human interferons or phorbol ester tumor promoters. Anticancer Res 9:1639-47, 1989.
42. Michalek MT, Benacerraf B, Rock KL. The class II MHC-restricted presentation of endogenously synthesized ovalbumin displays clonal variation, requires endosomal/lysosomal processing, and is up-regulated by heat shock. J Immunol 148:1016-24, 1992.
43. Clements VK, Baskar S, Armstrong TD, Ostrand-Rosenberg S. Invariant chain alters the malignant phenotype of MHC class II$^+$ tumor cells. J Immunol 149:2391-6, 1992.
44. Baskar S, Ostrand-Rosenberg S, Nabavi N et al. Constitutive expression of B7 restores immunogenicity of tumor cells expressing truncated major histocompatibility complex class II molecules. Proc Natl Acad Sci U S A 90:5687-90, 1993.
45. Damle NK, Klussman K, Linsley, PS et al. Differential regulatory effects of intercellular adhesion molecule-1 on costimulation by the CD28 counter-receptor B7. J Immunol 149:2541-8, 1992.
46. Damle NK, Klussman K, Leytze G et al. Costimulation with integrin ligands intercellular adhesion molecule-1 or vascular cell adhesion molecule-1 augments activation-induced death of antigen-specific CD4$^+$ T lymphocytes. J Immunol 151:2368-79, 1993.
47. Barth RJ, Mulé JJ, Spiess PJ et al. Interferon gamma and tumor necrosis factor have a role in tumor regressions mediated by murine CD8$^+$ tumor infiltrating lymphocytes. J Exp Med 173:647-58, 1991.
48. Barth RJ, Bock SN, Mulé JJ, Rosenberg SA. Unique murine tumor-associated antigens identified by tumor infiltrating lymphocytes. J Immunol 144:1531-7, 1988.
49. Barth RJ, Mulé JJ, Asher AL et al. Identification of unique murine tumor associated antigens by tumor infiltrating lymphocytes using tumor specific secretion of interferon-gamma and tumor necrosis factor. J Immunol Methods 140:269-79, 1991.
50. Yang JC, Mulé JJ, Rosenberg SA. Murine lymphokine-activated killer (LAK) cells: Phenotypic characterization of the precursor and effector cells. J Immunol 137:715-22, 1986.
51. Phillips JH, Lanier LJ. Dissection of the lymphokine-activated killer phenomenon:

relative contribution of peripheral blood natural killer cells and T lymphocytes to cytolysis. J Exp Med 164:814-825, 1986.
52. Fogler WE, Fidler IJ. Nonselective destruction of murine neoplastic cells by syngeneic tumoricidal macrophages. Cancer Res 45:14-8, 1985.
53. Fidler IJ. Macrophages and metastasis—a biological approach to cancer therapy: presidential address. Cancer Res 45:4714-26, 1985.
54. Keller R. Abrogation of antitumor effects of Corynebacterium Parvum and BCG by antimacrophage agents. J Natl Cancer Inst 59:1751-3, 1977.
55. Mulé JJ, Rosenstein M, Shu S, Rosenberg SA. Eradication of a disseminated syngeneic mouse lymphoma by systemic adoptive transfer of immune lymphocytes and its dependence upon a host component(s). Cancer Res 45:526-31, 1985.
56. Baldwin RW, Pimm MW. BCG in tumor immunity. Adv Cancer Res 28:91-147, 1978.
57. Cohen MH, Jessup JM, Felix EL et al. Intralesional treatment of recurrent metastatic cutaneous malignant melanoma. Cancer 41:2456-63, 1978.
58. Matis LA, Ruscetti SK, Longo DL et al. Distinct proliferative T cell clonotypes are generated in response to a murine retrovirus-induced syngeneic T cell leukemia: viral gp70 antigen-specific MT4+ clones and Lyt-2+ cytolytic clones which recognize a tumor-specific cell surface antigen. J Immunol 135:703-13, 1985.
59. Kahn M, Sugawara H, McGowan P et al. CD4+ T cell clones specific for the human p97 melanoma-associated antigen can eradicate pulmonary metastases from a murine tumor expressing the p97 antigen. J Immunol 146:3235-341, 1991.
60. Yoshizawa H, Chang AE, Shu S. Specific adoptive immunotherapy mediated by tumor-draining lymph node cells sequentially activated with anti-CD3 and IL-2. J Immunol 147:729-37, 1991.
61. Yoshizawa H, Chang AE, Shu SY. Cellular interactions in effector cell generation and tumor regression mediated by anti-CD3/interleukin 2-activated tumor-draining lymph node cells. Cancer Res 52:1129-36, 1992.
62. Shu S, Krinock R, Matsumura T et al. Specific immune T cells generated from tumor-draining lymph nodes by activation with bacterial superantigenic toxins. J Cellular Biochem 17D: 99, 1993.
63. Schwartzentruber DJ, Stetler-Stevenson M, Rosenberg SA, Topalian SL. Tumor-infiltrating lymphocytes derived from select B-cell lymphomas secrete granulocyte-macrophage colony-stimulating factor and tumor necrosis factor-alpha in response to autologous tumor stimulation. Blood 82:1204-11, 1993.
64. Hom SS, Rosenberg SA, Topalian SL. Specific immune recognition of autologous tumor by lymphocytes infiltrating colon carcinomas: analysis by cytokine secretion. Cancer Immunol Immunother 36:1-8, 1993.
65. Schwartzentruber DJ, Solomon D, Rosenberg SA, Topalian SL. Characterization of lymphocytes infiltrating human breast cancer: specific immune reactivity detected by measuring cytokine secretion. J Immunother 12:1-12, 1992.
66. Schwartzentruber DJ, Topalian SL, Mancini M, Rosenberg SA. Specific release of granulocyte-macrophage colony-stimulating factor, tumor necrosis factor-alpha, and IFN-gamma by human tumor-infiltrating lymphocytes after autologous tumor stimulation. J Immunol 146:3674-81, 1991.
67. Cohen, PA, Kim H, Fowler, DJ et al. Use of interleukin-7, interleukin-2 and γ-interferon to propagate CD4+ T cells in culture with maintained antigen-specificity. J Immunother 14:242-52, 1993.
68. Topalian SL, Rivoltini, Mancini M et al. Melanoma-specific CD4+ T lymphocytes recognize human melanoma antigens processed and presented by Epstein-Barr virus-transformed B cells. Int J Cancer 58:69-79, 1994.
69. Cohen PJ, Cohen PA, Rosenberg SA et al. Murine epidermal Langerhans cells and splenic dendritic cells present tumor-associated antigens to primed T cells. Eur J Immunol 24:315-319, 1994.
70. Cohen PA, Cohen PJ, Rosenberg SA, Mulé JJ. CD4+ T cells from mice immunized to

syngeneic sarcomas recognize distinct, non shared tumor antigens, Cancer Res 54:1055-1058, 1994.
71. Chou T, Chang AE, Shu S. Generation of therapeutic T lymphocytes from tumor-bearing mice by in vitro sensitization. Culture requirements and characterization of immunologic specificity. J Immunol 140:2453-61, 1988.
72. Cohen PA, Fowler DJ, Kurasawa K et al. Manuscript in preparation,
73. Fraker DL, Thom AK, Doherty GM et al. Tumour necrosis factor mediates the survival benefit of interleukin 2 in a murine pulmonary metastases model. Surg Oncol 1:1-9, 1992.
74. Sibille C, Gould K, Hämmerling, G Townsend A. A defect in the presentation of intracellular viral antigens is restored by interferon-gamma in cell lines with impaired major histocompatibility complex class I assembly. Eur J Immunol 22:433-40, 1992.
75. Gattoni-Celli S, Kirsch K, Timpane R, Isselbacher KJ. Beta 2-microglobulin gene is mutated in a human colon cancer cell line (HCT) deficient in the expression of HLA class I antigens on the cell surface. Cancer Res 52:1201-4, 1992.

CHAPTER 5

Anti-CD3-Stimulated T Cells and IL-2 Liposomes in Adoptive Immunotherapy

**Augusto C. Ochoa, Brendan D. Curti,
Arnold H. Zea, Peter M. Anderson,
Mark Saxton, Susan S. Strobl,
William C. Kopp, Walter J. Urba, Dan L. Longo**

Adoptive immunotherapy initially centered around the use of IL-2-activated peripheral blood lymphocytes (lymphokine activated killer cells—LAK cells) followed by the infusion of high doses of IL-2.[1,2] The treatment of tumor-bearing mice with LAK cells and IL-2 resulted in marked reductions in the number of metastases and produced some antitumor effects in patients with melanoma and renal cell carcinoma. These early results expanded the research efforts in adoptive immunotherapy from LAK cells (comprised mainly of activated NK cells) to the use of activated T lymphocytes. The initial adoptive immunotherapy clinical trials also demonstrated two major difficulties with this therapeutic approach: (1) the high level of toxicity produced by IL-2, and (2) the failure of adoptively transferred cells to home to tumor sites.

Initial work identifying and isolating the effector subsets in the LAK cultures demonstrated that the cells which developed most of the cytotoxic activity were natural killer (NK) cells.[3,4] However, immunohistology of tumors regressing after immunotherapy with LAK cells and IL-2 failed to show infiltration by NK cells and instead demonstrated infiltration by T cells. It was also shown that T cells could infiltrate tumors (tumor-infiltrating lymphocytes, TILs), especially immunogenic tumors, and that these TILs had an increased response (lytic activity or lymphokine production) to the malignant cells.[5,6] The latter findings suggested that T cells might indeed be recognizing some form of tumor antigen.

Immunotherapy of Cancer with Sensitized T Lymphocytes, edited by Alfred E. Chang and Suyu Shu.

COMBINED USE OF ANTI-CD3-STIMULATED T CELLS AND IL-2-LIPOSOMES

These findings prompted us to use a polyclonal stimulus as a means of expanding T cells to large numbers for their use in adoptive immunotherapy with the aim of increasing the number of tumor specific cells. In addition, if tumor specific cells were not increased to high numbers by this approach, it would still be possible that the infusion of highly activated T cells would drive the tumor specific response present in the host and result in tumor reduction. The binding of anti-CD3 monoclonal antibody OKT3 to the ε chain of the T-cell receptor induces the upregulation of high affinity IL-2 receptors, the production of cytokines and cellular proliferation; all hallmarks of T-cell activation. A similar effect was observed with murine cells stimulated with murine anti-CD3 (145-2C11). Cells activated with anti-CD3 (T-cell receptor activated T cells-T-AC) + IL-2 resulted in a rapid expansion of T cells.[7] The phenotype of the rapidly expanding T cells was mostly $CD3^+CD8^+$. Intravenous infusion of anti-CD3-stimulated T cells in mice bearing pulmonary metastases of MCA-106 sarcoma, followed by five days of intraperitoneal IL-2, induced decreases in the number of pulmonary metastases[8] in a manner comparable to that of LAK cells (Fig. 5.1).

Another major difficulty encountered in IL-2-based adoptive immunotherapy was the toxicity produced by the use of high doses of IL-2. Even though IL-2 is a cytokine central to the function of the immune system, it is produced in small amounts at the site of an ongoing immune response. However, when administered intravenously and at high doses, it produces considerable toxicity ranging from chills and fevers to hypotension and, in a few cases, death.[9-11] The cause of this clinical toxicity appears to be the production of other lymphokines such as IL-1, interferon and tumor necrosis factor by cells of the immune system, and the production of nitric oxide by the endothelial cells and macrophages leading to vasodilatation, capillary leak and hypotension.[12] Low doses of IL-2 tend to produce minor toxicity; however, the animal models demonstrated and the clinical trials suggested that the best anti-tumor responses were obtained with the higher doses of IL-2. A strategy tested in other drugs to decrease their toxicity has been to encapsulate them into liposomes.[13] In some cases, for example amphotericin B, liposome encapsulation has resulted in increased therapeutic efficacy. The encapsulation of IL-2 provided a new IL-2 formulation with novel characteristics including a prolonged release and preferential delivery to the reticuloendothelial system (liver, spleen, peribronchial lymph nodes). IL-2-

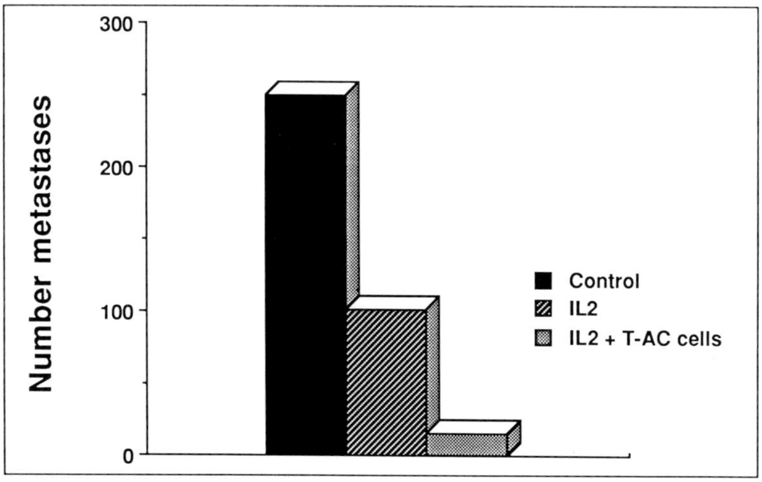

Fig. 5.1. C57Bl/6 mice bearing three-day lung metastasis of MCA-106 sarcoma received an infusion of 5 million cells activated with anti-CD3 and IL-2 (25,000 units/8 hours x 3 days). Lung metastasis were counted on day 15 after tumor inoculation.

liposomes in animal models was significantly more efficacious in inducing an anti-tumor effect and less toxic than unencapsulated IL-2, as determined by the capillary leak assay.[14] Preliminary Phase I data suggest that IL-2-liposomes is less toxic in humans than free IL-2 (data not shown).

The combined effect of the activated T lymphocytes (T-AC) and IL-2-liposomes was tested using the murine MCA-38 colon carcinoma model. Splenic injection of MCA 38 results in liver metastases after three days and death of the animals from progressive tumor growth after 17 days. When C57Bl/6 mice bearing MCA 38 liver metastases were treated with T-AC and IL-2-liposomes (50,000 units/day IP), there was a marked reduction in the number of metastases.[15] Neither component of the therapy given separately had any significant anti-tumor effect. Even when T-AC cells were given in combination with IL-2 mixed with empty liposomes, only a minimal reduction in the numbers of metastases was observed (Fig. 5.2). Both T-AC cells and IL-2-liposomes were essential to obtain a maximal anti-tumor effect since a dose-response curve can be demonstrated for each component of this therapy.

CLINICAL EXPERIENCE WITH HUMAN T-AC CELLS

These murine models formed the basis for the development of Phase I trials at the Biological Response Modifiers Program (BRMP) of the National Cancer Institute. These trials evaluated the toxicity of IL-2 plus T-AC obtained by stimulating peripheral blood lymphocytes in vitro with anti-CD3. A second Phase I study is examining the toxicity of IL-2-liposomes. Previous experience at the BRMP with intravenous infusion of anti-CD3 (Orthoclone OKT3) revealed the rapid development of dose-limiting toxicities, particularly severe headache associated with aseptic meningitis, at doses of anti-CD3 as low as 3 mcg/m[16] without achieving any demonstrable activation of

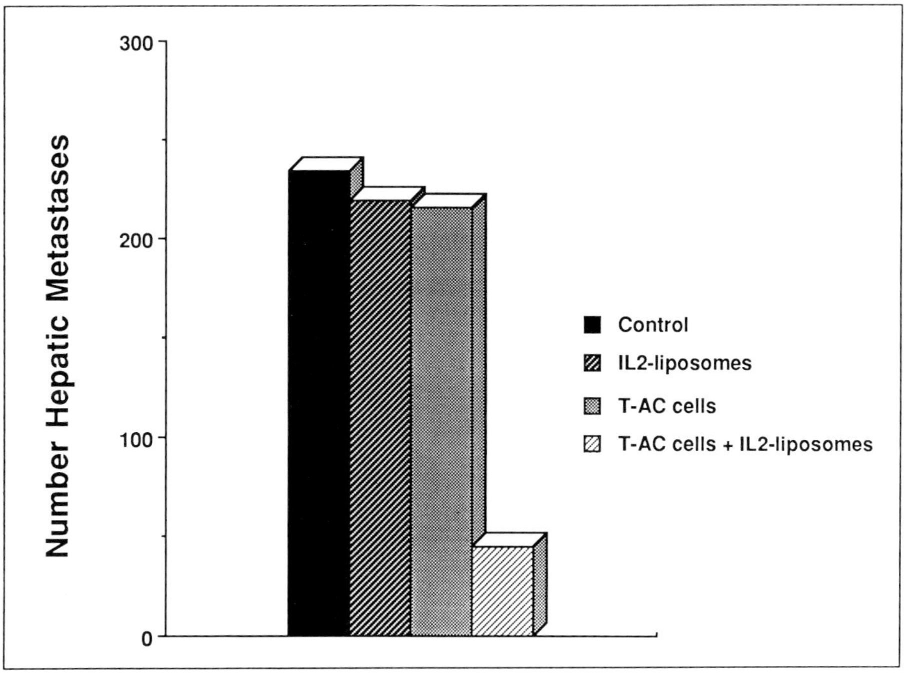

Fig. 5.2. C57Bl/6 mice bearing three-day liver metastasis of MCA-38 colon adenocarcinoma received 50 million T cells activated with anti-CD3 (T-AC) by tail vein injection and 5 days of intraperitoneal IL-2-liposomes or free IL-2 (50,000 U/day). On day 14 after tumor inoculation mice were sacrificed and the liver metastasis were counted.

the peripheral blood T cells. In addition, there was a rapid development of human anti-mouse antibodies. The stimulation of these T cells in vitro circumvents both these problems to a large degree.

In vitro activation of a large number of T cells presents significant logistical problems. T cells obtained from a leukapheresis (approximately 5×10^9), stimulated with anti-CD3 + IL-2 and cultured for a period of 14 days to obtain maximal expansion of cell numbers requires several hundred liters of tissue culture medium with an appropriate large amount of IL-2, similar to the expansion of TIL cells. To circumvent this problem, T cells were stimulated with anti-CD3 in vitro for short periods of time (18-96 hours) in the absence of IL-2 resulting in the expression of high affinity IL-2 receptors with a minimal increase in the number of cells. These highly activated T cells were then infused into patients who concomitantly started receiving an IV infusion of IL-2. As shown in Figure 5.3, this approach resulted in a substantial leukocytosis approximately 7 days after receiving the T-AC cells and a continuous (3×10^6 IU/m^2/day) plus bolus

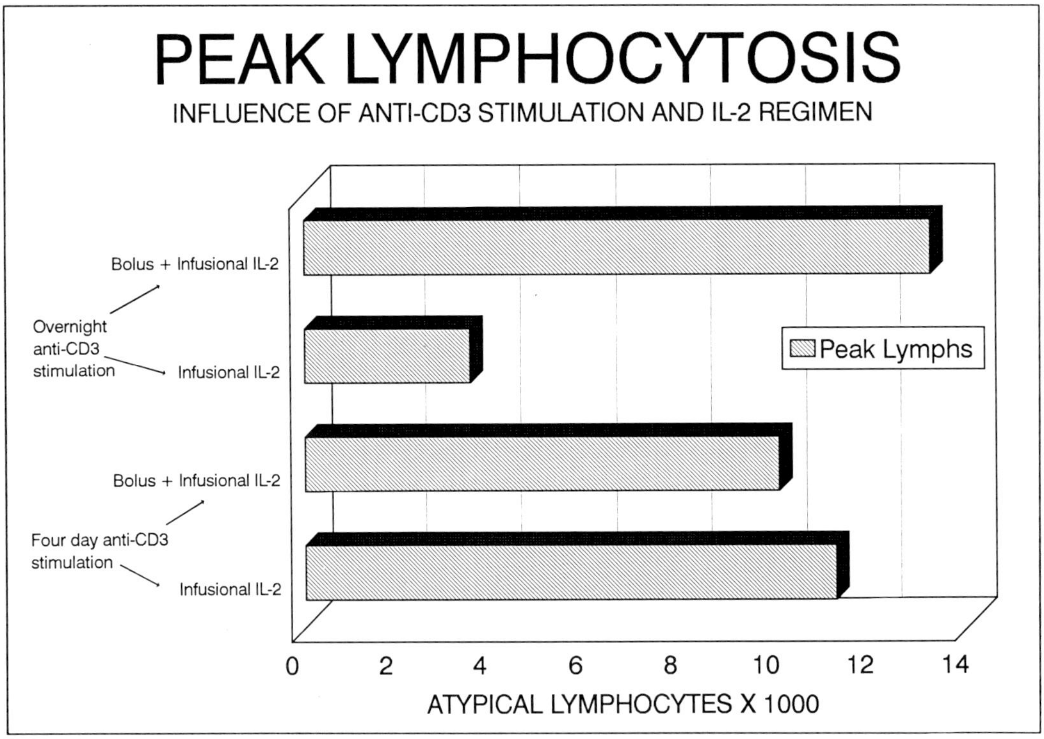

Fig. 5.3. Patients received 5×10^{10} autologous peripheral blood lymphocytes activated with anti-CD3 for 18 hours or for 96 hours followed by the infusion IL-2 (Bolus 1.5 million U/m^2/day once a day, Continuous infusion 3 million Um^2/day) for a total of seven days. Leucocyte numbers were determined on the day of the initiation of therapy and on day 8 of therapy (one day after the end of the IL-2 infusion).

Table 5.1. Surface phenotype of peripheral blood lymphocytes

	% Positive				CD3$^+$ Cells		
	CD3	CD4	CD8	CD56	CD25	CD38	HLA-Dr
Day 0	76	49	28	10	6	31	3
Day 7	83	39	43	16	31	82	55

(1.5 x 10^6 IU/m^2/day) infusion of IL-2. A marked increase in the leukocyte count was observed in every patient with some developing counts as high as 300,000 cells/mm.[3] The T-cell proliferation in vivo was closely related to the time of incubation with anti-CD3. Lymphocytes stimulated overnight (approximately 18 hours), required continuous infusion plus a daily bolus of IL-2 to proliferate in vivo. However, a similar increase in white blood cells could be achieved by continuous infusion without the bolus doses of IL-2 in the patients where the T cells were stimulated in vitro for a period of 4 days before transfer into the adoptive host. This major difference might be explained by the higher percentage of T cells expressing the IL-2 receptor in the cultures which were stimulated in vitro for 4 days. The phenotypic analysis of the leukocytes at the peak of proliferation (Table 5.1) demonstrated them to be mostly activated T cells as inferred by the co-expression of CD3 and activation markers such as CD25, CD38, HLADr and CD69 (Table 5.1).

T-AC cells not only proliferate in the peripheral blood, but also can infiltrate the sites of tumors, as shown by comparing a limited number of biopsies of subcutaneous melanoma nodules before and after treatment. Immunohistology demonstrated these infiltrating cells to be mainly $CD8^+$ cells. The toxicities observed in this clinical trial were unique. Patients experienced a metabolic acidosis at the peak of T-cell proliferation 5-7 days after treatment. The acidosis was characterized by rapidly falling levels of $HCO3^-$ and increasing levels of lactic acid. In addition, a coagulopathy characterized by a moderate decrease in the vitamin K-dependent clotting factors II, VII, IX, X and antithrombin III was observed. Finally, some of the traditional IL-2 toxicities were also seen. Ultimately however, there were few clinical responses.[17]

LOSS OF THERAPEUTIC ACTIVITY IN T CELLS FROM TUMOR-BEARING INDIVIDUALS

Of the several potential explanations for the lack of anti-tumor effects of T-AC plus IL-2 in spite of the massive T-cell response in vivo, two were chosen for further research. First was the possibility that the T cells from patients with cancer had lost their therapeutic efficacy as a result of the suppression created by the tumor. The therapeutic efficacy of T cells from normal or tumor bearing animals was tested using the MCA 38 murine colon carcinoma. T cells from mice bearing tumors (subcutaneous MCA 38) for different periods of time (<14 days or > 20 days) or from normal donors were used to treat mice bearing liver metastases of the same tumor. As shown in Figure 5.4, the T cells from mice bearing tumor for prolonged periods of time (>20 days) showed a marked decrease in their in vivo anti-tumor efficacy as compared to T cells from normal mice or from mice bearing tumor for 14 days or less (short-term tumor-bearers). These results

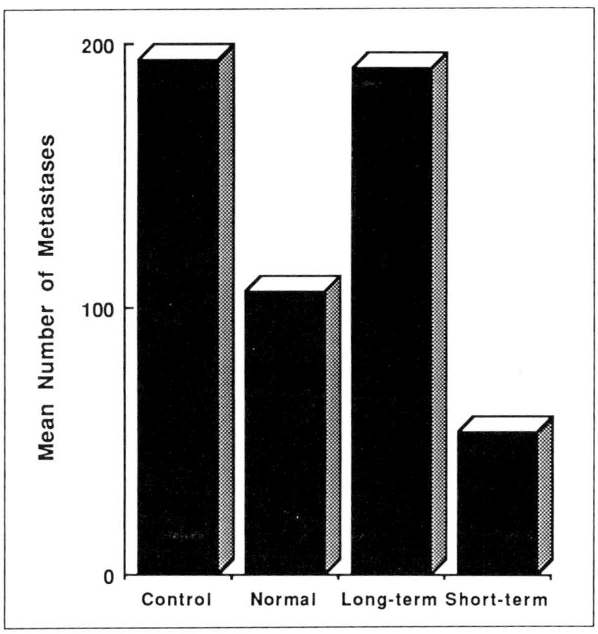

Fig. 5.4. Mice bearing MCA-38 liver metastasis were treated with 20 million activated T cells obtained from normal (non-tumor bearing) mice or mice bearing tumor for <14 days (short term tumor bearing) or >20 days (long-term tumor bearing).

suggested that there might be an initial recognition and immune response against the tumor, which confers the moderately higher therapeutic efficacy of the T cells from short-term tumor-bearing mice. However, with tumor progression, as represented in the long-term tumor-bearing mice, this therapeutic activity was lost or suppressed.

A series of in vitro cellular functions including 3H-thymidine incorporation, lymphokine production and cytotoxicity were tested 48 hours after stimulating the T cells from long-term tumor-bearing mice with anti-CD3 in vitro. The only major difference observed was a decreased cytotoxic function in the T cells of long-term tumor bearing mice. Further testing of proteins involved in the lytic mechanism demonstrated that the expression of the genes encoding for perforin and for TNF-α were markedly decreased in T cells from long-term tumor bearing mice.[18] With these changes in T-cell function, a careful evaluation of T-cell signal transduction was done. Tyrosine kinase phosphorylation and Ca^{2+} flux, two early events occurring after activation, were markedly decreased in the T cells from long-term tumor-bearing mice. These changes suggested that major alterations could be occurring in the T-cell antigen receptor (TCR). The study of the TCR by flow cytometry using antibodies against the TCRαβ and the CD3ε chains did not demonstrate any significant difference between the T cells of normal mice and those of long-term tumor-bearing mice. However, this approach only evaluated the surface expression of three of the seven chains forming the TCR-CD3 structure. Surface labeling of the T cells with I^{125}, followed by immunoprecipitation using anti-CD3, demonstrated that the T cell antigen receptor ζ chain (TCRζ), a major element in signal transduction was markedly decreased and in some cases totally absent.[19] A similar observation could be seen in T cells from melanoma patients using a Western blot technique (Figure 5.5). In contrast, chains such as CD3ε were not decreased, explaining why flow cytometry analysis with anti-CD3 (which binds the CD3 ε chain) or anti-TCR αβ antibodies of the T cells from long-term tumor bearing mice had not shown any clear abnormalities. The alterations in signal transduction in the T cells from tumor-bearing mice does not seem to be circumscribed only to alterations in the T-cell antigen receptor. Indeed signaling changes and alterations in the receptor isoform could be late or secondary effects. Recent work by P. Ghosh and collaborators[24] has also shown that the nuclear form of certain NFκB fam-

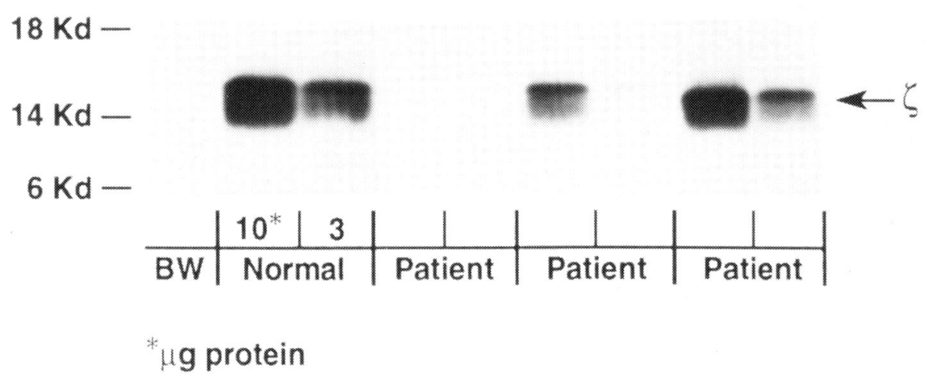

Fig. 5.5. T cells were purified from a normal donor and from 3 melanoma patients prior to receiving any immunotherapy, and at least 30 days after having received any other form of therapy. The T cells were lysed, and 10 and 3 ng of protein (equivalent to 0.5 million cells) were tested for the presence of the TCRζ chain by Western blot. TCR h chain is undetectable in the first patient, decreased in the second and normal in the last patient.

ily proteins, which are transcription factors that mediate the activation of cytokine genes, are also markedly altered. It is therefore possible that these changes in signal transduction in the T cells from tumor-bearing mice could, in part, explain the loss of therapeutic efficacy in the T cells from long-term tumor-bearing mice.

When human cancer patients were tested, major decreases (<50% of the normal expression) in the TCR ζ chain were observed in the tumor-infiltrating lymphocytes of renal cell carcinoma,[20] colon carcinoma,[21] in approximately 50% of the cases in the peripheral blood lymphocytes of patients with melanoma (Zea, manuscript in preparation), and in some patients with other tumors. The correlation between these observations and the clinical course of the patients is not known at this time. A larger number of patients, and a prospective study of signal transduction over the time of treatment will be required to determine the clinical significance of changes in signal transduction.

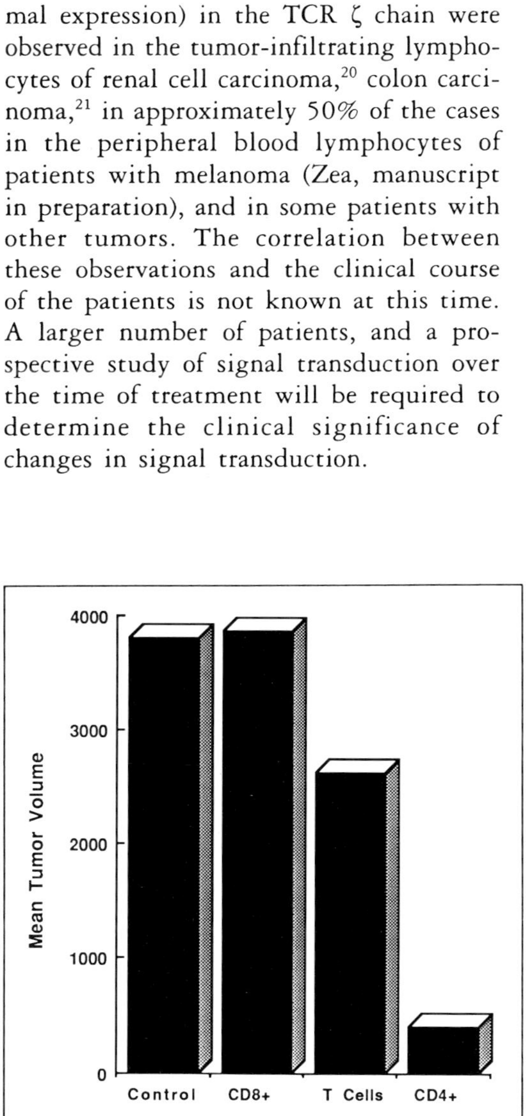

Fig. 5.6 and Table 5.2. Mice with subcutaneous MCA-38 tumors received an intravenous infusion of unseparated T cells, CD8⁺ or CD4⁺ T cells activated with anti-CD3 for 18 hours, and an intraperitoneal infusion of IL-2-liposomes (50,000 U/mouse/day x 5 days).

THE ROLE OF CD4⁺ T CELLS ACTIVATED WITH ANTI-CD3 IN ADOPTIVE IMMUNOTHERAPY

The in vivo or in vitro stimulation of whole peripheral blood lymphocytes (PBL) with anti-CD3 and IL-2 results in the preferential expansion of CD8⁺ T cells. It was possible that the CD8⁺ effector cells in the subset were not the anti-tumor activity observed in vivo in the murine model and could in part explain the lack of therapeutic efficacy in patients receiving anti-CD3 stimulated T cells. To test this hypothesis, mice bearing subcutaneous MCA-38 were treated with purified CD4⁺ or CD8⁺ T cells, which had been stimulated with anti-CD3 for 24 hours, and IL-2-liposomes (50,000 U/mouse/day x 5 days). All of the mice were pre-treated with cyclophosphamide (2 mg/mouse) 4 days before the infusion of activated T cell subsets. As shown in Figure 5.6, most of the anti-tumor effects were seen in mice receiving CD4+ T cells. In addition, a major proportion of the mice receiving CD4+ T cells showed total regression of the tumor while none of those receiving CD8⁺ T cells showed a complete response (Table 5.2). These results do not rule out a role for CD8⁺ host cells in the development of the anti-tumor response in vivo; however, they strongly suggest that CD4⁺ T cells stimulated with anti-CD3 may play an important role in initiating this process. Mice cured from the tumor by CD4⁺ T cells were resistant to further challenge with the original tumor, but not to an unrelated tumor, suggesting the development of a tumor-specific memory response (data not shown). These data sug-

Table 5.2. Anti-tumor effect of activated CD4⁺ T cells

Treatment Group	Tumor Free
1. Control	0/14
2. Unseparated T cells	3/13
4. CD8⁺ T cells	0/6
5. CD4⁺ T cells	4/7

gest, as has been shown by others,[22,23] that $CD4^+$ T cells could drive the host response to eradicate established tumor in vivo. The major difference in this model is that the initial stimulus to the $CD4^+$ T cells is not a tumor specific antigen. However, the final outcome seems to be a tumor specific response.

In summary, the work presented here demonstrated the following:

1. T cells with anti-tumor activity can be expanded by the use of anti-CD3. Short-term ex-vivo stimulation followed by their infusion into patients receiving IL-2 results in a marked in vivo expansion.
2. IL-2 entrapped in liposomes appears to be less toxic than the free lymphokine, which could facilitate its use in an outpatient setting. The therapeutic efficacy of IL-2-liposomes is not yet determined.
3. T cells from cancer patients present major alterations in the process of signal transduction and might therefore explain the decreased therapeutic efficacy observed in the human immunotherapy trials as compared to the work done in mice.
4. $CD4^+$ T cells stimulated with anti-CD3, an antigen nonspecific signal, induce the development of an anti-tumor response and the development of immunological memory both of which are tumor-specific.

References

1. Grimm EA, Mazumder A, Zhang H, Rosenberg S. Lymphokine activated killer phenomenon: lysis of natural killer resistant fresh solid tumor cells by interleukin-2 activated autologous human peripheral blood lymphocytes. J Exp Med 155:1823-1841, 1982.
2. Rosenberg SA, Lotze MT, Muul LM, Leitman SE, Chang AE, Ettinghausen SE, Matory YL, Skibber JM, Shiloni E, Vetto JT, Seipp CA, Simpson C, Reichert CM. Observations on the systemic administration of autologous lymphokine-activated killer cells and recombinant interleukin-2 to patients with metastatic cancer. N Engl J Med 313:1485-1492, 1988.
3. Ortaldo JR, Mason A, and Overton R. Lymphokine activated killer cells: analysis of progenitors and effectors. J Exp Med 164:1193-1205, 1986.
4. Phillips JH, Lanier LL. Dissection of the lymphokine activated killer phenomenon. Relative contribution of peripheral blood natural killer cells and T lymphocytes to cytolysis. J Exp Med 164:814-825, 1986.
5. Slingluff CL, Darrow TL, Seigler HF. Human T cells specifically activated against autologous melanoma. Arch Surg 122:1407-1411, 1987.
6. Skornick Y, Topalian S, Rosenberg SA. Comparative studies of the long-term growth of lymphocytes from tumor infiltrates, tumor draining lymph nodes and peripheral blood by repeated in vitro stimulation with autologous tumor. J Biol Response Modif 9:431-438, 1990.
7. Ochoa AC, Gromo G, Alter BJ, Sondel PM, Bach FH. Long-term growth of lymphokine activated killer (LAK) cells: role of anti-CD3 β-IL-1 interferon γ and β. J Immunol 138:2728-2733, 1987.
8. Anderson PM, Blazar B, Bach FH, Ochoa AC. Anti-CD3 + IL-2 stimulated murine killer cells in vitro generation and in vivo anti-tumor activity. J Immunol 142:1383-1394, 1989.
9. Matory YL, Change AE, Lipford EH, Braziel R, Hyatt CL, McDonald HD, Rosenberg SA. Toxicity of recombinant human interleukin-2 in rats following intravenous infusion. J Biol Response Mod 4:377-390, 1985.
10. Lotze MT, Matory YL, Ettinghausen SE, Rainier AA, Sparrow SO, Seipp CAY, Caster MC, Rosenberg SA. In vivo administration of purified interleukin 2. J Immunol 135:2865-2875, 1985.
11. Anderson TD, Hayes TJ, Gatley MK, Bontempo JM, Stern LL, Truitt GA. Toxicity of human recombinant interleukin-2 in mouse is mediated by interleukin-activated lymphocytes. Lab Invest 59:598-612, 1988.
12. Ochoa JB, Curti B, Peitzman AB, Simmons RL, Biliar TR, Hoffman R, Rault R, Longo

DL, Urba WJ, Ochoa AC. Increased circulating nitrogen oxides after human tumor immunotherapy correlate with toxic hemodynamic changes. J Natl Cancer Inst 84:864-867, 1992.

13. Brenner DE. Liposomal encapsulation: making old and new drugs do new tricks. J Natl Cancer Inst 81:1436-1438, 1989.
14. Anderson PM Hasz D, Drickell L, Senser S. Interleukin-2 in liposomes: Increased intravenous potency and less pulmonary toxicity in the rat. Drug Development Res 27:15-31, 1992.
15. Loeffler CM, Platt JL, Anderson PM, Katsansis E, Ochoa JB, Urba WJ, Longo DL, Leonard, AS. Ochoa AC. Anti-tumor effects of Interleukin 2 liposomes and anti-CD3-stimulated T-cells against murine MCA-38 hepatic metastasis. Cancer Res 51:2127-2132, 1991.
16. Urba WJ, Ewel C, Kopp W, Smith II JW, Steis RG, Ashwell JD, Creekmore SP, Rossio J, Sznol M, Sharfman WH, Fenton RG, Janik J, Conlon K, Watson T, Beveridge J, Longo DL. Anti-CD3 monoclonal antibody treatment of patients with CD3-negative tumors: A phase Ia/b study. Cancer Res 52:2394-2401, 1992.
17. Curti BD, Longo DL, Ochoa AC, Conlon KC, Smith JW, Alvord WG, Creekmore SP, Fenton RG, Gause BL, Holmlund J, Janik JE, Ochoa J, Rice PA, Sharfman WH, Urba WJ. Treatment of cancer patients with ex vivo anti-CD3-activated killer cells and interleukin-2. J Clin Oncol 11:652-660, 1993.
18. Loeffler CM, Smyth MJ, Longo DL, Kopp WC, Harvey LK, Tribble HR, Tase JE, Urba WJ, Leonard AS, Young HA, Ochoa AC. Immunoregulation in cancer-bearing hosts: Down regulation of gene expression and cytotoxic function in $CD8^+$ T cells. J Immunol 149:949-956, 1992.
19. Mizoguchi H, O'Shea JJ, Longo DL, Loeffler CM, McVicar DW, Ochoa AC. Alterations in signal transduction molecules in T lymphocytes from tumor-bearing mice. Science 258:1795-1798, 1992.
20. Finke JH, Zea AH, Stanley J, Longo DL, Mizoguchi H, Tubbs RR, Wiltrout RH, O'Shea JJ, Kudoh S, Klein E, Bukowski RM, Ochoa AC. Loss of T-cell receptor ζ chain and $p56^{lck}$ in T-cells infiltrating human renal cell carcinoma. Cancer Res 53:5613-5616, 1993.
21. Nakagomi H, Petersson M, Magnusson I, Juhlin C, Matsuda M, Mellstedt H, Taupin J-L, Vivier E, Anderson P, Kiessling R. Decreased expression of the signal transducing ζ chains in tumor-infiltrating T cells and NK cells of patients with colorectal carcinoma. Cancer Res 53:5610-5612, 1993.
22. Greenberg PD, Cheever MA. Treatment of disseminated leukemia with cyclophosphamide and immune cells Tumor immunity reflects long-term persistence of tumor-specific donor T cells J Immunol 133:3401-3407, 1984.
23. Bookman MA, Swerdlow R, Matis LA. Adoptive chemoimmunotherapy of murine leukemia with helper T lymphocyte clones. J Immunol 139:3166-3170, 1987.

CHAPTER 6

Lymphocyte Cytokine Secretion in Response to Tumors

Richard J. Barth, Jr.

HUMAN STUDIES

Immunohistologic studies have revealed that many human tumors are infiltrated by mononuclear cells, the main component of the infiltrate being $CD3^+$ cells.[1,2] The degree of infiltration varies, with some tumor histologies often being well infiltrated (e.g. melanomas and head and neck carcinomas[3,4]). Since the tumors are progressively growing in the presence of these lymphoid infiltrates, the function of tumor-infiltrating lymphocytes (TIL) in vivo comes into question.

In Situ Human Lymphocyte Cytokine Secretion

One way to assess the in vivo function of TIL is to examine their pattern of cytokine secretion in situ. Using ^{35}S-labeled cDNA probes for cytokine mRNA, in situ hybridization has been performed on human ovarian, breast and head and neck cancers.[5] In this study, a high proportion of the lymphocytes from the head and neck carcinomas expressed mRNA for IL-2, IFNγ and TNF. In contrast, the ovarian and breast carcinoma infiltrates expressed very little mRNA for IL-2, IFNγ and TNF.

Others have approached this question by amplifying the cytokine mRNA from ovarian tumors, cell lines and normal ovary using PCR.[6] Ten of 11 tumors biopsied expressed mRNA for TNFα and IL-10; 8 tumors expressed IL-1α, IFNγ and GM-CSF; 7 exhibited IL-6 and 1 biopsy expressed mRNA for G-CSF and IL-3. Message for IL-2 and IL-4 was not found in any of these biopsies. In contrast, when the biopsies of eight normal ovaries which were also infiltrated with a similar number of T cells were examined, TNFα was found in five, IL-6 in three and

Immunotherapy of Cancer with Sensitized T Lymphocytes, edited by Alfred E. Chang and Suyu Shu.

IFNγ in two. This qualitative assessment suggests that GM-CSF, IFNγ, TNFα, IL-1α and IL-10 are being selectively expressed in the ovarian tumors as compared to normal ovary. These cytokine messages are most likely originating from the infiltrating cells, rather than the neoplastic cells, since two tumor cell lines were only found to express message for IL-1α and IL-6.

The lack of any detectable message for IL-2 in these tumor biopsies, if found to be a generalized deficit when other tumor histologies are studied using similar methods, may help explain why human TIL, which in many cases have been antigen exposed (as evidenced by the activation marker CD45RO), fail to proliferate and have an anti-tumor effect. Clearly, this finding supports the rationale for the use of systemic IL-2 as an anti-tumor therapy. The presence of detectable amounts of mRNA for IFNγ and TNFα is also intriguing, since in murine systems tumors transduced with the genes for IFNγ and TNFα have been shown to elicit a prompt and vigorous T-cell mediated anti-tumor response.[7,8]

One study of freshly isolated human melanoma TIL indicated that cells with the capability to secrete IFNγ when stimulated with IL-2 are present in tumors at a higher concentration than in peripheral blood.[9] In this report, freshly isolated melanoma TIL and peripheral blood mononuclear cells (PBMC) were incubated for 18 hours. No significant IFNγ was detected in the absence of stimulation; the addition of IL-2 to the culture resulted in a marked increase in IFNγ secretion by TIL when compared to PBMC.

Cytokine Secretion by Established Human T Cell Lines

Most studies of cytokine secretion by human TIL have examined the cytokine secretion patterns of established TIL lines or clones. One of the earliest studies was by Belldegrun et al.[10] Twelve long-term TIL cultures, from melanoma, renal and breast tumors, were found to express the mRNA for TNFα; five of these cultures expressed GM-CSF mRNA.

Further investigation by Schwartzentruber et al[11] revealed that cytokine secretion by human TIL cultures can be specifically induced by autologous tumor cell stimulation. Two of four melanoma TIL cultures, which were specifically cytolytic, specifically secreted GM-CSF, TNFα and IFNγ when stimulated by autologous tumor (Fig. 6.1). Fractionation of these polyclonal TIL on antibody coated flasks revealed that the $CD8^+$ fraction was responsible for the specific cytokine secretion. Anti-MHC class I mAb inhibited this response, providing further evidence that the cytokine secretion resulted directly from T-cell receptor recognition of antigen.

Somewhat different results were obtained in another study of 12 bulk melanoma TIL cultures and 14 melanoma clones, by Itoh et al.[9] They found that melanoma bulk TIL could be induced to secrete IFNγ upon tumor stimulation, but such secretion was not specific for the autologous tumor. IL-2 was secreted by bulk TIL when stimulated with anti-CD3 mAb, but not autologous tumor. Many clones, although specifically cytotoxic, did not specifically secrete IFNγ or IL-2.

The demonstration, using cytotoxicity assays, that melanoma-derived CTL may lyse other melanomas which share the same HLA type implies that common melanoma tumor antigens exist.[12] Therefore, analysis of the specificity of cytokine secretion by melanoma TIL requires that the autologous stimulators be HLA typed. Such an analysis was done by Hom, et al.[13] In this study, seven melanoma TIL were stimulated with autologous and HLA-matched melanomas. Indeed, for six of the seven TIL cultures, some HLA-matched allogeneic melanomas also stimulated significant cytokine release. An anti-MHC class I mAb could block the cytokine secretion induced by both the autologous and the allogeneic melanomas, suggesting that a shared melanoma antigen was being presented by a class I antigen in these cases. However, in many cases, HLA-matched melanomas failed to induce TIL to secrete cytokines; this may be due to expression of unique melanoma antigens.

Analysis of the pattern of cytokine secretion induced by a panel of HLA-A2 restricted TIL indicated that at least two melanoma antigens exist.

Specific recognition of human breast cancer tumor antigens has also been demonstrated by analyzing cytokine secretion patterns of breast cancer TIL. In a study of 12 TIL cultures, 7 from the breast tumor and 5 from tumor-containing draining lymph nodes, it was found that none of these predominantly CD4⁺ TIL displayed significant in vitro cytotoxicity.[14] Three of these TIL cultures secreted IFNγ, TNFα and GM-CSF in response to autologous tumor stimulation and failed to secrete when stimulated by at least two allogeneic, class II expressing, partially HLA-matched stimulators. The cytokine secretion by these breast TIL was inhibited by anti-MHC class II mAb (but not by an anti- MHC class I mAb), indicating that the MHC restriction for these CD4⁺ cells was a class II molecule, as expected. Of interest, two of these CD4⁺ TIL were cultured from tumors which expressed class II on only 16% and 2% of the cells, demonstrating that low levels of class II expression are sufficient to allow immune recognition by CD4⁺ TIL. Of further interest, the cytokine secretion pattern of these CD4⁺ TIL (i.e. TNFα, IFNγ and GM-CSF) was analogous to that secreted by the CD8⁺ fraction of the melanoma TIL cultures.[11] In the past, much emphasis has been placed on determining which class of lymphocytes (CD4 versus CD8) was most effective for tumor eradication; it may prove to be that the more important determinant is the pattern of cytokine secretion by the lymphocytes

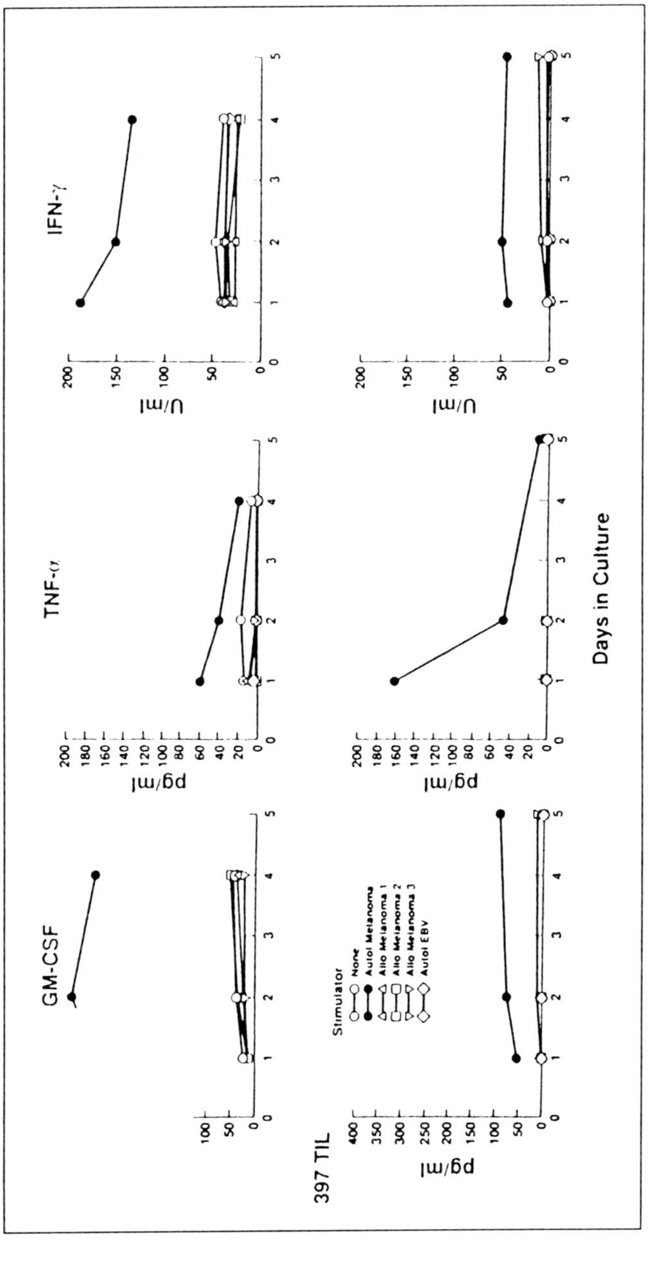

Fig. 6.1. Specific cytokine production by melanoma TIL over time. TILS (1 x 10⁶/ml) were cultured with irradiated stimulator cells (2 x 10⁵/ml) in the presence of 20 U/ml IL-2. Supernatants from replicate experiments were harvested on days 1, 2, and 4 or 5. GM-CSF and TNF-α were measured by ELISA and IFN-γ by RIA. Cytokine release was specific for autologous melanoma at every time point assayed.

(this will be discussed in greater detail in the section on cytokine secretion by murine lymphocytes).

It has been difficult to demonstrate a specific anti-tumor cellular immune response in human colon carcinoma due to the low level of in vitro cytotoxicity seen when colon TIL are challenged with autologous tumor.[15] However, assaying for cytokine secretion has enabled one group[16] to identify 3 of 10 colon TIL cultures which specifically secreted IFNγ, TNFα and/or GM-CSF. Two of these TIL cultures secreted significant amounts of cytokines only when stimulated with autologous tumor and not when stimulated with 9 or 10 allogeneic, partially HLA-matched stimulators, suggesting the presence of unique colon carcinoma antigens. One TIL secreted cytokines when stimulated both by the autologous tumor as well as by an HLA-matched allogeneic tumor, implying that shared colon cancer antigens may also exist.

Human Lymphocyte Cytokine Secretion: Summary and Implications

In summarizing cytokine secretion by human TIL, the results of in situ analyses on ovarian carcinomas has revealed that messages for IFNγ, TNFα and GM-CSF are present at the tumor site. The results of analysis of long term TIL cultures from melanoma, breast and colon adenocarcinomas reveal that IFNγ, TNFα and GM-CSF are in some cases specifically secreted by TIL in response to autologous tumor stimulation. Renal TIL were found to express mRNA for TNFα and GM-CSF. The secretion of other lymphokines has, to date, not been extensively examined. One breast TIL, 3 melanoma TIL and some renal TIL did not secrete IL-1, IL-4 or IL-6;[14,16,17] IL-6 was nonspecifically secreted by some melanoma TIL.[11]

It has been proposed that human CD4⁺ and CD8⁺ cells can each be separated into two distinct classes based on their pattern of cytokine secretion.[18] Studying T cell clones from patients with leprosy and normal volunteers, CD4⁺ cells could be separated into "Type 1" cells which secrete IFNγ, IL-2, GM-CSF, and TNFα; and "Type 2" cells which secrete IL-4, IL-5, IL-2, GM-CSF and TNFα when stimulated with anti-CD3 mAb. Functional cytotoxic CD8⁺ cells could be distinguished from functional suppressor CD8⁺ lymphocytes by the secretion of IL-4 and IL-5 by the T suppressor (Ts) cells. Thus, viewed in this framework, cultures of human TIL secrete a pattern of cytokines consistent with "Type 1" CD4⁺ cells and non-suppressor CD8⁺ cells.

The demonstration of tumor specific cytokine secretion by human lymphocytes has provided an assay which has facilitated the analysis of tumor antigens important in the T cell immune response. A cytokine secretion assay was used in the identification and cloning of the MAGE (melanoma antigen) gene family.[19] The MAGE1 gene codes for an antigen, MZ2-E, that is recognized by immune CTL in the context of HLA-A1. The MAGE1 gene appears to be commonly expressed in human melanomas (in one study 9 of 17 melanomas expressed MAGE1) and as such may be a useful antigen for use in active immunization of melanoma patients.[20]

The relationship between cytokine secretion by human TIL and therapeutic effectiveness is currently under study.[21] One approach designed to enhance the effectiveness of adoptive immunotherapy with T cells involves transducing tumor-reactive T cells with the gene for a particular cytokine so that it is constitutively expressed, and then rely on the ability of these cells to home to the tumor so that the cytokine will be secreted in high concentrations at the tumor site. Theoretically, a therapeutic dose of cytokine could be delivered locally to the tumor and systemic toxicity could be avoided. It is unclear whether TIL which are concentrated in normal organs (e.g. liver) will cause toxicity in these sites. Rosenberg has initiated a therapeutic trial of TNF transduced TIL in melanoma patients. In a preliminary report on the in vitro characteristics of TNF transduced human TIL, it was noted that in 11 of 16 cultures, more TNF was detected in the media of transduced TIL than in non-transduced controls.[22] In this report, none of the TIL were stimulated with tumor. It will be interesting to see whether the transduced gene will be transcribed in response to tumor stimulation, and whether the magnitude of stimulated cytokine expression will be significantly higher in the transduced TIL.

MURINE STUDIES

MURINE CD4⁺ LYMPHOCYTE CYTOKINE SECRETION

Murine T cells are divided into two subsets; one set expresses the antigen CD4 and recognizes peptide antigens in the context of class II MHC molecules, while the other set of lymphocytes express the antigen CD8 and recognizes peptides presented by class I MHC molecules. $CD4^+$ T cells have recently been further subdivided into two groups based on their pattern of cytokine secretion: Th1 cells secrete IL-2 and IFNγ, but not IL-4, IL-5 or IL-10. Th2 cells secrete IL-4, IL-5 and IL-10, but not IL-2 or IFNγ.[23] Functionally, Th1 cells mediate delayed type hypersensitivity reactions while Th2 cells provide help for B lymphocyte differentiation.

Once the antibodies capable of depleting the $CD8^+$ T cell subset became available, it was soon shown that the resultant $CD4^+$ cells were very capable of eradicating tumors in multiple murine models.[24,25] In contrast to many $CD8^+$ T cell cultures, most $CD4^+$ T cells, when challenged with tumor cells in vitro, are non-cytolytic. The possibility that these helper $CD4^+$ cells were activating host cytolytic $CD8^+$ lymphocytes to mediate tumor regression was investigated by using mice that were thymectomized, lethally irradiated, and then reconstituted with T cell-depleted, syngeneic bone marrow (B mice). The adoptive transfer of CD8-depleted splenocytes from tumor-immune mice to such B mice still eradicated the established tumor and prevented the growth of a subsequent tumor challenge.[26] Although no cells that were cytotoxic to tumor could be cultured from the splenocytes of these cured mice, they were able to mediate a tumor-specific delayed type hypersensitivity reaction when rechallenged with a tumor. These observations led investigators to propose that $CD4^+$ lymphocytes may convey tumor resistance by initiating a DTH reaction; thus implicating macrophages, the cytotoxic cells in DTH reactions, as the final effectors of tumor killing. Further support for this hypothesis came from the observation that macrophage-activating factor (IFNγ) was secreted in vitro in response to tumor stimulation by a $CD4^+$ lymphocyte line that demonstrated anti-tumor efficacy in vivo.[27] The secretion of IFNγ by these $CD4^+$ lymphocytes was implicated in the mechanism of tumor regression when it was found that concurrent treatment with a mAb against IFNγ blocked the effectiveness of these cells in vivo.[28]

Other investigators have studied the pattern of cytokine secretion by $CD4^+$ antitumor T cells more extensively. The tumor reactive $CD4^+$ lymphocytes responsible for eradication of a murine lymphoma after BCNU treatment secrete the Th1 pattern of lymphokines: IL-2 and IFNγ, but not IL-4, are secreted after tumor-specific stimulation.[29] These Th1 type tumor reactive lymphocytes were capable of initiating a DTH reaction in response to tumor challenge.

MURINE CD8⁺ LYMPHOCYTE CYTOKINE SECRETION

Cytolytic $CD8^+$ T cell clones and lines, when administered with IL-2, have been shown to very effectively cause the regression of established tumors. The observation that a non-cytolytic, $CD8^+$ TIL culture also eradicated tumor metastases led our laboratory to investigate the mechanism by which $CD8^+$ TIL caused tumor regressions. We found that many murine $CD8^+$ TIL rapidly secrete IFNγ and TNF specifically in response to autologous tumor stimulation, but not when they are stimulated by other syngeneic sarcomas.[30] Cytokine secretion was considered specific if the response to autologous tumor was at least three times the amount secreted in response to other syngeneic tumor stimulators. One such experiment is shown in Table 6.1.

To analyze what role, if any, lymphokine secretion by TIL had in their in vivo efficacy, we simultaneously tested TIL for lymphokine secretion and cytolysis in vitro and adoptively transferred these TIL into mice bearing pulmonary metastases. Twenty-six paired in vitro and in vivo tests were done on 14 different CD8+ TIL cultures from 3 different sarcomas.[31] In 15 of these tests, TIL therapy was effective in causing tumor reductions; in 11 tests, treatment with TIL did not cause a significant reduction in tumor metastases. The relationship between in vivo effectiveness and the in vitro parameters of cytotoxicity and cytokine secretion are shown in Table 6.2. Specific secretion of IFNγ was associated with in vivo effectiveness in 14 of 15 tests. There was only one case of an effective TIL that did not specifically secrete IFNγ; in this case, secretion of IFNγ in response to autologous tumor was twice that seen in response to non-autologous tumor. In 10 of 11 tests on ineffective TIL, there was low or nonspecific IFNγ secretion. Since 9 of 15 effective TIL did not specifically secrete TNF and 7 of 15 effective TIL were marginally lytic or non-lytic, neither specific secretion of TNF nor specific cytolysis ap-

Table 6.1. Specific secretion of INF-γ by TIL in response to tumor stimulation

TIL Culture	Tumor of origin of TIL	None	MCA tumor stimulator* 105	233	205
				U/2.5 x 10⁵ TIL/ml	
105-53	105	2	44	6	3
233-92B	233	0	7	50	2
233-90D	233	3	9	45	6

*All TIL cultures at 2.5 x 10^5 cells/ml were stimulated simultaneously with 5 x 10^5 tumor cells/ml. Supernatants were collected at 18 h and assayed by ELISA.

Table 6.2. Relationship between lymphokine secretion and cytolysis in vitro and efficacy of TIL in vivo

In vitro parameter		In vivo effectiveness: Effective* (No. of Tests)	Ineffective (No. of Tests)
IFN-γ secretion	Specific‡	14	1
	Nonspecific	1	10
TNF secretion	Specific‡	6	0
	Nonspecific	9	11
Cytolysis secretion	Specific§	8	0
	Nonspecific	7	11

* The mean number of pulmonary metastases in mice treated with effective TIL + rIL-2 was significantly less than those treated with rIL-2 alone by Wilcoxon rank sum test.
‡ Secretion of IFN-γ (and TNF) was considered specific if the amount secreted in response to relevant tumor stimulation was greater or equal to three times the amount secreted by two irrelevant tumors and ≥15 U/2.5 x 10^5 cells/ml (and > 100pg/2.5 x 10^5 cells/ml).
§ Cytolysis was considered specific in a 4-h 51 Cr release assay if relevant tumor lysis was ≥20% and irrelevant tumor lysis was <10% at an E/T ratio of 50:1.

peared to be necessary for in vivo effectiveness. However, if an IFNγ-secreting culture also specifically secreted TNF or was specifically cytolytic, this appeared to be sufficient for in vivo effectiveness (in six of six tests that showed specific TNF secretion, the TILs were effective; TILs were effective in eight of eight tests that showed cytolytic specificity).

To further investigate the role of IFNγ secretion in the therapeutic effectiveness of murine lymphocytes, TILs that specifically secreted IFNγ were adoptively transferred into metastasis bearing mice that had been treated with an anti-IFNγ mAb. In each of 5 such experiments, using 4 different TILs cultures from 3 different sarcomas, anti-IFNγ mAb significantly inhibited the in vivo effectiveness of TIL. These experiments and the in vitro characteristics of the cells at the time of transfer are shown in Figure 6.2. Concurrent experiments were done using an anti-TNF antibody; in 2 of the 5 tests, anti-TNF abolished the TIL response, but no significant effect was observed in the other three tests.

These experiments strongly support the hypothesis that secretion of IFNγ is an essential part of the mechanism whereby both cytolytic and non-cytolytic $CD8^+$ lymphocytes mediate tumor regressions. Recently, another laboratory has independently reported similar experiments using draining lymph node cells (DLN) as effectors, with analogous results.[32] DLN cells, when activated by the protein kinase C activator, Bryostatin 1, and the calcium ionophore, ionomycin, will proliferate in vitro in the presence of IL-2 and cause tumor regressions when adoptively transferred to tumor bearing hosts. These DLN cells, like DLN cells activated by anti-CD3 mAb,[33] are commonly non-lytic in vitro. Stimulation of DLN cells with tumor in vitro resulted in secretion of IFNγ. Although these cultures were a mixture of $CD4^+$ and $CD8^+$ cells, depletion experiments revealed that the $CD8^+$ cells were responsible for the IFNγ secretion. In three separate experiments, pretreatment with anti-IFNγ mAb significantly diminished the therapeutic effectiveness of these DLN cells when they were transferred to mice bearing metastases.

Evans et al have provided evidence that the IFNγ which is secreted in vitro by TIL in response to tumor stimulation is also being synthesized in vivo at the tumor site at the time of tumor regression.[34] Ten day old intramuscular murine sarcomas were treated with cytoxan and immune splenocytes. Eight days later T cells were separated from the tumor by panning and their mRNA was analyzed by Northern blotting. Substantial mRNA for IFNγ was detected in the $CD8^+$ fraction from these regressing tumors. Further experiments demonstrated that the supernatant obtained when the $CD8^+$ cells were incubated for three days had IFNγ activity in a bioassay.

Summary and Implications

In summary, studies of murine $CD4^+$ and $CD8^+$ tumor reactive lymphocytes have revealed that certain lymphokines, in particular IFNγ, are secreted in response to tumor stimulation both in vitro and at the site of regressing tumors. The in vitro secretion of IFNγ correlates with TIL effectiveness in vivo. Antibody blocking studies reveal that the injection of an anti-IFNγ mAb markedly inhibits the anti-tumor efficacy of both $CD8^+$ and $CD4^+$ tumor reactive lymphocytes. One group has shown that a CTL clone transduced with the gene for IFNγ was more effective than the parent clone in causing tumor regressions in vivo.[35] Collectively, these experiments indicate that IFNγ secretion is an important part of the mechanism by which TIL eradicate tumor cells in mice.

There are several mechanisms by which the local secretion of IFNγ at the tumor site might lead to tumor regressions. Although IFNγ is toxic to some tumors, no appreciable cytotoxicity was observed when the tumors used in these experiments were incubated in IFNγ.[31] Tuttle et al demonstrated that high doses of IFNγ inhibited the in vitro proliferation of tumor MCA 105.[32] IFNγ has been shown in vitro and in vivo to upregulate MHC class I anti-

LYMPHOKINE SECRETION, CYTOLYSIS *IN VITRO*

EXP. # MCA Tumor Stimulator or Target

1. TIL 105-53

	None	105	233	205
IFN-γ	2	70	19	8
TNF	10	480	0	0
% Lysis	-	52	9	2

2. TIL 105-53

	None	105	205	207
IFN-γ	1	53	6	17
TNF	20	905	140	200
% Lysis	-	45	0	4

3. TIL 205-93B

	None	205	105	233
IFN-γ	1	21	3	2
TNF	150	0	0	0
% Lysis	-	12	-8	ND

4. TIL 233-92B

	None	233	105	205
IFN-γ	0	41	9	2
TNF	250	75	75	10
% Lysis	-	16	-5	-1

5. TIL 205-87

	None	205	105	203
IFN-γ	4	80	17	11
TNF	50	1020	45	40
% Lysis	-	24	ND	-6

IN VIVO EFFICACY

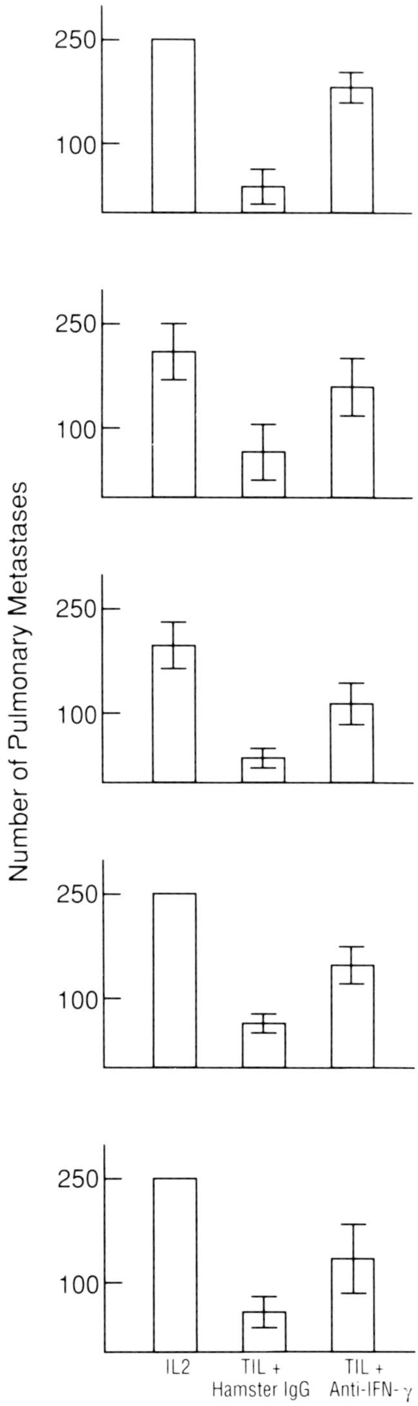

Fig. 6.2.

Fig. 6.2. (opposite) Inhibition of TIL effectiveness by anti-IFN-γmAb. On day - 1, TIL were tested for lymphokine secretion and cytolysis as described in Materials and Methods. IFN-γ is expressed as units per 2.5 x 10^5 cells/ml; TNF is expressed as picograms per 2.5 x 10^5 cells/ml; percent lysis is measured in a 4-h ^{51}Cr release assay at an E/T ratio of 50:1. Pulmonary metastases were induced by intravenous injection on day 0. On day 2, 200 μg of anti-IFN-γ mAb or hamster IgG control was injected intraperitoneally. 5 x 10^6 TIL were adoptively transferred on day 3, and 10,000 U rIL-2 was given intraperitoneally twice a day on days 3-7. The mean ± SEM number of metastases on day 15 is plotted. Treatment of mice that received control hamster IgG with TIL + rIL-2 in all experiments significantly decreased the number of pulmonary metastases compared with the group receiving rIL-2 alone (Exp. 1, p = 0.002; Exp. 2, p = 0.03; Exp 3, p = 0.003; Exp. 4, p = 0.002; Exp. 5, p = 0.002). In Exps. 2, 3, and 5, anti-IFN-γmAb completely inhibited the TIL (TIL + anti-IFN-γ versus IL-2, p = NS). In Exps. 1 and 4, anti-IFN-γ inhibited TIL effectiveness when compared with TIL + hamster IgG control (TIL + anti-IFN-γ versus TIL + hamster IgG: Exp. 1, p = 0.02; Exp. 4, p = 0.025).

gens.[36] A compelling hypothesis is that the local secretion of IFNγ at a tumor site may lead to tumor regression by mediating a DTH reaction. The importance of IFNγ in the initiation of DTH has been established through the use of anti-IFNγ mAbs to block DTH in several animal models.[37] Local secretion of IFNγ (macrophage activating factor) and TNF at a tumor site may induce the priming and triggering steps necessary for the activation of cytotoxic macrophages.[38] The availability of mice with disrupted IFNγ and IFNγ receptor genes may offer models to test these hypotheses.[39]

References

1. Rowe DJ, Beverly PCL. Characteristics of breast cancer infiltrates using monoclonal antibodies to human leukocyte antigens. Br J Cancer 49:149-160, 1984.
2. Svennevig J-L, Svaar H. Content and distribution of macrophages and lymphocytes in solid human malignant tumors. Int J Cancer 24:754-758, 1979.
3. Poppema S, Brocker EB, DeLeij L. In situ analysis of the mononuclear cell infiltrate in primary malignant melanoma of the skin. Clin Exp Immunol 51:77-82, 1983.
4. Whiteside TL, Heo DS, Chen K, Adler A, Johnson JT, Herberman RB. Expansion of tumor-infiltrating lymphocytes from human solid tumors in interleukin 2. In: Truitt RL, Gale RP, Bortin MM, eds. Cellular Immunotherapy of Cancer. New York:Alan R Liss 1987:213-222.
5. Whiteside TL, Jost LM, Herberman, RB. Tumor-infiltrating lymphocytes. Critical Rev Hem/Onc12:25-47, 1992.
6. Pisa P, Halapi E, Pisa EK, Gerdin E, Hising C, Bucht A, Gerdin B, Kiessling R. Selective expression of interleukin 10 interferon γ and GM- CSF in ovarian cancer biopsies. Proc Natl Acad Sci USA 89:7708-7712, 1992.
7. Gansbacher B, Bannerji R, Daniels B, Zier K, Cronin K, Gilboa E. Retroviral vector-mediated interferon γ gene transfer into tumor cells generates potent and long lasting anti-tumor immunity. Cancer Res 50:7820-7825, 1991.
8. Asher AL, Mule JJ, Kasid A, Restifo NP, Salo JC, Reichert CM, Jaffe G, Fendly B, Kreigler M, Rosenberg SA. Murine tumor cells transduced with the gene for TNFα. J Immunol 146:3327-3234, 1991.
9. Salmeron MA, Morita T, Seki H, Platsoucas CD, Itoh K. Lymphokine production by human melanoma tumor-infiltrating lymphocytes. Cancer Immun Immunother 35:211-217, 1992.
10. Belldegrun A, Kasid A, Uppenkamp M, Topalian SL, Rosenberg SA. Human tumor infiltrating lymphocytes. Analysis of lymphokine mRNA expression and relevance to cancer immunotherapy. J Immunol 142:4520-4526, 1989.
11. Schwartzentruber DJ, Topalian SL, Mancini M, Rosenberg SA. Specific release of GM-CSF TNFα and IFNγ by human tumor infiltrating lymphocytes after autologous tumor stimulation. J Immunol 146:3674-3681, 1991.
12. Darrow TL, Slingluff CL, Seigler HF. The role of HLA class I antigens in recognition of melanoma cells by tumor-specific cytotoxic T lymphocytes. J Immunol 142:3329-3335, 1989.

13. Hom SS, Schwartzentruber DJ, Rosenberg SA, Topalian SL. Specific release of cytokines by lymphocytes infiltrating human melanomas in response to shared melanoma antigens. J Immunother 13:18-30, 1993.
14. Schwartzentruber DJ, Solomon D, Rosenberg SA, Topalian SL. Characterization of lymphocytes infiltrating human breast cancer: specific immune reactivity detected by measuring cytokine secretion. J Immunother 12:1-12, 1992.
15. Yoo Y, Heo DS, Hata K, Van Thiel DH, Whiteside TL. Tumor-infiltrating lymphocytes from human colon carcinomas. Gastroenterology 98:259-268, 1990.
16. Hom SS, Rosenberg SA, Topalian SL. Specific immune recognition of autologous tumor by lymphocytes infiltrating colon carcinomas: analysis by cytokine secretion. Cancer Immun Immunother 36:1-8, 1993.
17. Koo AS, Tso C, Shimabukuro T, Peyret C, deKernion JB, Belldegrun A. Autologous tumor-specific cytotoxicity of tumor infiltrating lymphocytes derived from human renal cell carcinoma. J Immunother 10:347-354, 1991.
18. Salgame P, Abrams JS, Clayberger C, Goldstein H, Convit J, Modlin RL, Bloom BR. Differing lymphokine profiles of functional subsets of human CD4 and CD8 T cell clones. Science 254:279-282, 1991.
19. van der Bruggen P, Traversari C, Chomez P, Lurquin C, De Plaen E, Van den Eynde B, Knuth A, Boon T. A gene encoding an antigen recognized by cytolytic T lymphocytes on a human melanoma. Science 254:1643- 1647, 1991.
20. Zakut R, Topalian SL, Kawakami Y, Mancini M, Eliyahu S, Rosenberg SA. Differential expression of MAGE-1 -2 and -3 mRNA in transformed and normal human cell lines. Cancer Res 53:5-8, 1993.
21. Doug Schwartzentruber personal communication.
22. Hwu P, Yannelli J, Kriegler M Anderson WF, Perez C, Chiang Y, Schwarz S, Cowherd R, Delgado C, Mule JJ, Rosenberg SA. Functional and molecular characterization of tumor infiltrating lymphocytes transduced with TNFα cDNA for the gene therapy of cancer in humans. J Immunol 150:4104-4115, 1993.
23. Mosmann TR, Coffman RL. Th1 and Th2 cells: different patterns of lymphokine secretion lead to different functional properties. Ann Rev Immunol 7:145-173, 1989.
24. Greenberg PD, Cheever MA, Fefer A. Eradication of disseminated murine leukemia by chemoimmunotherapy with cytoxan and adoptively transferred immune syngeneic Lyt-1+2- lymphocytes. JExp Med 154:952-960, 1981.
25. Bhan, AK, Perry LL, Cantor H, McCluskey RT, Benacerraf B, Greene MI. The role of T-cell sets in the rejection of MCA induced sarcoma (S1509a) in syngeneic mice. Am J Pathol 102:20-30, 1981.
26. Greenberg PD, Kern DE, Cheever MA. Therapy of disseminated murine leukemia with cyclophosphamide and immune Lyt-1+2- T cells. J Exp Med 161:1122-1130, 1985.
27. Prat M, DiRenzo MF, Comoglio P. Characterization of T lymphocytes mediating in vivo protection against RSV induced murine sarcomas. Int J Cancer 31:757-765, 1983.
28. Prat M, Bretti S, Amedeo M, Landolfo S, Comoglio P. Monoclonal antibody against IFNγ abrogates in vivo tumor immunity against RSV-induced murine sarcomas. J Immunol 138:4530-4536, 1987.
29. Nagarkatti M, Clary S, Nagarkatti P. Characterization of tumor infiltrating CD4⁺ cells as Th1 cells based on lymphokine secretion and functional properties. J Immunol 144:4898-4905, 1990.
30. Barth RJ Jr, Mule JJ, Asher A, Sanda M, Rosenberg SA. Identification of unique murine tumor associated antigens by tumor infiltrating lymphocytes using tumor specific secretion of IFNγ and tumor necrosis factor. J Immunol Methods 140:269-279, 1991.
31. Barth RJ Jr, Mule JJ, Spiess P, Rosenberg SA. Interferon γ and tumor necrosis factor have a role in tumor regressions mediated by murine tumor infiltrating lymphocytes. J Exp Med 173:647-658, 1991.
32. Tuttle TM, McCrady CW, Inge T, Salour M, Bear HD. Interferon γ plays a key role in T-cell induced tumor regression. Cancer

Res 53:833-39, 1993.

33. Yoshizawa H, Chang AE, Shu S. Specific adoptive immunotherapy mediated by tumor-draining lymph node cells sequentially activated with anti-CD3 and IL-2. J Immunol 147:729-737, 1991.
34. Evans R, Kamdar SJ, Duffy T, Edison L. Intratumor gene expression after adoptive immunotherapy in a murine tumor model. J Immunol 150:177-184, 1993.
35. Miyatake S, Nishihara K, Kikuchi H, Yamashita J Namba Y, Hanaoka M, Watanabe Y. Efficient tumor suppression by glioma-specific murine cytotoxic T lymphocytes transfected with IFNγ gene. J Natl Cancer Inst 82:217-220, 1990.
36. Weber JS, Rosenberg SA. Modulation of murine tumor MHC antigens by cytokines in vivo and in vitro. Cancer Res 48:5818-5823, 1988.
37. Fong TAT, Mosmann TR. The role of IFNγ in DTH mediated by Th1 clones. J Immunol 143:2887-2892, 1989.
38. Pace JL, Russell BA, Torres BA, Johnson HM, Gray PW. Recombinant mouse IFNγ induces the priming step in macrophage activation for tumor cell killing. J Immunol 130:2011-2017, 1983.
39. Huang S, Hendriks W, Althage A, Hemmi S, Bluethmann H, Kamijo R, Vilcek J, Zinkernagel R, Aguet M. Immune response in mice that lack the Interferon γ receptor. Science 259:1742-1745, 1993.

CHAPTER 7

TRAFFICKING AND SURVIVAL OF EFFECTOR T CELLS IN VIVO

Bernard A. Fox, John J. Osterholzer, Vikram Mali, Mark Schomogyi

INTRODUCTION

The movement of lymphocytes from one organ to the next has been referred to as lymphocyte recirculation or trafficking. This trafficking of lymphocyte subpopulations integrates tissues of the body and provides a basis for the systemic nature of the immune response. The concept of lymphocyte recirculation was hypothesized by Davis and Carlson in 1909 as an explanation for their experimental observations in the dog.[1] Their extensive studies of leukocytes present in the blood and lymphatics suggested that lymphocytes were replaced at least once and possibly 3 to 4 times per day. They proposed that lymphocytes "may circulate from lymph to blood and from blood, through the capillary endothelium, into the tissue lymph, and thence back into lymph, of the larger lymphatic trunks."

Fifty years later, James Gowans, with the benefit of radioactive labels, elegantly demonstrated that labeled lymphocytes infused into the venous blood quickly migrated to the lymph and could be recovered from the thoracic duct.[2,3] Furthermore, he correctly identified that the small lymphocytes were truly resting cells and were not being rapidly synthesized since less than 2% incorporated ^{3}H-thymidine into their nuclei. Therefore, he argued that the small lymphocytes must be recirculating, because his previous studies suggested that the daily flow of lymphocytes in the thoracic duct was sufficient to replace the total number of lymphocytes in the blood 11 times each day.

In the 85 years since the report of Davis and Carlson, numerous studies have firmly supported their original hypothesis and documented the longevity and recirculatory nature of lymphocytes.[4,5] Unfortunately, the mechanism(s) responsible for the lymphocyte migration from blood

Immunotherapy of Cancer with Sensitized T Lymphocytes, edited by Alfred E. Chang and Suyu Shu.

into tissue and subsequent exit via afferent lymphatics have not been well characterized. Over the past decade, a considerable amount has been written characterizing the molecules and receptors present on lymphocytes, and their corresponding ligands, which play a role in the adhesion to endothelium.[6-12] Recently, Shimizu and colleagues concisely summarized these molecules into four groups based on structure and molecular sequence.[13]

These four groups are:

1. *Selectins* include L-selectin (MEL-14/LECAM-1), E-selectin (ELAM-1), and P-selectin.[14,15] The ligands for both E- and L-selectin are specifically sialyated carbohydrates which have been referred to as 'vascular addressins,' because of their capacity to participate in tissue-specific adhesion of lymphocytes.
2. *Integrins* include LFA-1, VLA-4, LPAM-1, and LPAM-2.[14] These molecules bind to members of the Immunoglobulin Supergene family and to components of the extracellular matrix.
3. *Immunoglobulin supergene family* includes ICAM-1, ICAM-2, VCAM-1, and CD 31.[13] Members of this family serve as endothelial cell ligands for the class of integrins found on T cells.
4. *Other molecules* include CD 44. This molecule binds to hyaluronic acid and possibly other members of the glycosaminoglycans and plays a role in adhesion to high endothelial venules (HEV) and endothelial cells.[9,16,17]

While these categories aid in simplifying our understanding of interactions involved in trafficking, it is critical that we continue to appreciate the complexity inherent to this process, as well as the potential for additional molecules to play a role in lymphocyte migration. The remainder of this manuscript will focus at the cellular level, primarily on in vivo studies of lymphocyte trafficking in tumor bearing hosts and discuss new strategies for designing experiments which may identify the cells that traffic to tumor sites and mediate, either directly or indirectly, tumor regression.

TRAFFICKING OF LYMPHOCYTES IN NAIVE ANIMALS

In vivo analysis of lymphocyte trafficking has generally been attempted by radioactive tagging of specified cells. More recently, studies have employed congenic mouse strains or used fluorescent markers to label lymphocytes. Using these techniques, investigations of lymphocyte trafficking have been undertaken in a variety of animal models. One common observation in these models is the accumulation of labeled cells in the lungs of experimental subjects. Results have suggested that after intravenous (IV) injection, up to 40% of in vitro labeled lymphocytes are found in the lung within the first few minutes.[18,19] In the following 24-48 hours this percentage may fall to 10% or less of the total cells injected. Similar observations have been reported in clinical studies.[20] The rapid accumulation of labeled cells within the lung has generally been interpreted as microembolization or retention of lymphocytes traumatized by in vitro cell separation and labeling, trapped because the lung is the first capillary bed encountered by iv. injected cells. In 1987 Pabst and colleagues directly addressed the issue when labeled cells were injected either IV. or into the left heart. The cells injected via the cardiac route had to pass through another capillary bed before reaching the lung, and yet comparable numbers of labeled lymphocytes had trafficked to the lung within 30 minutes.[21] This intriguing result suggests that the lung probably plays an important yet underappreciated role in the trafficking of some populations of lymphocytes.

Similarly, lymphocyte trafficking to the liver and spleen is more than simple trapping of damaged or dying cells. Experiments from a number of investigators suggest that homing to these sites is physiological. An extensive review of the literature pertinent to "normal" lymphocyte trafficking to lymphoid and non-lymphoid organs has been reviewed recently.[5] Therefore, we will focus on the selective trafficking patterns of immune T-cell populations.

TRAFFICKING PATTERNS OF IMMUNE T CELLS IN ANIMAL MODELS

In 1979, Mulé and colleagues demonstrated that adoptively transferred immune spleen cells, labeled with a radioactive marker, traffic to syngeneic MCA-induced sarcoma implants.[22] In "criss-cross" experiments, they identified that immune spleen cells selectively localized to the tumor implants they were sensitized against. Furthermore, tumor-specific trafficking could only be demonstrated in recipients which had been sublethally radiated prior to adoptive transfer. Also in 1979, Chang and Sugarbaker used ^{3}H or ^{14}C to differentially label populations of spleen cells immune to distinct MHC alloantigens.[23] Spleen cells immune to one alloantigen were labeled with ^{3}H, while spleen cells immune to another alloantigen were labeled with ^{14}C. These two populations of labeled immune spleen cells were mixed and adoptively transferred into recipient animals bearing five-day-old skin grafts expressing one of the alloantigens used to generate the immune cells. Two days later, skin grafts were biopsied, lymph nodes were excised, and tissue was counted to generate a ratio of ^{3}H to ^{14}C. Preferential localization of immune spleen cells to the graft expressing the immunizing alloantigen was detected without evidence of selective trafficking to draining lymph nodes. Taken together, these two early reports presented clear evidence that, following adoptive transfer, fresh (non-cultured) immune spleen cells could recognize the antigen to which they had been sensitized and localize at sites of the "specific" antigen deposition in vivo.

Later de Jong and colleagues demonstrated similar observations using cultured cells and line 10 hepatocarcinoma in guinea pigs.[24] Immune spleen cells were restimulated in vitro with 3M KCl extracted line 10 soluble proteins, labeled with ^{3}H-thymidine, and adoptively transferred into animals bearing either specific tumor (line 10) or an immunologically distinct hepatocarcinoma (line 1). Labeled Line 10 immune spleen cells preferentially localized to line 10 tumor when compared to a contralateral line 1 tumor, further demonstrating a propensity of short-term cultured immune spleen cells to localize to sites of specific tumor. In 1989, Ames and colleagues compared the ability of spleen cells, NK, LAK and TIL cells to preferentially accumulate in mice bearing mammary adenocarcinoma.[25] In this study, only ^{111}In-TIL exhibited selective accumulation in tumor when compared to normal mammary tissue.

Recently, Wallace and colleagues utilized two lipophilic cell tracking compounds to follow immune T cells in vivo.[26] Incorporation of an ^{125}I-labeled lipophilic compound, PKH95, into cell membranes allowed for the detection of marked cells by radioactive counting methods. Cells tagged with the fluorescent compound, PKH26, were detectable using flow cytometric analysis and fluorescent microscopy. After adoptive transfer of labeled TIL into tumor bearing and control mice, the investigators were able to demonstrate increased accumulation of TIL in the lungs of tumor-bearing animals. However, in contrast to other studies reported here, they were unable to show increased accumulation of TIL in mice bearing autologous tumors compared to mice with non-autologous lung tumors. Flow cytometric analysis on populations of cells recovered from tumor bearing animals suggested that there was not preferential proliferation of TIL in animals bearing autologous tumor versus non-autologous tumors. Analysis of frozen tissue sections by fluorescent microscopy did not conclusively demonstrate a pattern of higher TIL density in either tumor or normal parenchyma, or in autologous versus non-autologous tumor. Their results suggested that differential accumulation, selective retention, or proliferation at the tumor site cannot account for the observed pattern of therapeutic efficacy.

Using a similar technical approach, and performing the analysis with clonal populations of effector T cells, Matsumura and colleagues came to a different conclusion.[27] T cell clones were isolated from lymph nodes draining progressively growing tumors, fluorescently labeled, and adoptively transferred into mice bearing pulmonary metastases. The T cell clones studied were generated by anti-CD3/IL-2 stimulation of lymph node cells draining intradermal MCA 106 sarcomas, with repeated in vitro stimulation with irradiated MCA 106 tumor cells and IL-2, and subsequent limiting dilution culture to isolate clonal populations. Two clones, 5A2 and 9H6 were well characterized and studied for their in vivo and in vitro anti-tumor activity. Clone 5A2 mediated specific anti-tumor activity towards MCA 106 both in adoptive immunotherapy and in vitro cytotoxicity experiments whereas clone 9H6 demonstrated partial cross reactivity in vivo and in vitro against the antigenically distinct MCA 205 sarcoma. Fluorochrome labeling of clones with H333421 allowed investigators to study, by fluorescent microscopy, the localization of these cells in the lungs of animals bearing 14 day established MCA 106 or 205 metastases. Results demonstrated that adoptively transferred immune T cell clones accumulated at tumor deposits, and that patterns of localization correlated with observed in vivo and in vitro anti-tumor properties. The 5A2 clone accumulated only in the lungs of animals bearing MCA 106 tumor. The 9H6 clone localized in both tumor metastases of MCA 106 and 205, which parallels its cross reactive nature observed in adoptive immunotherapy and in vitro cytotoxicity.

In contrast to the findings reported by Wallace et al, the study of Matsumura et al demonstrated a selective homing ability of tumor-specific immune T cells. A possible explanation for these differences is that the transferred TIL population used by Wallace et al, was composed of heterogeneous cell populations which may have interfered with the detection of immune T cell localization at sites of tumor. The use of specific clones by Matsumura et al, may have reduced the amount of interference caused by nonspecific interactions and cell trafficking. Alternatively, differences in culture conditions, in vitro stimulation, or time in culture, could be responsible for the variation between these two reports.

SURVIVAL OF ADOPTIVELY TRANSFERRED THERAPEUTIC T CELLS IN ANIMAL MODELS

Persistence of functional, tumor-specific T cells following adoptive transfer is a goal of immunotherapy. However, it is unclear how long cultured T cells survive following adoptive transfer. Cheever et al, Klarnet et al, and Alexander and Rosenberg, have utilized flow cytometric analysis in congenic mice to examine the survival of adoptively transferred, therapeutic T cells.[28-30] These congenic mice are "essentially syngeneic" to the mouse strain being used, but they differ from each other at one independently segregating genetic locus. This single difference at Thy 1, which is not seen by the hosts immune system, can be identified by immunofluoresence with a fluorescein-labeled antibody. Using this reagent, congenic T cells were identified in the lung or lymphoid organs of recipient animals at periods as long as 6 to 16 weeks following adoptive transfer. In all three series of experiments, recipient animals were "pretreated" with an immunosuppressive agent. This strategy of pretreating recipients with lymphocyte-depleting agents prior to adoptive transfer has been employed by many investigators in hopes of facilitating engraftment of transferred T cells. This effect is theoretically due to the elimination of host suppressor T cells and/or the creation of space in the lymphoid organs.[31-34]

In the first study, Cheever et al demonstrated that after 120 days in vivo, transferred T cells could respond to antigenic stimulation in vitro and mediate tumor-specific cytotoxicity.[28] In the study by Klarnet et al, a clone of T cells derived from immune animals, was administered and recovered from lymphoid organs 125 days after adoptive transfer and shown to retain its pattern of specific cytolytic activity following antigenic stimulation in vitro.[29] In the study of Alexander and Rosenberg, congenic TIL were recovered from the lung 6 weeks following adoptive transfer.[30] Their mice were challenged with an IV. dose of tumor cells 5 weeks after adoptive transfer and 1 week prior to harvesting lungs. Cells isolated from the lung were then selected by flow cytometry and expanded with IL-2 in vitro. These studies suggest that the number of transferred T cells surviving in the lung or lymphoid organs are presumably very small prior to stimulation and expansion, but are detectable using flow cytometric or functional (cytolytic) analysis. Whether these few surviving cells mediate the rejection of subsequent tumor challenges, or whether regression of tumor challenges is due to host memory T cells sensitized during initial tumor regression remains an open question which may be addressed in clinical trials with "gene marked" effector T cells.

TRAFFICKING AND SURVIVAL OF ADOPTIVELY TRANSFERRED T CELLS IN PATIENTS WITH CANCER

The adoptive transfer of TIL combined with the administration of IL-2 is capable of mediating the regression of established tumors in selected patients.[35] Extensive studies from Fisher et al and Griffiths et al using ^{111}In-labeled TIL clearly demonstrated that TIL can traffic to and accumulate at sites of tumor metastases in patients pretreated with cyclophosphamide.[20,36] Initially, Fisher and colleagues identified TIL localization as early as 24 hours following infusion in 6 of 6 patients; however, not all the sites imaged. Subsequently, Griffiths et al expanded on this and reported TIL localization in 13 of 18 patients. In this second study, Griffiths et al included a comparison of ^{111}In-labeled PBL in four patients. In one patient previously treated with ^{111}In-TIL, which localized at multiple tumor sites, ^{111}In-PBL demonstrated transient localization at one site and failed to accumulate at other tumor sites. Subsequent infusion of ^{111}In-TIL again imaged tumor at multiple sites, confirming that TIL can preferentially localize to tumor sites and that the propensity to localize at areas of tumor deposits is greater for TIL than for PBL. In an update of the NCI trial, Pockaj and colleagues recently reported results from 38 patients treated with ^{111}In-labeled TIL and high-dose IL-2.[37] All patients had metastatic melanoma and some received a single treatment of cyclophosphamide 24-36 hours prior to TIL infusion. Cyclophosphamide administration was associated with a significantly increased ($p = 0.026$) incidence of tumor imaging in a univariate analysis of factors, and tumor imaging was also associated with a significant ($p2 = 0.022$) response to treatment. Ten of 26 patients who demonstrated imaging of their tumor sites exhibited a partial response, while there were no responses in 12 patients who failed to image. However, other factors, including number of TIL injected and number of ^{111}In-labeled TIL administered were also associated with a significant increase ($p2 = 0.0052$ and $p2 = 0.0049$ respectively) in TIL localization to tumor. Unfortunately, the interpretation of these important studies are seriously handicapped by the heterogeneity of these bulk populations and our inability to identify which cell subpopulations are trafficking to tumor sites.

Additional studies by others suggest that peripheral blood T cells, activated in vitro by culture with autologous tumors and IL-2, can also traffic to and accumulate at tumor sites. Mukherji and colleagues identified localization of ^{111}In-labeled tumor-sensitized T cells in four of seven patients studied.[38] Swift and colleagues, using a similar system, reported visualization of tumor metastases in 6 of 6 patients examined;[39] identifying tumor metastases with the transfer of as few as 5×10^6 ^{111}In-tumor-activated PBL While these five reports concluded that TIL or tumor-sensitized/activated T cells can demonstrate a propensity to traffic to tumor disseminated throughout the body, localization of T cells has only been associated with tumor regression in the study of Pockaj and colleagues.[37] Still, the mechanism or functional activities associated with the cells which mediate regression of tumor in vivo is largely unknown.

Recently, Aebersold and colleagues identified a significant correlation between tumor specific cytotoxicity of TIL administered to the patient and clinical response, suggesting that anti-tumor activity in vitro appears to correlate with therapeutic efficacy.[40] In a murine tumor model, Barth et al observed a correlation between tumor necrosis factor-α or IFNγ release by TIL in vitro, following tumor stimulation, and a capacity to mediate a therapeutic effect in a murine tumor model.[41] Subsequently, Schwartzentruber and colleagues observed similar tumor-specific release of GM-CSF, TNFα and IFNγ by human TIL, but have not reported on whether this in vitro activity correlates with therapeutic efficacy.[42]

These observations and associations between in vitro functions and therapeutic activity represent important steps in understanding the immunobiology of T cell-tumor interactions and help to analyze the mechanisms of tumor regression by immune cells. However, this approach represents an indirect or "black box" approach to the analysis of tumor regression. Certainly, these efforts can identify anti-tumor properties associated with individual populations of T cells present in heterogeneous TIL cultures, and identify that some component of these TIL localize at tumor sites in vivo. Unfortunately, it does not allow the identification of the specific anti-tumor properties of those cells that do traffic to tumor deposits.

GENE-MARKED T CELLS FACILITATE STUDY OF TRAFFICKING IN PATIENTS WITH CANCER

The advent of clinically approved gene transfer afforded the opportunity to genetically label TIL with a marker gene. The gene selected for the initial clinical trial was a bacterial gene encoding for resistance to the antibiotic, Neomycin (Neo^R).[43] Advantages of this approach included the potential to follow cells long term since unlike radioactive labels, the marker would not decay or become diluted as cells divided in vivo. Additionally, extremely sensitive detection of the Neo^R marker was possible using the polymerase chain reaction (PCR). Finally, the selective isolation of Neo^R cells from other host lymphocytes becomes possible by exploiting the functional activity encoded by the Neo^R gene.

In 1990 Rosenberg and colleagues reported on the first clinical application of adoptively transferred, genetically-marked TIL.[43] Using PCR analysis, Neo^R marked cells were found to circulate in the peripheral blood for at least three weeks and as long as two months. Gene marked T cells were observed in tumor biopsies of two patients where multiple tumor-biopsy specimens could be obtained. In one patient, TIL grown from the tumor biopsy could be selected by culture in the neomycin analog, G418; demonstrating expression of the Neo^R gene. In another patient, Neo^R T cells were isolated from a resected regrowth of tumor 64 days after cell infusion. This capability to transduce a marker gene into a heterogeneous population of TIL and then administer these cells to a patient affords a unique opportunity to probe the phenomenon of tumor regression. However, before this can be exploited, improved methods to isolate, expand, and select these cells must be developed. The mouse model provides a system for the development of these methods which may be applicable to the study of cancer in humans.

DEVELOPMENT OF A METHOD TO RECOVER TRANSDUCED T CELLS FOLLOWING ADOPTIVE TRANSFER

Recently we developed T cell clones from murine TIL to study the immunobiology of T cell-tumor interactions in vitro and in vivo. One of these T cell clones, BF-1, was specifically cytotoxic in vitro against the murine colon adenocarcinoma-38 (MC-38) tumor of origin and capable of mediating significant regression of established tumor burdens in vivo.[44] This T cell clone was transduced with a retroviral vector which encoded the genes for Neo^R and human adenosine deaminase (ADA).[45] This transduced T cell clone maintained a pattern of specific cytotoxicity and expressed some therapeutic efficacy, but was generally less effective than the non-transduced parental counterpart. Following adoptive transfer into animals, these cells were identified by PCR in the organs of recipients. Utilizing cell culture and selection techniques transduced cells were recovered from recipient animals and shown to express the ADA gene product, and a pattern of specific cytotoxicity against the MC-38 tumor. Certain recipients of these cells were followed long-term without demonstrating toxicity.[46] The key finding of these experiments was the demonstration that retroviral-mediated transduction of a selectable marker gene into TIL could be utilized to recover Neo^R T cells following adoptive transfer and characterize their functional activity. However, given the limitations of PCR, a drawback to this approach was the inability to reproducibly and accurately quantitate the number of Neo^R T cells present in the freshly isolated population. More importantly, there was no opportunity to assess the frequency of cells which exhibited a particular functional activity or immunological phenotype. Only the activity of the Neo^R T cell population as a whole could be identified.

In an attempt to quantitate the Neo^R T cells present in tissues following adoptive transfer, we examined whether the selective pressure of culture with G418 could be combined with the analytical power of limiting dilution analysis (LDA) culture conditions. LDA is a well established method for the detection and evaluation of immune-reactive cells present in single cell suspensions.[47] Briefly, the methodology was developed as follows: Single cell suspensions containing known or unknown numbers of Neo^R T cells were plated by limiting dilution into 96 well microtiter plates in media containing the neomycin analog, G418. As early as 8 days later neomycin resistant colonies were observed growing in isolated wells, predominantly at the higher dilution. Microscopic analysis revealed healthy, dividing colonies in those wells containing the gene-modified Neo^R T cells. No viable or dividing cells were observed in control wells which did not contain Neo^R cells. Studies demonstrated that no new colonies arose beyond day 14. After 2-3 weeks, tissue culture plates were observed by light microscopy and the number of viable colonies per dilution enumerated. This data was analyzed by chi square minimization analysis (using a computer program developed by Dr. Larry Sirinek and kindly provided by Dr. Charles Orosz) which yielded a minimal frequency estimate and provided 95% confidence limits of the frequency estimates.[48] Analysis of LDA by chi square minimization has been reported to be the most accurate interpretation of the data.[49] This frequency was then used to estimate the number of Neo^R T cells present in the original culture by multiplying the total number of cells by the observed frequency of Neo^R cells. In multiple experiments, LDA with G418 provided a good approximation to the actual number of Neo^R T cells present in the cell suspension.

In order to utilize Neo^R as a selectable marker it is critical to ascertain the sensitivity of the non-transduced cell population to G418. Therefore, 10,000 non-transduced BF-1 T cells were cultured in microtiter wells with an increasing concentration of G418 (none, 200, 400, 600, 800 or 1000 μg/ml G418). As little as 200 μg/ml of G418 was sufficient to prohibit colony formation, thereby establishing the sensitivity to G418 of the non-transduced T cell clone (data not shown). As the transduced T cells grew equally well in 400 μg/ml of G418, experiments were performed at that concentration. Other studies examined the ability of normal tissue cell populations isolated from the spleen, liver or lung to grow in microtiter plates with 400 μg/ml G418. No colonies were ever observed under these conditions (data not shown). Having established conditions which were selective for a series of Neo^R T cell clones, we investigated the effect of different culture conditions and feeder cell treatments on the development of colonies in LDA. Four subclones of the BF-1.50 T cell clone

(BF-1.50-1A, BF-1.50-2B, BF-1.50-4B, and BF-1.50-8A), transduced with a retroviral construct containing both Neo^R and human IL-1β (hIL-1β) genes, were used in these experiments. Transduced T cells were serially diluted and cultured with different feeder cell conditions; including fresh spleen cells + G418, BF-1 T cells + G418, irradiated BF-1 T cells + G418 or irradiated BF-1 T cells without G418. Results of these experiments using transduced T cell clones demonstrated that all conditions, except irradiated T cells without G418, were adequate to support a high frequency of colony formation (Fig. 7.1). Interestingly, the most variable condition was the combination of irradiated feeders without G418. In several experiments LDA under these conditions did not support the growth of G418 resistant colonies. As presented in Figure 7.1, LDA of transduced Neo^R T cells with G418 and either fresh spleen cells or T cell clones as feeder cells provided a good approximation to the number of transduced cells plated. For the remainder of these experiments LDA was generally performed using either fresh spleen or non-transduced T cell clones as a feeder cell layer with 400 μg/ml G418.

A major problem in the clinical studies of Neo^R human TIL has been the difficulty in recovering G418 resistant T cells. One hypothesis suggests that the death of non-transduced cells, sensitive to culture with G418, is toxic to the small percentage of transduced T cells present in the culture. To test this hypothesis, cell suspensions were prepared from liver or spleen and added at various concentrations to the LDA cultures. Mechanically isolated prepa-

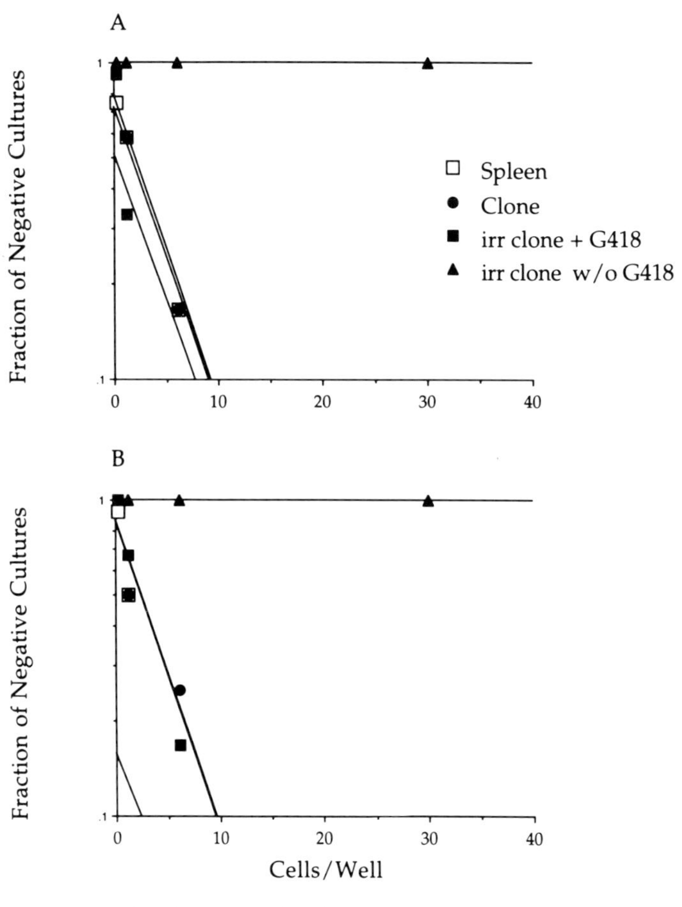

Fig. 7.1. The BF-1.50-1A (A) or BF-1.50-2B transduced Neo^R T cells (B) were plated in 24 replicates for each dilution (5 fold serial dilution's starting at 30 cells/well) in CM containing 150 IU/ml IL-2 and 400 μg/ml active G418. The following four culture conditions were evaluated: 10,000 fresh C57BL/6 spleen cells/well + 400 ug/ml G418; 10,000 non-transduced BF-1 T cells/well + 400 μg/ml G418; 10,000 irradiated (3000R) BF-1 T cells/well + 400 μg/ml G418; and 10,000 irradiated (3000 R) BF-1 T cells/well without G418. LDA cultures were incubated at 37°C for 14-21 days and evaluated for colony formation. The data were analyzed by Chi Square minimization analysis which plotted the results, yielded a minimal frequency estimate, and provided 95% confidence limits of the frequency estimates. Data were plotted as the number of transduced T cells plated/ well (linear X axis) versus the fraction of microwells per dilution which failed to show colony formation (logarithmic y axis).

rations of hepatic cells were highly toxic to the growth of colonies; generally preventing colony formation (CF) when as few as 15,000 cells were added to the culture (Fig. 7.2A). This inhibitory effect on cell growth was lessened when enzymatically isolated hepatic preparations were added to the LDA cultures. In a simultaneous study presented in Figure 7.2B, 30,000 enzymatically isolated hepatic cells had no significant impact on CF while 15,000 mechanically isolated hepatic cells eliminated CF. However, increasing the number of enzymatically isolated hepatic cells to 100,000 impaired CF such that no colonies were identified. Clearly, using enzymatic digestion to obtain hepatic cells for LDA increases the sensitivity of detection, allowing for the recovery of as few as 1 transduced T cell in 15,000 hepatic cells. LDA detection of G418 re-

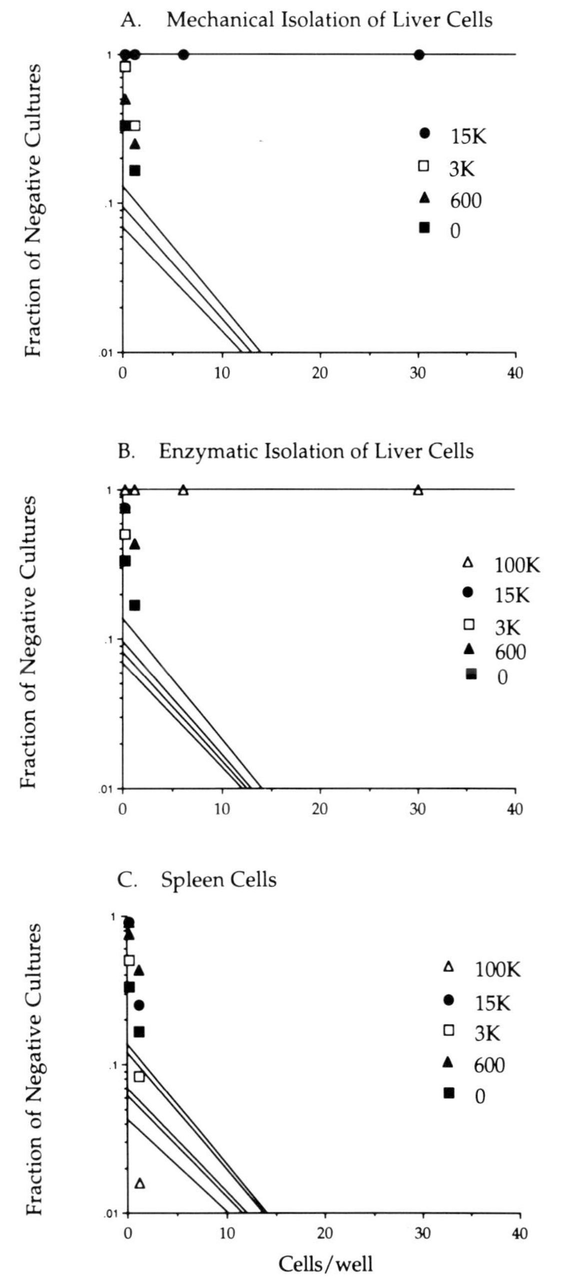

Fig. 7.2. BF-1.50 transduced Neo^R T cells were plated in 24 replicates for each dilution (5 fold serial dilution's starting at 30 cells/well) in CM with 150 IU/ml IL-2 and 400 µg/ml active G418. LDA cultures were incubated at 37°C for 14-21 days and then evaluated for colony formation. The data were analyzed by Chi Square minimization analysis which plotted the results, yielded a minimal frequency estimate, and provided 95% confidence limits of the frequency estimates. Data was plotted as the number of BF 1.50 1A cells plated/well (linear axis) versus the fraction of microwells per dilution which failed to show colony formation (logarithmic y axis). The following culture conditions were evaluated: (A.) Freshly harvested livers from C57BL/6 mice were minced with scissors, disassociated with syringe plungers, filtered with nytex gauze, washed, and the number of single cells enumerated. These single cell suspensions of liver cells were plated into the LDA cultures at 15,000 (15K), 3,000 (3K), or 600 freshly harvested liver cells/well. Control cultures had no liver cells added to the LDA. (B.) Surgically resected livers were processed as above except that cells were disassociated by incubation with a triple enzyme solution containing collagenase, DNAse and Hyaluronidase for 2 hours. Resulting single cell suspensions were washed, counted, and plated into the LDA cultures at 100,000 (100K), 15,000 (15K), 3,000 (3K) or 600 cells/well. Control cultures had no liver cells added to the LDA. C.) Fresh spleen cells were isolated, washed, counted and plated into the LDA cultures at 100,000 (100K), 15,000 (15K), 3,000 (3K), or 600 cells/well. Control cultures had no liver cells added to the LDA.

sistant T cells in a population of spleen cells was even more effective. As presented in Figure 7.2C, the addition of 100,000 normal spleen cells in this experiment, and up to 300,000 spleen cells in other experiments has not prevented CF. These results clearly demonstrate the potential of this approach to quantitate and recover Neo^R T cells which have trafficked to organ sites.

It is envisioned that recovery of transduced T cells which have infiltrated a regressing tumor might provide substantial information on the mechanism of immune-mediated tumor regression following adoptive transfer. To determine whether tumor cells would interfere with LDA, graded numbers of freshly isolated tumor cells were added to LDA cultures. Figure 7.3 presents two experiments using different T cell clones. In one experiment the addition of up to 10,000 MCA-106 tumor cells had no significant inhibitory effects on CF (Fig. 7.3A). However, the addition of 30,000 tumor cells/well completely inhibited CF. This analysis was simultaneously repeated (Fig. 7.3B) using a second Neo^R T cell subclone and adding graded numbers of the same freshly isolated tumor cell preparation used in Figure 7.3A. In this experiment, increasing the number of tumor cells to 10,000-30,000 had a variable (but insignificant) effect on recovery of G418 resistant colonies. Similar results were obtained in studies using the B16BL6 tumor where 15,000 tumor cells failed to inhibit CF in some experiments but exhibited some decrease in CF with 10,000 tumor cells/well in other experiments (data not shown). These results demonstrate that while high concentrations of tumor cells/well may inhibit CF of some Neo^R T cells, culture with G418 can be used to recover these T cells by further diluting the tumor cell concentration used for LDA. This level of inhibition may only interfere with testing this strategy in a clinical situation when the

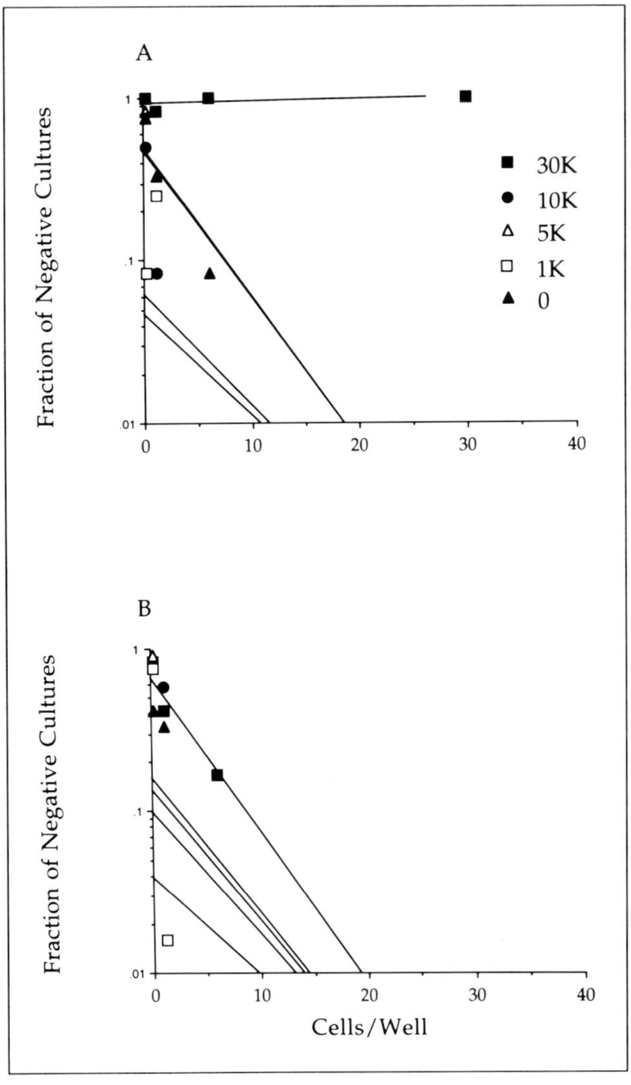

Fig. 7.3. BF 1.50-1A (A) or BF 1.50-4B (B) transduced Neo^R T cells were plated in replicate 96 microwells for each dilution (5 fold serial dilution's starting at 30 cells/well) in CM with 150 IU/ml IL-2 and 400 μg/ml active G418. Tumor cells was added to LDA cultures at either 30,000, 10,000, 5,000, or 1,000 tumor cells per well. Control plates received CM without tumor cells. LDA cultures were incubated at 37°C for 14-21 days and then evaluated for colony formation. The data were analyzed by Chi square minimization analysis which plotted the results, yielded a minimal frequency estimate, and provided 95% confidence limits of the frequency estimates.

concentration of Neo^R lymphocytes infiltrating a tumor is less than 1 T cell for every 10,000 tumor cells. It might be anticipated that during T cell-mediated tumor regression, the percentage of Neo^R T cells at the tumor site may be significantly higher than 1 in 10,000. This may increase the likelihood of successfully recovering gene-marked T cells from the tumor site and allow for analysis of their specific phenotype and immunological functions.

RECOVERY OF NEO^R T CELLS FOLLOWING ADOPTIVE TRANSFER

LDA methodology was next used to assess the survival, trafficking, and functional properties of Neo^R T cells following adoptive transfer into mice. Two x 10^7 Neo^R T cells were adoptively transferred into syngeneic mice that were sacrificed 2, 4, or 8 days later. All animals received 90,000 IU IL-2 q8h for 5 days. The lung, liver, spleen and mesenteric lymph nodes were removed from each animal, cell suspensions prepared, and LDA cultures initiated. Control animals, which had not received Neo^R T cells were also sacrificed and LDA performed. Cultures were inspected at regular intervals and final enumeration of colonies performed between 14-21 days. Frequencies and estimates of Neo^R T cell numbers were generated for all four organs at each time point.

Results of these experiments demonstrated that small numbers of Neo^R T cells could be recovered from multiple organs (Fig. 7.4A). This allowed for the determination of the frequency of gene-marked T cells in the population and allowed for an extrapolation of the absolute number present in each organ. Changes in frequencies of Neo^R T cells over time correlated approximately with changes in the estimated number of Neo^R cells per organ. Both the frequencies and total numbers of Neo^R T cells appeared to increase between days 2 and 4 in all organs, suggesting that cells surviving the initial transfer were able to expand to some extent in vivo. Consistent with our previous study and that of Klarnet and colleagues, results of these experiments demonstrated that transferred, gene-modified T cells did not survive in the intact host much beyond one week.[29,46]

One parameter believed critical for the long-term success of adoptive immunotherapy regimens is the ability of the transferred cells to survive and circulate throughout the host. Numerous studies, reviewed in the introduction, generally demonstrate that immunosuppression of the host is required to facilitate the survival of adoptively transferred T cells. Similarly, investigators have demonstrated that chemo-immunotherapies increase the therapeutic efficacy of transferred cells. It is hypothesized that drugs such as cyclophosphamide (Cy) not only affect the tumor directly but enhance the ability of transferred cells to survive and traffic in the host. Several mechanisms have been postulated to account for the effect of cyclophosphamide on transferred cells. One possibility is that Cy is capable of reducing the number of host lymphocytes,[50] such that transferred cells have more "space" in which to migrate and take up residence. Others have suggested that radiation or Cy treatment selectively eliminates or prevents the development endogenous suppressor cells that may inhibit the expansion of newly introduced cells,[31,32] Also, the recovery of granulocytes from chemotherapy correlates with a release of a variety of colony stimulating factors.[51,52] Cells adoptively transferred into such an environment may also positively respond to the numerous factors involved in the host's recovery.

IMMUNOSUPPRESSION OF HOST PROMOTES SURVIVAL OF NEO^R T CELLS

In order to evaluate the effect of immunosuppression in this model, mice receiving various doses of Cy prior to the transfer of Neo^R T cells were compared with mice receiving the gene-modified T cells only. Cy was administered at doses of either 100, 80, or 50 mg/kg 6-8 hours prior to the adoptive transfer of 2 x 10^7 Neo^R T cells (BF-1.50 T cells). Control

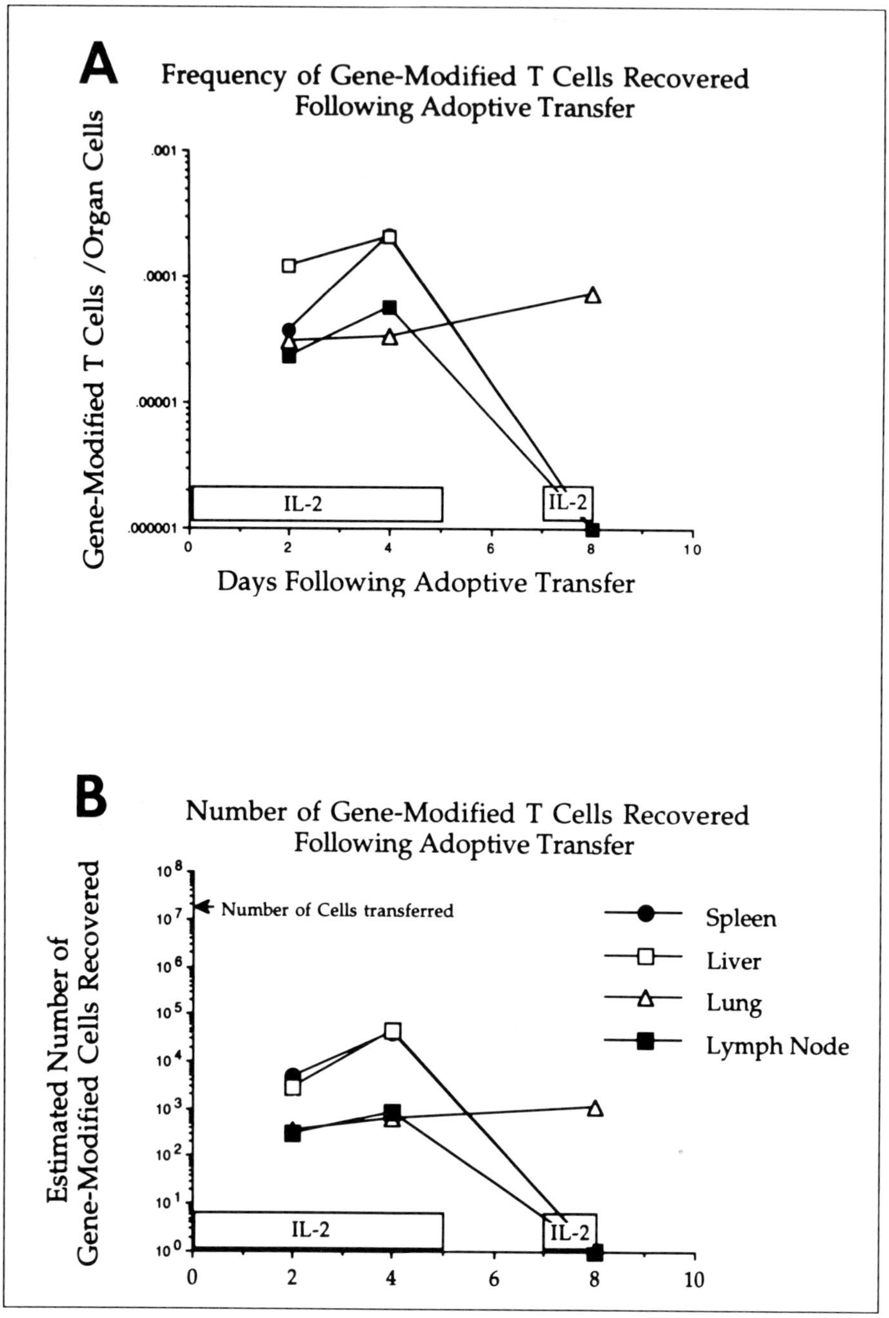

Fig. 7.4. Twenty million BF-1.50-1A Neo^R T cells were adoptively transferred into normal C57BL/6 mice. Animals received 180,000 IU IL-2 IP q8h. At 2, 4, and 8 days following adoptive transfer animals were sacrificed and spleen, lung, liver and MLN removed. Single cell suspensions were generated and placed into LDA culture containing 400 μg/ml active G418 and 150 IU/ml IL-2. Cultures were incubated at 37°C for 14-21 days and evaluated for colony formation. The data were analyzed by Chi Square minimization analysis to yield a minimal frequency estimate of Neo^R T cells present in each organ population. The frequencies of Neo^R T cells residing per organ were then compared at consecutive time points (A). These frequencies were then used to estimate the total number of Neo^R T cells/organ by multiplying the frequency of Neo^R T cells/organ by the total number of cells isolated from that organ (B).

animals received cells only. Animals received rIL-2 q8h for 5 days after which they went 2 days without IL-2 treatment. This cycle was repeated until animals were sacrificed. On days 2, 4, 7, 8, and 15 post adoptive transfer, mice were sacrificed, cell suspensions prepared from the spleen, lung, liver, and mesenteric lymph nodes, and LDA with G418 was performed. The frequency of Neo^R cells recovered per organ was determined for both control animals and animals pretreated with Cy (100, 80, or 50 mg/kg). These comparisons demonstrated that Cy significantly ($p < 0.05$) increased the ratio of gene modified cells per organ on days 2 and 4 for the spleen, lung, and liver (significance determined by chi square minimization). No significant difference in recovery of Neo^R T cells was noted between the mesenteric lymph nodes of Cy treated or control animals. By day 8, all organs demonstrated significantly ($p < 0.05$) increased frequencies in Cy treated animals. Having obtained the frequency of T cells present in the specified organ, the number of Neo^R T cells recovered per organ was extrapolated (using actual organ cell yields from each experiment) and compared for animals receiving high dose Cy (100 mg/kg), low dose Cy (50-80 mg/kg), and control animals which did not receive Cy treatment (Fig. 7.5). Results demonstrated that treatment of animals with Cy prior to adoptive transfer increased the number of Neo^R T cells recovered from all organs, most notably by day 7/8.

To evaluate the effect of Cy treatment on the survival of transferred cells in the entire animal, the numbers of Neo^R cells recovered in the spleen, lung, liver, and mesenteric lymph nodes were totaled for each animal. Averages of the number of modified cells recovered per animal were compiled for each treatment group (100 mg/kg Cy, 80-50 mg/kg Cy, no Cy), at each time point (2, 4, 7/8, and 15 days). This data was used to observe trends in the survival of gene-modified T cells following transfer into control or Cy treated animals. Figure 7.6, demonstrates that the administration of Cy prior to the adoptive transfer of T cells promotes the survival and expansion of these cells in the entire animal.

Analysis of comparisons between Cy treated and control animals demonstrated that Cy treatment increased the number of donor cells residing per organ at early time points, and enhanced their ability to expand and survive in vivo. The number of donor cells recovered at all time points, most notably day 7/8, appeared dependent upon the dose of Cy administered. This translated into a 4-to-5 log difference in the number of cells recovered when the 100 mg/kg dose of Cy was compared to mice that were not immunosuppressed. Since all experimental models of adoptive immunotherapy for cancer show increased efficacy when greater numbers of therapeutic cells are administered, it seems likely that the capacity to expand cells in vivo and extend their survival would be advantageous. Interestingly, while Cy treatment prior to adoptive transfer significantly increased the survival of Neo^R T cells, engraftment did not extend beyond 2 weeks. This result, while consistent with the observed inability of long-term cultured IL-2-dependent T cells to survive for an extended length of time in vivo, may not be relevant to T cells generated and maintained under culture conditions that are more "immunological" (i.e. antigen driven). Overall, these results support the hypothesis that an important factor contributing to the therapeutic benefits of Cy treatment in adoptive immunotherapy strategies is its ability to facilitate the survival and expansion of transferred immune T cells.

RECOVERED T CELLS MAINTAIN SPECIFIC IMMUNOLOGIC FUNCTION AND hIL-1β EXPRESSION

The functional properties of Neo^R T cells recovered by LDA from different organs were evaluated. Representative colonies from lung, liver and spleen were recovered, expanded in media containing G418, and analyzed for cytolytic activity against either their specific tumor (MC 38)

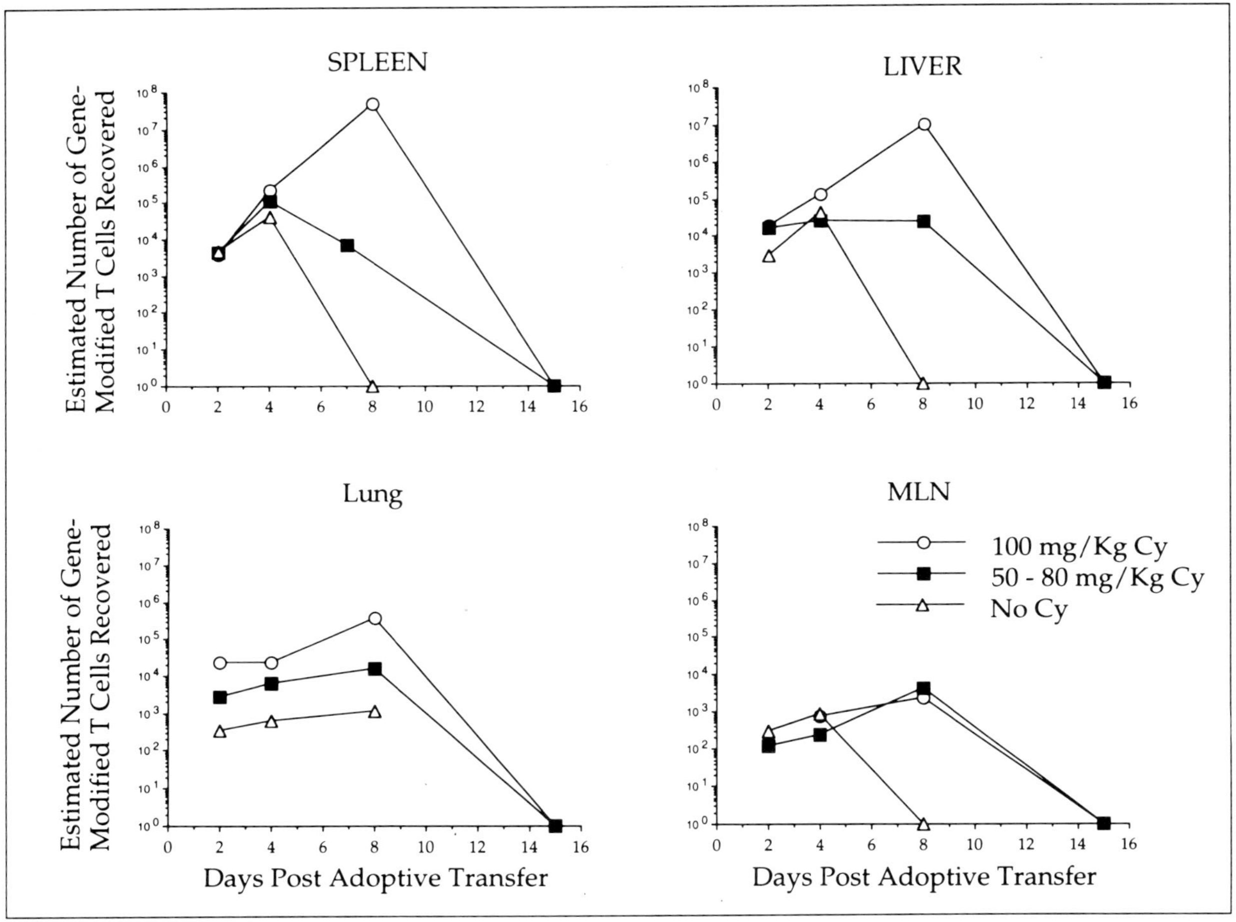

Fig. 7.5. Animals received 100, 80, or 50 mg/kg cyclophosphamide 4-6 hours prior to adoptive transfer of 2 x 10^7 BF-1.50-1A Neo^R T cells. Animals receiving 80 or 50 mg/kg cyclophosphamide were combined for the purpose of these analyses. Control animals received cells only. All animals received 180,000 IU IL-2 IP tid in 5 day cycles followed by 2 days without IL-2 treatment. At 2, 4, 7/8 and 15 days post adoptive transfer animals were sacrificed and LDA cultures in media containing 25 u/ml IL-2 and 400 µg/ml G418 were initiated from cultures derived from spleen, liver, lungs, and mesenteric lymph nodes. Plates were incubated for 14-21 days and then assessed for colony formation. Results were analyzed by Chi Square minimization analysis which yielded a minimal frequency estimate of Neo^R T cells present in the population. The total number of Neo^R T cells residing per organ was extrapolated by multiplying the frequency of Neo^R T cells/organ by the total number of cells isolated from that organ.

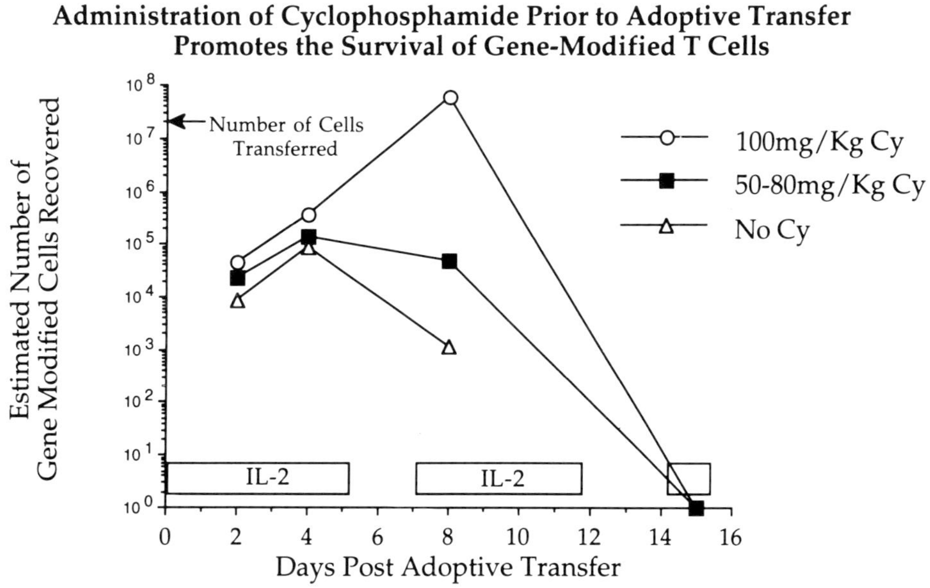

Fig. 7.6. Animals received either 100 mg/kg cyclophosphamide, 80 or 50 mg/kg cyclophosphamide, or no cyclophosphamide prior to the adoptive transfer of 2 x 10^7 BF-1.50-1A Neo^R T cells. All animals received 180,000 IU IL-2 IP q8h in 5 day cycles, with 2 days off of IL-2. Animals were sacrificed and LDA performed 2, 4, 7/8, and 15 days following adoptive transfer. The frequency of Neo^R T cells recovered from each organ, was multiplied by the total number of cells isolated from that organ to yield an estimate of the total number of Neo^R T cells in that organ. Results from each organ (spleen, liver, lung and MLN) were combined for each animal to yield an estimate of the total number of NeoR T cells present in those organs. This number was used as an estimate of the total number of gene-modified T cells in that animal. Each point is the mean of at least two animals.

or an unrelated syngeneic tumor (B16BL6). Results of two LDA experiments utilizing two different T cell clones are presented in Table 7.1. These results clearly demonstrated that the isolated colonies uniformly expressed cytotoxicity against the MC-38 tumor but not the B16 BL6 tumor. LAK cells efficiently killed both MC-38 and B16 BL6 targets, demonstrating the lysability of both tumor lines. These results are consistent with the pattern of cytotoxicity expressed by the BF-1.50-1A/8A T cell clones which were not passaged in vivo (data not shown) and suggests that transduced T cells which have been adoptively transferred and recovered by LDA selection in G418 retain specific immunologic reactivity. Since the BF-1.50 series of T cell subclones were transduced with a vector containing both Neo^R and hIL-1β, colonies recovered by LDA were analyzed for expression of hIL-1β protein. Results of this analysis, which is non-reactive with murine IL-1β, demonstrated expression of the human gene product in 3 of 3 isolates (data not shown). These results further confirm that colonies recovered by LDA were derived from gene-modified T cells.

ISOLATION OF T CELLS WITH ORGAN-SELECTIVE TRAFFICKING CAPACITY

The selective growth advantage imparted by the neomycin resistance gene may also be used to study the selective homing capacity of T cells following adoptive transfer. This is similar to a concept proposed by Rosenberg and colleagues, to use selection in G418 as a method to recover Neo^R T cells that have trafficked to the

Table 7.1. T cells recovered by LDA maintain specific cytotoxicity for MC-38 tumor

Effector[a]	Tissue	Cytotoxic Activity of Recovered T Cells Against their Specified Tumor Target Lytic $Units_{20}$ / 10^6 Effectors	
		MC-38	B16-BL6
BF-1.50 8A	Lung	244	< 4
	Lung	175	< 4
	Spleen	71	< 4
	Liver	85	< 4
			< 4
BF-1.50 1A	Lung	400	< 4
	Liver	> 200	< 4
LAK		160	53

[a] Colonies were isolated from LDA of tissue (lung, spleen, or liver) preparations taken from mice which had received 20 million transduced T cells (BF-1.50 -1A and 8A) two days earlier. Colonies were isolated, expanded and tested for cytotoxicity against MC-38 or B16-BL6. Cytotoxicity was evaluated in Lytic Units / 10^6 Effectors (LU /10 effectors = 10^6 effectors/E:T ratio which generates 20% lysis x number of tumor targets used)

tumor site.[43] They reasoned that recovered Neo^R T cells could then be expanded in vitro and reinfused back into the patient providing a source of T cells selected for their capacity to traffic to the tumor. We sought to determine whether the selective recovery and subsequent expansion of Neo^R T cells recovered from a specific organ could enrich for cells capable of homing to that organ upon repassage into other animals. Following adoptive transfer and LDA, Neo^R T cells were recovered from specific organs, and expanded to high enough numbers to allow for another adoptive transfer. This cycle of culture with G418 to select Neo^R T cells following adoptive transfer, was repeated multiple times. Results demonstrated that for non-lymphoid organs (lung or liver), after four consecutive passages, there was an increase in the frequency with which cells trafficked to their specific organ, as compared to animals that received Neo^R cells that had not been previously passaged (data not shown). In a similar series of experiments, we attempted to select for cells capable of homing to the lymph nodes. While variable, the frequency of Neo^R T cells homing to lymph nodes did not increase following five consecutive passages. Suggesting that we had not enriched for cells capable of homing to the lymph node. This approach to study trafficking may prove valuable to investigators seeking to identify specific "tissue-homing" receptors.

There are likely multiple factors that influence a given cell's trafficking properties. The most important factors are likely the expression of particular cell adhesion molecules, such as the ones reviewed previously in this chapter, or the state of cellular activation. Certain patterns of adhesion molecule expression may result in the entrapment of cells in specific organs. The BF-1.50-1A Neo^R T cell clone expresses heterogeneous levels of the various adhesion molecules (data not shown), which potentially allowed for distinct sets of cells to localize in different organs following adoptive transfer. That we could enrich for cells capable of trafficking to the lung or liver suggests that for these organs, there may be selective factors which regulate the homing of adoptively transferred cells. Our inability to select for cells capable of localizing in lymph nodes may imply that there were not selective factors involved which could be detected in this study. Alternatively, it is possible that the cells capable of trafficking to the lymph nodes remain there more transiently than in other non-lymphoid organs; making it more difficult to demonstrate increased localization of these cells after multiple selective passages.

In summary, we are exploring imaginative techniques to study the phenomenon of T cell-mediated tumor regression. That the development of these new methodologies will aid our understanding of which types of T cells are essential for tumor regression. This information may lead to alternative new strategies for the effective generation of effector T cells ex vivo. Ultimately, this information will be critical to the development of vaccine strategies for the treatment of cancer.

References

1. Davis BF, Carlson AJ. Contributions to the physiology of lymph. IX. Notes on the leucocytes in the neck lymph, thoracic lymph and blood of normal dogs. AM J Physiol 25:173, 1909.
2. Gowans JL. The effect of the continuous re-infusion of lymph and lymphocytes on the output of lymphocytes from the thoracic duct of unanesthetized rats. Br J Exp Pathol 38:67-78, 1957.
3. Gowans JL. The recirculation of lymphocytes from blood to lymph in the rat. J Physiol (London) 146:54, 1959.
4. Butcher EC. The regulation of lymphocyte traffic. Current Topics in Microbiology and Immunology 128:85-122, 1986.
5. Pabst R, Binns RM. Heterogeneity of Lymphocyte homing physiology: Several mechanisms operate in control of migration of lymphoid and non-lymphoid organs in vivo. Immunological Reviews 108:87-109, 1989.
6. Mackay CR, Marston WL, Dudler L, et al. Tissue specific migration pathways by phenotypically distinct subpopulations of memory T cells. Eur Jour Immunol 22:887-895, 1992.
7. Streeter PR, Berg EL, Rouse BTN, et al. A tissue specific endothelial cell molecule involved in lymphocyte homing. Nature 331:41-46, 1988.
8. Mobley JL, Daily MO. Regulation of adhesion molecule expression by CD8 T cells in vivo. J Immunol 148:2348-2356, 1992.
9. Oppenheimer-Marks N, Davis LS, Lipsky PE. Human T lymphocyte adhesion to endothelial cells and transendothelial migration: Alteration of receptor use relates to the activation status of both T cells and the endothelial cell. J Immunol 145:140-148, 1990.
10. Tamatani T, Kotani M, Tanaka T, Miyasaka M. Molecular mechanisms underlying lymphocyte recirculation II: Differential regulation of LFA-1 in the interaction between lymphocytes and high endothelial cells. Euro Jour Immunol 21:855-858, 1991.
11. Nickoloff BJ, Griffiths CEM. Lymphocyte trafficking in Psoriasis: A new perspective emphasizing the dermal dendrocyte with active dermal recruitment mediated via endothelial cells followed by intra-epidermal T cell activation. Jour Investig Derm 95:35s-37s, 1990.
12. Siegelman MH, van de Rijn M, Weissman IL. Mouse lymph node homing receptor cDNA clone encodes a glycoprotein revealing tandem interaction domains. Science 243:1165-1172, 1989.
13. Shimizu Y, Newman W, Tanaka Y, Shaw S. Lymphocyte interactions with endothelial cells. Immunol Today 13:106-112, 1992.
14. Springer TA. Adhesion receptors of the immune system. Nature 346:425-434, 1990.
15. Brandley BK, Swiedler SJ, Robbins PW. Carbohydrate ligands of the LEC cell adhesion molecules. Cell 63:861-863, 1990.
16. Aruffo A, Stamenkovic I, Melnick M, Underhill CB, Seed B. CD44 is the principal cell surface receptor for hyaluronate. Cell 61:1303-1313, 1990.
17. Jalkanen S, Bargatze RF, de los Toyos J, Butcher EC. Lymphocyte recognition of high endothelium: antibodies to distinct epitopes of an 85-95-kD glycoprotein antigen differentially inhibit lymphocyte binding to lymph node, mucosal, or synovial endothelial cells. Jour. Cell Biol 105:983-990, 1987.
18. Binns RM and Licence ST. Patterns of migration of labelled blood lymphocyte subpopulations; evidence for two types of peyer's patch in the young pig. Adv Exp Med Biol 186:661-668, 1985.

19. Rannie GH, Donald KJ. The migration of thoracic duct lymphocytes to non lymphoid tissues. A comparison of the distribution of radioactivity at intervals following IV transfusion of cells labelled with ^{3}H, ^{14}C, ^{75}Se, ^{99m}Tc, ^{125}I and ^{51}Cr in the rat. Cell Tissue Kinet 10:523, 1977.
20. Fisher B, Packard BS, Read EJ, Carrasquillo JA, Carter CS, Topalian SL, Yang JC, Yolles P, Larson SM, Rosenberg SA. Tumor localization of adoptively transferred indium-111 labeled tumor infiltrating lymphocytes in patients with metastatic Melanoma. Jour Clin Oncol 7:250-261 1989.
21. Pabst R, Binns RM, Licence ST, Peter M. Evidence of a selective major vascular marginal pool of lymphocytes. Am Rev Respir Dis 136:1213-1218, 1987.
22. Mule JJ, Jones FR, Hellstrom I, Hellstrom KE. Selective localization of radiolabeled immune lymphocytes into syngeneic tumors. J Immunol 123 (2):600-6 1979.
23. Chang AE, Sugarbaker PH. Preferential homing of passively transferred T cells into skin allografts of mice. Transplantation 28 (3):247-52, 1979.
24. de Jong WH, wan de Plas MM, Steerenberg PA, Kruizinga W, Ruitenberg EJ. Selective localization of tumor-immune spleen cells at the tumor challenge site after adoptive transfer of line 10 tumor immunity in strain 2 guinea pigs. J Immunol 134 (3):2032-40, 1985.
25. Ames IH, Gagne GM, Garcia AM, Hohn PA, Scatorchia GM, Tomar RH, McAfee JG. Preferential homing of tumor-infiltrating lymphocytes in tumor-bearing mice. Cancer Immunology, Immunotherapy 29 (2):93-100, 1989.
26, Wallace PK, Palmer LD, Perry-Lalley D, Bolton ES, Alexander RB, Horan PK, Yang JC, Muirhead KA. Mechanisms of adoptive immunotherapy: improved methods for in vivo tracking of tumor-infiltrating lymphocytes and lymphokine-activated killer cells. Cancer Research 53 (10 Suppl):2358-67, 1993.
27. Takafumi M, Sussman JJ, Krinock RA, Chang AE, Shu S. Characteristics and in vivo homing of long-term T cell lines and clones derived from tumor draining lymph nodes. (in press).
28. Cheever MA, Thompson DB, Klarnet JP, Greenberg PD. Antigen-driven long term cultured T cells proliferate in vivo, distribute widely, mediate specific tumor therapy, persist long-term as functional memory T cells. J Exp Med 163:1100-1112, 1986.
29. Klarnet JP, Matis LA, Kern DE, Mizuno MT, Peace DJ, Thompson JA, Greenberg PD, Cheever MA. Antigen-driven T cell clones can proliferate in vivo, eradicate disseminated leukemia, provide specific immunologic memory. J Immunol 138:4012-4017, 1987.
30. Alexander RB, Rosenberg SA. Long term survival of adoptively transferred tumor infiltrating lymphocytes in mice. J Immunol 145:1615-1620, 1990.
31. North RJ, Cyclophosphamide-facilitated adoptive immunotherapy of an established tumor depends upon elimination of tumor-induced suppressor T cells. J Exp Med 155:1063, 1982.
32. North RJ. Gamma-irradiation facilitates the expression of adoptive immunity against an established tumor by eliminating suppressor T cells. Cancer Immunol Immunother 16:175, 1984.
33. Chang AE, Shu S, Chou T, Lafreniere R, Rosenberg SA. Differences in the effects of host suppression on the adoptive immunotherapy of subcutaneous and visceral tumors. Cancer Res 46:3426, 1986.
34. Papa MZ, Yang JC, Vetto JT, Shiloni E, Eisenthal A, Rosenberg SA. Combined effects of chemotherapy and interleukin-2 in the therapy of mice with advanced pulmonary tumors. Cancer Res 48:122, 1988.
35. Rosenberg SA, Packard BS, Aebersold PM, Solomon D, Topalian SL, Toy ST, Simon P, Lotze MT, Yang JC, Seipp CA, Simpson C, Carter C, Bock S, Schwartzentruber D, Wei JP, White DE. Special report: use of tumor-infiltrating lymphocytes and interleukin-2 in the immunotherapy of patients with metastatic melanoma. A preliminary report. N Engl J Med 319:1676, 1988.
36. Griffiths KD, Read EJ, Carrasquillo JA, Carter CS, Yang JC, Fisher B, Aebersold P, Packard BS, Yu MY, Rosenberg SA. In vivo distribution of adoptively transferred Indium-111-labelled tumor infiltrating lym-

phocytes in patients with metatatic melanoma. Jour Natl Can Inst 81:1709-1717, 1989.

37. Pockaj BA, Sherry RM, Wie JP, Yannelli JR, Carter CS, Leitman SF, Carassquillo JA, Steinberg SM, Rosenberg SA, Yang JC. Localization of ^{111}Indium-labelled tumor infiltrating lymphocytes to tumor in patients receiving adoptive immunotherapy: Augmentation with cyclophosphamide and correlation with response. Cancer 73:1731-1737, 1994.
38. Mukherji B, Arnbjarnarson O, Spitznable LA, Kalish RI, Hoffman J, Ergin MT, Spencer RP. Imaging pattern of previously in vitro sensitized and interleukin-2 expaneded autologous lymphocytes in human cancer. International Journal of Radiation Applications & Instrumentation - Part B, Nuclear Medicine & Biology 15 (4):419-27, 1988.
39. Swift RI, Danpure HJ, Osman S, Gaer J, Tsikos C, Peters AM, Lavender JP, Tebbut S, Habib NA, Wood CB. Imaging of metaqstatic colorectal cancer with tumour-activated killer lymphocytes. Lancet 337:1511-1512, 1991.
40. Aebersold P, Hyatt C, Johnson S, Hines K, Korcak L, Sanders M, Lotze MT, Topalian SL, Yang JC, Rosenberg SA (1991) Lysis of autologous melanoma cells by tumor infiltrating lymphocytes is associated with clinical response. Jour Natl Cancer Inst 83:932.
41. Barth RJ, Mule JJ, Spiess PJ, Rosenberg SA. Interferon g and tumor necrosis factor have a role in tumor regressions mediated by murine CD8^{+} tumor-infiltrating lymphocytes. J Exp Med 173:647-658, 1991.
42. Schwartzentruber DJ, Topalian SL, Mancini M, Rosenberg SA. Specific release of granulocyte-macrophage colony-stimulating factor, tumor necrosis factor-α and IFN-γ by human tumor-infiltrating lymphocytes after autologous tumor stimulation. Jour Immunol 146:3674-3681, 1991.
43. Rosenberg SA, Aebersold P, Cornetta K, Kasid A, Morgan RA, Moen R, Karson EM, Lotze MT, Yang JC, Topalian SL, Merino MJ, Culver K, Miller AD, Blaese RM, Anderson WF. Gene transfer into humans—Immunotherapy of patients with advanced melanoma, using tumor-infiltrating lymphocytes modified by retroviral gene transduction. New Eng Jour Med 323:570-578, 1990.
44. Fox BA, Spiess PJ, Kasid A, Puri RK, Mule JJ, Rosenberg SA. In vitro and in vivo antitumor properties of a T-cell clone generated from murine tumor infiltrating lymphocytes. J Biol Resp Mod 9(5):499-511, 1990.
45. Fox BA., Culver KW., Cornetta K, Morgan RA, Spiess PJ, Mule JJ., Kasid A, Blaese RM, Anderson WF, Rosenberg SA. Retroviral gene transduction of murine tumor infiltrating lymphocytes: A new approach to study trafficking in vivo. FASEB Journal 3:(3) 3496, 1989.
46. Fox BA, Culver KW, Cornetta K, Kasid A, Morgan RA, Mule JJ, Blaese RM, Anderson WF, Rosenberg SA. Biological and immunological properties of a murine tumor infiltrating lymphocyte clone transduced with human adenosine deaminase and neomycin resistance genes. (submitted for publication).
47. Sharrock CEM, Kaminski E and Man S. Limiting dilution analysis of human T cells: a useful clinical tool. Immunol Today 11:281-285, 1990.
48. Tzeng JJ, Barth RF, Orosz CG. Quantitation of glioma-rteactive cytolytic T lymphocyte precursors by means of limiting dilution analysis. Jour Immunol Meth 146:177-184, 1992.
49. Taswell C. Limiting dilution assays for the determination of immunocompetent cell requencies. J Immunol 126:1614-1619, 1981.
50. Quesenberry P, Cohen H, Levin J, Sullivan R, Bealmear P, Ryan M. Effects of bacterial infection and irradiation on serum colony-stimulating and colony-inhibitory factor levels in tolerant and non-tolerant CF1 mice. Blood 51:229-244, 1978.
51. Zidar BL, Shadduck RK. Serum colony-stimulating and colony-inhibitory activity in response to neutropenia. J Lab Clin Med 91:584-591, 1978.
52. Goto M, Mitsuoka A, Sugiyama M, Kitano M. Enhancement of delayed hypersensitivity reaction with varieties of anti-cancer drugs. A common biological phenomenon. J Exp Med 154:204-209, 1981.

CHAPTER 8

TUMOR-INDUCED SUPPRESSION OF T CELLS

Jon M. Hain, Vernon K. Sondak

INTRODUCTION

Neoplastic growth is a dynamic interaction between the growth characteristics of a cancer and the immunologic defenses of the host. Tumor-induced suppression (TIS) of the anti-tumor immune response shifts the equilibrium in favor of the neoplasm, allowing for the progressive growth of a tumor and the eventual death of the host, as well as limiting the usefulness of adoptive immunotherapy. The suppression of the immune response is a complex tumor-host interaction involving both cellular and soluble factors. Its enigmatic nature continues to elude a firm understanding; further exacerbating the difficulty in studying this phenomenon is our current dependence on animal tumor models rather than direct analysis of the human anti-tumor immune response.

The concept of tumor-induced suppression of the cellular immune response has long been hinted at in the immunology literature. A historical look at this concept seems appropriate as the notion of cellular dysfunction has strong roots in the efforts of early researchers. The depression of the immune system seen in end-stage malignancy sparked germinal studies into the field of tumor suppression. The experimentally observed phenomena of "sneaking through" and concomitant immunity added further credence to the idea of a cellular basis for tumor-induced suppression. Many investigations, including studies from our own laboratory, have produced results which document the presence of tumor-induced T cell dysfunction.

It has long been known that the presence of tumor induces a nonspecific suppression of the immune system. Eilber and Morton's pioneering study suggested a correlation between inoperability, early tumor recurrence, or metastasis and the inability to exhibit a delayed cutaneous hypersensitivity reaction to 2,4-dinitrochlorobenzene.[1] The development

Immunotherapy of Cancer with Sensitized T Lymphocytes, edited by Alfred E. Chang and Suyu Shu.

of anergy to common antigens was also noted to be associated with metastatic disease and a poor prognosis. The immune suppression demonstrated in the early human studies illustrates the degree to which a tumor may subvert the immune responses of the host to ensure its ability to proliferate.

HISTORICAL PERSPECTIVE

The ability of a tumor to "sneak through" the immune system and progressively grow is a remarkable phenomenon, which may have its roots in tumor-induced T cell suppression. "Sneaking through" can be defined as the ability of small tumor inocula to grow unimpeded, whereas larger doses are rejected by the host. Work by Gatenby and colleagues alluded to a preferential production of suppressor T cells (T_S) in small tumor inocula and the susceptibility of these cells to alkylating agents such as cyclophosphamide.[2] This was supported by the efforts of McBride and Howie using Meth-A tumor cells, who suggested that "low zone" tolerance was dependent on tumor-specific suppressor cells.[3] Haubeck and Kölsch demonstrated that ADJ-PC-5 plasmacytoma cells injected in low doses in syngeneic BALB/c mice induced T_S cells which were able to abrogate a cytotoxic T cell tumor response.[4,5] The "sneaking through" phenomenon illustrates the insidious and pervasive nature of tumor suppression; immunosuppression is not merely a consequence of end-stage disease with an overwhelming tumor burden.

The tumor and host form a unique compromise in the development of "concomitant immunity," defined as the ability of a tumor-bearing host to reject an homologous tumor graft. In 1906, Ehrlich described this phenomenon and hypothesized that "concomitant immunity" was mediated by the loss of essential nutrients.[6] Subsequent investigators studying this phenomenon have determined that concomitant immunity is tumor-specific, and is mediated at least in part through the generation of cytolytic T cells. The T cell basis for concomitant immunity is demonstrated by multiple in vitro and in vivo experiments in model systems where tumor-specific cytolytic T cells are capable of mediating tumor destruction.[7,8,9] The loss of these cells by radiation, thymectomy or anti-lymphocyte serum eliminates the beneficial effects of concomitant immunity, with a corresponding increase in metastatic disease and decrease in survival.[10,11]

As the initial tumor reaches a critical size, there is a rapid loss of the protective effect of concomitant immunity, manifest as unsuppressed tumor graft growth. This tumor-induced depression of concomitant immunity has been extensively studied by North and colleagues.[10] North hypothesized that progressive tumor growth induced the formation of suppressor T cells. Furthermore, he suspected these suppressor cells were responsible for another manifestation of immune suppression: the observed refractoriness of an immunogenic tumor to destruction by adoptively transferred tumor-sensitized effector T cells. These hypotheses were tested in a series of elegant experiments which demonstrated that otherwise immunocompetent tumor-bearing animals had a T cell dependent mechanism which interfered with the effectiveness of adoptive immunotherapy. Furthermore, this mechanism was abolished by rendering the animal T cell deficient. North pursued these results and discovered that suppression could be transferred to a previously immunocompetent host and that this suppression was mediated by $CD4^+$ T cells. Conversely, he established that $CD8^+$ T cells are responsible for the tumoricidal effects of concomitant immunity and that these cells could be used to successfully treat a suppressed animal after pretreatment with sublethal gamma radiation to break the suppression.[10,11]

TUMOR-INDUCED SUPPRESSION IN ADOPTIVE IMMUNOTHERAPY

Although the clinical use of adoptive immunotherapy has been a subject of great interest, the inherent problems tumor-induced suppression poses to this approach have been relatively ignored. In an effort to model tumor-induced suppression in the setting of adoptive immunotherapy, Sondak and coworkers investigated the effects of visceral tumor on the generation of effector cells using various techniques of in vitro lymphocyte activation and expansion.[12] In murine model systems, the progressive growth of subcutaneous weakly- or non-immunogenic methylcholanthrene-induced (MCA) sarcomas leads to the development of sensitized T lymphocytes within the tumor-draining lymph node (TDLN). These tumor-sensitized but not fully functional lymphocytes required in vitro activation to develop into specific anti-tumor effectors, and hence have been termed "pre-effector cells". Several different techniques for activating pre-effector cells within the TDLN have been employed, including co-incubation of TDLN cells with irradiated tumor cells and interleukin 2 (termed "in vitro sensitization" or IVS),[13] as well as sequential activation with a monoclonal antibody (mAb) to the CD3 molecule followed by expansion with IL-2.[14]

The generation of pre-effectors from tumor-draining lymph nodes (TDLN) is time-dependent; anti-tumor reactivity can be generated from TDLN after as little as four days of subcutaneous (sc) tumor growth, and is largely or completely lost by twenty-one days. Table 8.1 demonstrates the kinetics of the pre-effector cells in terms of their efficacy in adoptive immunotherapy experiments. The observed failure to generate therapeutically efficacious cells after three weeks of progressive tumor growth could be attributable either to the development of tumor-induced suppression or to the loss of pre-effector cells by migration out of the lymph node or cell death. To characterize the nature of tumor-induced immune suppression, the presence of pulmonary or visceral tumor was examined to determine its effect on the generation of pre-effector cells within lymph nodes draining sc tumor deposits. Multiple lung tumors induced by intravenous (iv) injection of tumor cell suspensions were used as the model for visceral tumor and were initiated simultaneously with the sc

Table 8.1. Kinetics of pre-effector cell development within lymph nodes draining a subcutaneous tumor deposit

Day of node harvest[a]	Tumor size	Mean no. of lung metastases ± SE[b]
--- (IL-2 only)	---	≥ 250
Day 0	2 mm	≥ 250
Day 4	4 mm	≥ 250
Day 6	5 mm	0[c]
Day 10	5.5 mm	0[c]
Day 13	6.5 mm	31 ± 12[d]
Day 17	8.5 mm	71 ± 36[d]
Day 22	12 mm	≥ 250

[a] Lymph node lymphocytes draining a sc deposit of MCA 106 were harvested at various times and sequentially activated in vitro with anti-CD3 monoclonal antibody and IL-2. The resultant cells were transferred (2×10^7 cells/mouse) to mice bearing 3-day established MCA 106 lung metastases. Days shown are duration of tumor growth at which lymph nodes were harvested. Mesenteric nodes from normal mice were used as day 0 lymph node controls. All mice received IL-2 (15,000 U ip bid for 4 days) commencing the day of adoptive transfer.

[b] Approximately three weeks after adoptive transfer of activated cells, all mice were sacrificed and the number of pulmonary metastases determined in a manner blinded as to the treatment received. Lungs with tumors too numerous to count were assigned an arbitrary value of 250, as this is the largest number that can be reliably enumerated. Groups in which all lungs contained tumors too numerous to count are represented as "≥ 250."

[c] $P \leq 0.05$ compared to the group that received IL-2 alone (two-sided Wilcoxon rank sum test).

[d] $P \leq 0.05$ compared to the Day 6 or 10 groups or the group that received IL-2 alone.

tumor injection. The concomitant presence of lung tumors markedly suppressed the activity of IVS cells generated from the TDLN in response to sc tumor (see Table 8.2).

The added tumor burden of the pulmonary tumor was not the critical factor in the observed suppression, as animals with equal tumor burdens restricted entirely to subcutaneous locations did not manifest any suppression. Additional experiments revealed that comparable suppression was induced by the presence of a solitary liver metastasis created at laparotomy by subcapsular injection of tumor cells. The same suppressive effect of visceral tumor on pre-effector cell development was manifest when the anti-CD3/IL-2 activation method (as described in chapter 1) was used (Table 8.2).[12]

In order to determine the kinetics of pre-effector cell suppression induced by visceral tumor, MCA 205 lung tumors were initiated at different time points in relationship to the establishment of MCA 205 sc tumors. Pre-effector cell activity was assessed after sequential activation and expansion of tumor-draining lymph nodes (TDLN) cells with anti-CD3 mAb and IL-2; the resultant cells were used in adoptive immunotherapy experiments against 3-day established pulmonary metastases. As shown in Table 8.3, when the lung tumors were initiated at the same time as the sc tumor (day 0), the anti-tumor efficacy of activated TDLN was suppressed compared to those from mice bearing only sc tumor. Lung tumors established 3 to 7 days *after* the sc tumor; however, had no suppressive effect on the activated TDLN cells. As pre-effector cells have been shown to develop within 3 to 4 days after sc tumor inoculation, the kinetic data suggest that the presence of visceral tumor has a systemic suppressive effect on the development of pre-effector cells, rather than inhibiting the function of such cells after their generation.[12]

To ascertain if the suppressive effect of visceral tumor was immunologically specific, a series of experiments were undertaken where mice bearing an MCA 205 sc tumor were given concomitant lung tumors of MCA 205, MCA 106 or MCA 203. As depicted in Table 8.4, the presence of autologous lung tumors led to suppression of the ability to generate pre-effector cells, but the presence of immunologically distinct lung tumors had no such effect. Iden-

Table 8.2. Suppressive effect of the presence of visceral tumor on anti-tumor efficacy of activated tumor-draining lymph nodes

	Mean no. of lung metastases ± SE	
Tumor site[a]	**IVS**	**Anti-CD3/IL-2**
--- (IL-2 only)	132 ± 41	≥ 250
SC only	3 ± 3[b]	4 ± 1[b]
SC and lung	157 ± 22[c]	≥ 250[c]
2 SC (footpad + flank)	2 ± 1[b]	---

[a] Subcutaneous tumor deposits of MCA 106 were established, and some mice also received concomitant iv injections to establish multiple lung tumors or a second sc tumor at a remote site. Ten days later, the lymph node draining the subcutaneous tumor deposit was harvested and the cells activated by one of two methods. In the IVS method, TDLN cells were incubated for 8 days along with irradiated autologous tumor cells in the presence of IL-2. In the anti-CD3/IL-2 method, TDLN cells were sequentially activated with anti- CD3 monoclonal antibody for 3 days followed by IL-2 for 2 days. In both experiments, the resultant cells were transferred to mice bearing 3-day established MCA 106 lung metastases. All mice received IL-2 (7500 U ip bid for 3 days for IVS experiment, 15,000 U ip bid for 4 days in anti-CD3/IL-2 experiment) commencing the day of adoptive transfer. Three weeks later, lung metastases were counted as described previously.

[b] $P \leq 0.05$ compared to the group that received IL-2 alone.

[c] $P \leq 0.05$ compared to the group that received sc only (or footpad plus flank) cells.

tical experiments using different strains of sc tumor yielded similar results: the suppression induced by visceral tumor was always immunologically specific.

To explore the effect of visceral tumor on established pre-effector cells, TDLN from control mice were incubated with an equal portion of TDLN from an animal bearing visceral tumor, and the mixture was activated using the anti-CD3/IL-2 method. The data presented in Table 8.5 suggest that TDLN from mice bearing both sc and lung tumors did not suppress already established pre-effector cells from differentiating into fully functional effector cells during in vitro activation. This result suggests that TIS affects the induction of pre-effector cells, but once formed, pre-effector cells are not subject to suppression.

Critical to an understanding of TIS is the development of techniques to transfer the suppression in vivo to naive mice. In a series of experiments, Sondak et al transferred splenocytes from mice bearing visceral tumor to naive animals at the time of sc tumor inoculation.[15] Activated TDLN of mice which received splenocytes from liver or lung tumor-bearers were ineffective, while similarly activated TDLN from

Table 8.3. Kinetics of the suppressive effect of visceral tumor on anti-tumor efficacy of activated tumor-draining lymph nodes

Tumor site[a]	Day of lung tumor inoculation	Mean no. of lung metastases ± SE IVS	Anti-CD3/IL-2
---	--- (IL-2 only)	180 ± 21	221 ± 16
SC only	---	45 ± 22[b]	92 ± 28[b]
SC and lung	Day 0	99 ± 20	191 ± 33[c]
SC and lung	Day +3	8 ± 3[b]	118 ± 33
SC and lung	Day +7	41 ± 22[b]	---

[a] Subcutaneous tumor deposits of MCA 106 were established, and some mice also received iv injections to establish multiple lung tumors at the same time or several days later. Fourteen days after the sc tumor inoculation, the lymph node draining the subcutaneous tumor deposit was harvested and the cells activated by one of two methods as previously described. In both experiments, the resultant cells were transferred to mice bearing 3-day established MCA 106 lung metastases. All mice received IL-2 (7500 U ip bid for 3 days for IVS experiment, 15,000 U ip bid for 4 days in anti-CD3/IL-2 experiment) commencing the day of adoptive transfer. Three weeks later, lung metastases were counted as described previously.

[b] $P \leq 0.05$ compared to the group that received IL-2 alone.

[c] $P \leq 0.05$ compared to the group that received SC only cells.

Table 8.4. Specificity of the suppressive effect of visceral tumor on anti-tumor efficacy of anti- CD3/IL-2 activated tumor-draining lymph nodes

SC Tumor	IV Tumor[a]	Mean no. of lung metastases ± SE
---	--- (IL-2 only)	≥ 250
MCA 205	---	20 ± 15[b]
MCA 205	MCA 205	≥ 250
MCA 205	MCA 106	21 ± 5[b]
MCA 205	MCA 203	3 ± 2[b]

[a] Lymph node lymphocytes draining a sc deposit of MCA 205, in the presence of concomitant lung tumors of various types, were harvested and activated with anti- CD3/IL-2. Control mice received no iv tumor at the time of sc tumor inoculation. The resultant cells were transferred (2×10^7 cells/mouse) to mice bearing 4-day established lung metastases from MCA 205. All mice received IL-2 (15,000 U ip bid for 4 days) commencing the day of adoptive transfer.

[b] $P \leq 0.05$ compared to the group that received IL-2 alone.

control animals displayed potent anti-tumor activity. To determine if this effect was mediated by T cells, splenocytes taken from visceral tumor-bearing animals were irradiated prior to transfer. As shown in Table 8.6, activated TDLN from mice which received no splenocytes or irradiated splenocytes were highly active, while activated TDLN from mice which received tumor-bearing splenocytes were relatively ineffective. Depletion of non-T cell elements from the tumor-bearer spleens by passage across nylon wool columns did not abrogate the ability to transfer suppression, further supporting the T cell-mediated nature of this phenomenon (unpublished data).

TIS is a reproducible phenomenon affecting the development of effector cells for adoptive immunotherapy. Studies in our laboratory have examined the ability of a variety of agents to overcome tumor-induced suppression and allow generation of highly active effector cells from "suppressed" hosts. From a variety of cytokines tested, Hammel et al found that the addition of IL-1α during the in vitro activation process with anti-CD3 mAb abrogated the

Table 8.5. Tumor-draining lymph nodes cells from mice bearing sc and lung tumors do not suppress established pre-effector cells

SC TDLN[a]	SC + Lung TDLN	Mean no. of lung metas-tases ± SE
--- (IL-2 only)	---	≥ 250
100%	---	47 ± 24[b]
---	100%	133 ± 39
50%	50%	11 ± 5[b]

[a] TDLN draining a subcutaneous deposit of MCA 205, from mice without or with concomitant MCA 205 lung tumors, were harvested on day 9. The TDLN cells were activated in anti-CD3/IL-2; in one case after mixing the two populations of cells in a 50:50 ratio. Equal numbers of lymphocytes were placed into anti-CD3/IL-2 activation in each group, hence the 50:50 mixture contained half the number of lymphocytes of each type as the corresponding pure groups. After activation, the resultant cells were transferred (2 x 10^7 cells/mouse) to mice bearing 4-day established lung metastases from MCA 205. Mice in group A received no cellular therapy and served as controls. All mice received IL-2 (15,000 U ip twice daily for 4 days) commencing the day of adoptive transfer.
[b] $P < 0.05$ compared to groups receiving IL-2 only or 100% SC+lung activated TDLN.

Table 8.6. Transfer of splenocytes from visceral tumor-bearers to naive mice abrogates the generation of pre-effector cells in the tumor-draining lymph nodes

Tumor site	In vivo treatment attime of sc tumor inoculation[a]	Mean no. of lung metastases ± SE 6 x 10^6 cells transferred	2 x 10^6 cells transferred
---	--- (IL-2 only)	≥ 250	
SC	HBSS	13 ± 7[b]	41 ± 15[b]
SC	Normal splenocytes	45 ± 16[b]	---
SC	Liver tumor-bearer splenocytes	122 ± 43[c]	250[c]
SC	Lung tumor-bearer splenocytes	166 ± 27[c]	---

[a] At time of sc tumor inoculation with MCA 106, mice received iv injections of: 2 x 10^8 splenocytes (2 organ equivalents) from normal mice 2 weeks after sham laparotomy; 2 x 10^8 splenocytes from mice bearing 2 week old solitary liver tumors; 2 x 10^8 splenocytes from mice bearing 2 week old multiple lung tumors; or HBSS. TDLN were harvested 2 weeks later and placed in IVS culture. After IVS culture, 6 x 10^6 or 2 x 10^6 cells were transferred to mice bearing 3-day established MCA 106 lung metastases. All mice received IL-2 (7500 U ip bid for 3 days) commencing the day of adoptive transfer.
[b] $P < 0.05$ compared to the group that received IL-2 alone.
[c] $P < 0.05$ compared to the group that received same dose of sc only IVS cells.

suppressive effects of concurrent visceral tumor on pre-effector cell development (see Table 8.7).[16] IL-1α appeared to upregulate the in vitro activation of tumor reactive lymphocytes derived from TDLN, both in the presence and absence of visceral metastases.

FUNCTIONAL AND PHENOTYPIC MARKERS OF SUPPRESSOR T CELLS

Despite the many studies of TIS, the very existence of a true suppressor T cell population remains controversial, and phenotypic markers of "suppressor" or "suppressed" T cells have been elusive. The CD4/CD8 phenotypical distinction alone does not help to distinguish suppressor T cell populations, as both phenotypes have been shown to participate in suppressive phenomena. Bloom and coworkers have attempted to address this thorny problem by classifying T cell populations based not only on CD4 and CD8 expression, but also on differing patterns of lymphokine production.[17] Type 1 cells are lymphocytes that produce predominantly interferon-γ, while type 2 cells produce IL-4 and IL-5 with little or no interferon-γ. These authors note that the different functional subsets of T cells appear to respond to antigen presented by different types of antigen presenting cells (APCs). Since IL-4 production in particular may lead to suppression of function of type 1 $CD4^+$ lymphocytes, they postulate that certain antigens—presented by appropriate APCs—may be more likely to result in "tolerance" or a suppressed T cell response.[17] It is easy to see how such a strategy of regulating the immune response based on the type of APC could have important implications in the prevention of autoimmunity. It remains unclear, however, whether T cells are committed to one type of lymphokine expression or are able to alter their lymphokine expression to suit the nature of the antigen and APC.

In addition to the production of suppressive lymphokines, there are at least two other documented methods by which T cells may suppress an immune response. The first method is by antigen-induced shedding of T cell receptor, in a fashion analogous to a B cell secreting antibody. The shed T cell receptor could act to block immune recognition either by binding antigen in a non-functional state, or by binding to activated T cells and inducing an anti-idiotypic response.[18,19,20] A second method involves anti-idiotypic T cells which may directly suppress or even destroy type 1 helper or cytolytic T cells required for an

Table 8.7. Addition of IL-1 during in vitro activation with anti–CD3 abrogates the suppression induced by visceral tumor

Tumor site[a]	IL-1 during activation	Mean no. of lung metastases ± SE Experiment 1	Experiment 2
– (IL-2 only)	---	247 ± 3	≥ 250
SC only	0	32 ± 10[b]	14 ± 7[b]
SC + lung	0	168 ± 38[c]	75 ± 36[b,c]
SC only	10,000 U/ml	21 ± 7[b]	8 ± 8[b]
SC + lung	10,000 U/ml	12 ± 3[b]	19 ± 10[b]

[a] TDLN were harvested from mice ten days after establishment of a subcutaneous deposit of MCA 205, without or with concomitant MCA 205 lung metastases induced by iv tumor injection at the time of sc inoculation. The TDLN cells were activated in vitro with anti–CD3 monoclonal antibody for 3 days followed by IL-2 for 2 days. Some groups also were exposed to IL-1α, 10,000 U/ml, during the 3 days of in vitro activation with anti–CD3 antibody. The resultant activated cells were transferred to mice bearing 3-day established lung metastases from MCA 205. All mice received IL-2 (15,000 U ip bid for 4 days) commencing the day of adoptive transfer.
[b] $P < 0.05$ compared to group receiving IL-2 only.
[c] $P < 0.05$ compared to groups receiving sc only cells or sc + lung cells treated with IL-1.

effective immune response to antigen.[17] Again, both these mechanisms may be of critical importance in preventing autoimmune responses. Precisely how they might be involved in tumor-induced immunosuppression remains to be elucidated.

SUPPRESSION OF T CELLS MAY BE MEDIATED VIA THE TCR/CD3 COMPLEX

While our ability to identify suppressor T cells, either through functional or phenotypic studies, is limited, almost nothing is known about what changes actually occur within the "suppressed" T cell. Recently, Mizoguchi and colleagues analyzed the structure of the T cell receptor/CD3 complex and the expression of CD3 complex-associated tyrosine kinases in T cells from normal and tumor-bearing mice.[21] The tumor-bearing mice had advanced (21-day) deposits of the MC38 or Renca adenocarcinomas, and were known from functional studies to be immunosuppressed. Using two-dimensional protein electrophoresis, they discovered that the CD3 complex of T lymphocytes from tumor-bearing mice contained low levels of CD3γ and completely lacked CD3ζ, which was replaced by the Fcεγ-chain. Furthermore, they noted reductions in expression of two protein tyrosine kinases, $p56^{lck}$ and $p59^{fyn}$, closely associated with the CD3 complex in tumor-bearers.[21] Protein tyrosine phosphorylation marks the germinal event in T cell receptor-mediated signaling; hence these observations strongly suggest that T cells from tumor-suppressed mice are deficient in their ability to respond to antigen binding. Still unclear is whether the observed changes are reversible, and what tumor-induced signals trigger the structural alterations.

Several groups have attempted to establish T cell lines as well as T cell hybridomas from tumor-induced suppressor cells in order to have a large supply of reagents to isolate and characterize. Koyama and workers generated an IL-2-dependent suppressor T cell line from the spleen of a mouse bearing an MCA fibrosarcoma.[22] These cells were able to inhibit the effect of tumor-induced cytolytic cells in an in vitro assay. Haubeck and Kölsch corroborated these findings by establishing a suppressor T cell clone, which bore $CD2^+$, $CD8^+$ phenotypes capable of blocking the in vitro primary cytotoxic response to the tumor.[23] It is hoped that further progress in the establishment and analysis of suppressor clones will allow significant expansion of our knowledge regarding the characteristics and mechanisms of action of these elusive cells.

CLINICAL OBSERVATIONS ON TUMOR-INDUCED SUPPRESSION

Virtually all of the above-mentioned data comes from animal models bearing experimental tumor inocula. What, if any, of this knowledge can be translated to the cancer patient in the clinical setting? To date, the mechanisms and cellular agents implicated in mediating human tumor-induced suppression are quite heterologous and appear to vary among individuals with the same malignancy. In an effort to provide a general representation of the cytotoxic and suppressor phenotypes for tumor-induced suppression, several investigators have attempted to characterize the T cell populations in patients with a variety of solid tumors. Previous reports have described decreased PHA-induced mitogenic responses in monocytes from cancer patients as compared to normal individuals.[24] In an attempt to demonstrate a phenotypical difference corresponding to this functional difference, Kaszubowski and colleagues analyzed T cells from cancer patients and found a higher level of T cells bearing receptors for the Fc of IgG (so-called Tγ cells) and a lower level of T cells bearing receptors for the Fc of IgM (Tμ) in cancer patients as compared to normal individuals.[25] In a similar report, the same findings were seen regarding patients with active non-Hodgkin's lymphoma and Hodgkin's lymphoma compared to patients in remission after radiation therapy.[26] Since in some experimental model systems Tγ cells represent a suppressor cell population, this may constitute evidence of increased T_S in human cancer patients. More recently, Dillman and associates demonstrated lower CD4:CD8 ratios in cancer patients.[27] Mizoguchi and coworkers noted that 7 of 12 patients with advanced cancers had a loss of CD3ζ and $p59^{fyn}$ proteins in T lymphocytes.[21] This finding mirrors their murine data and provides evidence that tumor-induced T cell suppression seen in animal models can be documented in humans.

While the experimental evidence for T cell-mediated TIS is clear, there is also a large body of evidence to support the existence of tumor-derived soluble factors which may directly mediate suppression. For example, Klajman and colleagues showed that supernatants from B-cell lymphoma cultures inhibited in vitro mitogenic stimulation, allogeneic immunization, and IL-2 induction in spleen cells. Characterization of the active factor(s) suggested a ganglioside or sialyated glycoprotein.[28] Floutis and coworkers studied gangliosides from human neuroblastoma and discovered that the gangliosides were highly inhibitory for in vitro human lymphoproliferative responses. Furthermore, gangliosides from clinically aggressive tumors were more immunosuppressive than those from slower-growing tumors.[29]

Tumor-derived soluble factors may also indirectly mediate suppression by interference with the host's ability to produce interleukins and other immunologically important cytokines. A recent report demonstrated a gradual increase in the amount of transforming growth factor-β (TGF-β) produced during progressive tumor growth of a CSA1M fibrosarcoma.[30] The addition of TGF-β to splenic cell cultures markedly decreased the ability of the splenocytes to produce IL-2 and other cytokines. Similarly, during tumor growth, the ability of $CD4^+$ T cells to produce IL-2 decreased. Li and colleagues observed that the $CD4^+$ cells in their model were normal in the early stages of tumor growth and that the observed dysfunction appeared to correlate with increasing levels of TGF-β.[30]

CONCLUDING REMARKS

The complex immunologic milieu of antagonistic and synergistic cytokines and lymphokines, antigens, and APCs collectively appear to determine which of the different functional T cell subsets responds to a given antigen stimulus, thereby influencing the final outcome—rejection/destruction or tolerance/suppression. The existence of tumor-induced T cell suppression cannot be questioned, yet the mechanisms remain an obscure part of the complex drama of the immune system. Clearly, given the immunologic imperative to prevent autoreactivity to self antigens, suppression of an immune response to certain antigens must be as fundamental to life as propagation of a response to other antigens. Could tumor cells merely be fooling the immune system into considering them as "self" and hence protected? As our understanding of the checks and balances of the immune system improves, we will be closer to unraveling one of the major mysteries of cancer: its subversive effect on the host's ability to defend itself immunologically.

ACKNOWLEDGMENTS

This work was supported in part by grant no. CA55299 from the National Institutes of Health, United States Public Health Service, Department of Health and Human Services, as well as a grant from the Boston Foundation, Boston, MA. Dr. Sondak is the recipient of a Career Development Award from the American Cancer Society. We wish to thank Melissa K. Tuck and Jeff Rado for expert assistance in performing many of the experiments described herein.

REFERENCES

1. Eilber FR, Morton DL. Impaired immunologic reactivity and recurrence following cancer surgery. Cancer 25:362-367, 1970.
2. Gatenby PA, Basten A, Creswick P. "Sneaking through": a T-cell-dependent phenomenon. Br J Cancer 44:753-756, 1981.
3. McBride WH, Howie SE. Induction of tolerance to a murine fibrosarcoma in two zones of dosage—the involvement of suppressor

cells. Br J Cancer 53:707-711, 1986.

4. Haubeck H-D, Kölsch E. Regulation of immune responses against the syngeneic ADJ-PC5 plasmacytoma in BALB/c mice. IV. Tumor-specific T suppressor cells, induced at early stages of tumorigenesis, act on the induction phase of the tumor-specific cytotoxic T cell response. Immunobiology 171:357-365, 1986.
5. Haubeck H-D, Kloke O, Kölsch E. Analysis of T suppressor cell-mediated tumor escape mechanisms. Curr Top Microbiol Immunol 126:225-230, 1986.
6. Ehrlich P. Experimentelle Karzinomstudien an Mäusen. Arb Inst Exp Ther Frankfurt/ Main 1:65-80, 1906.
7. Kearney R, Nelson DS. Concomitant immunity to syngeneic methylcholanthrene-induced tumours in mice. Occurrence and specificity of concomitant immunity. Aust J Exp Biol Med Sci 51:723-735, 1973.
8. North RJ, Kirstein DP. Activated macrophages as the expressors of nonspecific immunity to unrelated tumors and bacterial parasites. J Exp Med 145:275-292, 1977.
9. Tuttle RL, Knick VC, Stopford CR et al. In vivo and in vitro activity expressed by cells of concomitantly immune mice. Cancer Res 43:2600-2605, 1983.
10. North RJ. Down-regulation of the anti-tumor immune response. Adv Cancer Res 45:1-43, 1985.
11. Naor D. Suppressor cells: Permitters and promoters of malignancy? Adv Cancer Res 29:45-119, 1979.
12. Sondak VK, Wagner PD, Shu S et al. Suppressive effects of visceral tumor on the generation of anti-tumor T cells for adoptive immunotherapy. Arch Surg 126:442-446, 1991.
13. Shu S, Chou T, Rosenberg SA. In vitro sensitization and expansion with viable tumor cells and interleukin 2 in the generation of specific therapeutic effector cells. J Immunol 136:3891-3898, 1986.
14. Yoshizawa H, Chang AE, Shu S. Specific adoptive immunotherapy mediated by tumor-draining lymph nodes cells sequentially activated with anti-CD3 and IL-2. J Immunol 147:729-737, 1991.
15. Sondak VK, Tuck MK, Shu S et al. Transfer of specific tumor-induced immunosuppression by splenocytes from visceral tumor-bearing mice. Proc Am Assoc Cancer Res 33:323, 1992.
16. Hammel JM, Tuck MK, Chang AE et al. Effect of interleukin 1α on the in vitro activation tumor-draining lymph node cells for adoptive immunotherapy. J Immunother 16: 1-12, 1994.
17. Bloom RB, Padmini S, and Diamond B. Revisiting and revising suppressor T cells. Immunol Today 13:131-136, 1992.
18. Zheng H, Sahai BM, Kilgannon P et al. Specific inhibition of cell-surface T-cell receptor expression by antisense oligodeoxynucleotides and its effect on the production of an antigen-specific regulatory T-cell factor. Proc Natl Acad Sci USA 86:3758-3762, 1989.
19. Guy R, Ullrich SJ, Foo-Philips M et al. Antigen-specific helper function of cell-free T cell products bearing TCR V beta 8 determinants. Science 244:1477-1480, 1989.
20. Kuchroo VK, Byrne MC, Atsumi Y et al. T-cell receptor alpha chain plays a critical role in antigen-specific suppressor cell function. Proc Natl Acad Sci USA, 88:8700-8704, 1991.
21. Mizoguchi H, O'Shea JJ, Longo DL et al. Alterations in signal transduction molecules in T lymphocytes from tumor-bearing mice. Science 258:1795-1798, 1992.
22. Koyama S, Yoshioka T, Sakita T et al. Generation of T cell growth factor (TCGF)-dependent splenic lymphoid cell line with cell-mediated immunosuppressive reactivity against syngeneic murine tumor. Eur J Cancer Clin. Oncol 21:257-261, 1985.
23. Haubeck H-D, Kölsch E. Isolation and characterization of in vitro and in vivo functions of a tumor-specific T suppressor cell clone from a BALB/c mouse bearing the syngeneic ADJ-PC-5 plasmacytoma. J Immunol 135:4297-4302, 1985.
24. Wood GW, Neff JE, Stephens R. Relationship between monocytosis and T-lymphocyte function in human cancer. J Natl Cancer Inst 63:587-592, 1979.
25. Kaszubowski PA, Husby G, Tung KS et al. T-lymphocyte subpopulations in peripheral blood and tissues of cancer patients. Cancer

Res 40:4648-4657, 1980.

26. Romagnani S, Maggi E, Del Prete G et al. Short- and long-term effects of radiation on T-cell subsets in peripheral blood of patients with Hodgkin's disease. Cancer 46:2590-2595, 1980.
27. Dilman RO, Koziol JA, Zavanelli MI et al. Immunoincompetence in cancer patients. Assessment by in vitro stimulation tests and quantification of lymphocyte subpopulations. Cancer 53:1484-1491, 1984.
28. Klajman A, Drucker I, Zan-Bar I et al. Immunosuppression in vitro and in vivo by supernatants from murine lymphoma cell lines. Anticancer Res 12:741-748, 1992.
29. Floutsis G, Ulsh L, Ladisch S. Immunosuppressive activity of human neuroblastoma tumor gangliosides. Int J Cancer 43:6-9, 1989.
30. Li X-F, Takiuchi H, Zou JP et al. Transforming growth factor-β (TGF-β)-mediated immunosuppression in the tumor-bearing state: enhanced production of TGF-β and a progressive increase in TGF-β susceptibility of anti-tumor CD4+ T cell function. Jpn J Cancer Res 84:315-325, 1993.

CHAPTER 9

Adoptive Immunotherapy Utilizing IL-2 and IL-4 for Expansion of Tumor-Infiltrating Lymphocytes in Renal Cell Carcinoma

Patricia Rayman, James H. Finke, Thomas Olencki, Vicki Lorenzi, Laurie Tuason, Eric Klein, Raymond R. Tubbs, Denise McLain, Ronald M. Bukowski

INTRODUCTION

The host immune response to human tumors is currently being studied and the effector populations are being characterized. T-lymphocytes in the tumor bed (TIL) have been studied because they contain effector cells that are reactive to the autologous tumor.[1-10] Studies in different murine tumor models have documented that TILs have significant anti-tumor activity.[9-10] Additional animal studies suggested that TIL were more effective than lymphokine activated killer (LAKs) cells in producing a response to tumor.[9-10] Because of their anti-tumor activity, adoptive immunotherapy trials were performed in cancer patients using both lymphokine activated killers (LAKs) from peripheral blood and tumor-infiltrating lymphocytes (TILs).[9-14] Responses have been noted in patients with melanoma and renal cell carcinoma.[11-13] In a phase I study performed at the Cleveland Clinic, where TILs were grown in vitro with 1000 U/ml IL-2, there was no objective tumor regression in the RCC patients treated.[14] Phenotype analysis of the cultured TIL showed a very heterogeneous population with many of the cultures having a significant number of $CD56^+$ cells.[14] In addition, the cytolytic activity of the cultured

Immunotherapy of Cancer with Sensitized T Lymphocytes, edited by Alfred E. Chang and Suyu Shu.

TILs was MHC unrestricted and mediated by $CD3^-CD56^+$ NK cells. Here we report on a second trial that was conducted with the TILs cultured in both IL-2 and IL-4. IL-4 was combined with IL-2 in an attempt to potentiate T cell responses to RCC. IL-4 is known to enhance a specific T cell response including those derived from the tumor bed.[15-17] In the second trial, the majority of the TILs were $CD3^+$ with a very small percentage of $CD56^+$ cells. Of the 16 patients treated with TIL, four had a partial response, and one a minor response. From the cells cultured for this trial, studies were undertaken to find RCC specific T cells. To aid in the search, TIL were separated into $CD4^+$ and $CD8^+$ subsets with biomagnetic beads for positive selection. These cells were then tested for autologous tumor reactivity by measuring cytotoxicity, IFNγ production and proliferation. We were able to identify 5 RCC specific TIL lines from the patients' cell cultures and from one additional patient not on the trial.[18]

MATERIALS AND METHODS

Patient Population

Patients ≥ 18 years with objectively measurable metastatic renal cell carcinoma, which was surgically incurable and histologically confirmed, and who had tumor tissue (primary tumor or metastatic lesion) accessible for surgical removal, were eligible. A performance status of 0-1 (Eastern Cooperative Oncology Group), expected survival of ≥ three months and full recovery from surgery (≥ 14 days) was required. Patients had to have minimum tumor burden as defined by being post nephrectomy, ≤ 30% involvement of the liver, normal calcium levels if osseous metastases present, and no central nervous system involvement. No prior chemotherapy nor immunotherapy using IL-2 or IL-4 was allowed. Radiotherapy for control of pain from skeletal lesions must have been completed greater than 28 days prior to the start of therapy. Adequate organ function as defined by hematologic, biochemical, pulmonary and cardiac parameters previously described[14] was required. Institutional and National Cancer Institute guidelines were followed in obtaining informed consent.

Tumor tissue obtained from patients who met all eligibility criteria, was digested as described below and plated for TIL and tumor growth. TIL were cultured until ≥ 5 x 10^9 mononuclear cells were produced (28-42 days), and then therapy was initiated. Before therapy started, biochemical and hematologic baseline studies were repeated and the status of measurable disease determined.

Treatment and Study Design

rIL-2 was administered as an IV continuous infusion at a dose of 4.5 x 10^6 U/m^2 (Hoffmann La Roche units) on days 1-4, 8-11, and 15-18. TIL were given at doses ≥ 5x10^9 on days 1, 2, 3 and 4. The rIL-2 utilized was produced by Hoffmann La Roche, supplied by the NCI, and had specific activity between 5 and 15 x 10^6 U/mg protein. After reconstitution with sterile water, it was administered as a constant infusion via the CADD I ambulatory infusion pump in 100 ml of a 5% dextrose solution. The TILs were administered without a filter via a central intravenous catheter. Laboratory evaluations for hematologic and biochemical studies were performed throughout the course of therapy.

RCC TIL Isolation and Expansion In Vitro

Tissue obtained from nephrectomies and metastatic sites was digested as previously described.[18] Briefly, tissue was weighed, minced and treated with the following enzymes for 2 hours at 37°C on an orbital shaker; 20 ml of Collagenase Type III (1 mg/ml, Worthington Biochemical Freehold, NJ) and 1 ml of DNase type IV solution (2 mg/ml Sigma Chemical Co., St. Louis, MO) for every 10 g of tissue. The cell suspension was then washed twice and counted.

TILs were expanded by culturing cells (5x10^5/ml) in Aim V medium (Gibco, Gaithersburg, MD) supplemented with

1000 U/ml of IL-2 (Hoffmann La Roche, Nutley, NJ) and 1000 U/ml of IL-4 (patients 1-19 Sterling Drug, Malvern, PA; patients 20-21 Schering, Bloomfield, NJ). Cultures were incubated at 37°C in 5% CO_2 and 95% humidity in gas permeable bags (Terumo Medical Corp., Elkton, MD). The cell cultures were supplemented on day 10 and thereafter as needed with Aim V, IL-2 (1000 U/ml) and IL-4 (1000 U/ml) to maintain the cell concentration. The cell cultures were fed and harvested using the Stericell System (Terumo Medical Corp., Elkton, MD). The TILs were put through a 170 micron filter (Fenwal Blood Component Recipient Set, Deerfield, IL) before being placed in a 600 ml Fenwal transfer pack.

For research purposes, separate cultures were maintained in Aim V medium supplemented with 1000 U/ml IL-2 or 1000 U/ml IL-2 plus 1000 U/ml IL-4. These cultures were used to separate the cells into $CD4^+$ and $CD8^+$ subsets using antibody coated magnetic beads (AMAC, Westbrook, Maine). Briefly, the TIL were incubated with IOT8-coated and IOT4-coated beads and layered over Ficoll-Hypaque to enrich for $CD4^+$ and $CD8^+$ subsets respectively. The negatively selected cells were cultured overnight in Aim V with the appropriate cytokines. The cells were then positively selected using the IOT4-coated beads for $CD4^+$ subsets and IOT8-coated beads for $CD8^+$ subsets. The cells would grow off the beads within 24-48 hrs. After two days of culture, the subsets were tested by flow cytometry for purity. Subsets >90% pure were aliquoted and frozen for use in proliferation, cytotoxity, and cytokine assays.

Isolation of Tumor Targets

The cells isolated in the enzyme digest were plated on Primaria flasks (Falcon, Cockeyville, MD) in RPMI (complete) supplemented with 10% FCS, 200 mM L-glutamine, 25 mM Hepes, 100 mM sodium pyruvate and 10mM nonessential amino acids. After 24 hours, the medium containing all unattached cells was replaced with fresh complete RPMI. The cells cultured for two weeks were removed from the flasks using trypsin (Worthington Biochemical, Friehold, NJ) and replated. Immunohistology staining of cells with antibodies to RCC (Monosan, Inc., San Francisco, CA), Uro 2 (Signet, Dedham, MA) and AE1/3 (Boehringer Mannheim, Germany) demonstrated that they were epithelial cells of renal origin with the same phenotype as the fresh tumor. If the cultures grew to sufficient numbers, the TIL cultures were restimulated with these short term cultured tumor cells twice between day 17 and day 28 at TIL to tumor ratios between 20:1 and 50:1.

In Vitro Assays

The proliferative response of the TIL was assessed using a three day assay where the cells were pulsed with 1 µCi of ^{3}H-Thymidine (6.7 Ci/mmole; New England Nuclear, Dupont, Boston, MA) for 24 hrs prior to harvesting.[3] Cytotoxity was evaluated using a 4 hr ^{51}Cr (New England Nuclear, Dupont, Boston, MA) release assay as previously described.[18] IFNγ production was measured by using a radioimmunoassay kit (Centocor, Malvern, PA). Phenotypic analysis was performed with three color immunocytometry as we have previously described.[14] Proliferation and IFNγ production were examined in TIL cells that had been rested in medium for two days. Thereafter, TIL were stimulated with one of the following; medium, autologous tumor (7000 R), allogeneic RCC (7000 R), IL-2 (5 U/ml) or a combination of tumor and IL-2.

RESULTS

Twenty-one patients were entered, all were eligible, and 16 were ultimately treated. Of the five patients who did not receive TIL, two had inadequate TIL growth, two had disease progression while awaiting therapy initiation and one patient expired prior to therapy. Nine of the patients had a performance status of 0, and 12 had a performance status of 1 (Eastern Cooperative Oncology Group). The male to female ratio was 19:2 and the median age was 61 with a range of 45-74. The toxicity produced by the combination of rIL-2/TIL was moderate, rapidly reversible upon discontinuation of therapy and appeared to increase with continued IL-2 administration. All patients experienced flu-like symptoms consisting of fever and/or chills, and generalized malaise and fatigue were common. Gastrointestinal symptoms of nausea and/or vomiting, anorexia and diarrhea were common with the majority of the patients but were controlled symptomatically. Three of the patients needed 50% IL-2 dose reduction due to toxicity but were able to continue therapy without further reductions in the dose of IL-2. One patient expired during a second cycle of rIL-2 therapy (without TIL) related to possible rIL-2 toxicity. An autopsy revealed no residual renal cell carcinoma.

Hematologic studies included total WBC, differential, hemoglobin, hematocrit, and platelets. Total WBC and absolute lymphocyte counts demonstrated variable but consistent increases in all 16 patients. Mild-to-severe hepatotoxicity (elevation of SGOT and/or alkaline phosphatase) was evident in 14 patients. Mild-to-severe renal toxicity (elevation of serum creatinine and/or BUN) was also present in 14 of 16 patients.

Table 9.1 summarizes the patients who had a response to therapy. Thirty-one percent (95% CI 11 to 59%) or 5/16 patients had an objective response. Among the responders, there was one complete, three partial, and one minor response. The median length of response was 16 weeks with the longest response lasting 116 weeks.

In 19/21 patients, $\geq 5 \times 10^9$ TIL were produced. The average number of TILs infused was 1.88×10^{11} cells with 10/16 patients receiving greater than 1×10^{11} cells and only 2/16 receiving less than 1×10^{10} cells. A summary of the TIL expansion is given in Table 9.2.

Phenotyping of the cultured TIL infused on day 1 was performed on 16/16 patients and a summary of the results is presented in Table 9.3. In all 16 patients, the majority of the cells were $CD3^+CD56^-$ T cells. There were very few NK cells ($CD3^-CD56^+$), although 6/16 patients had between 10-26% $CD3^+CD56^+CD2^+$ cells. In 12/16 patients the percentage of $CD3^+CD4^+CD8^-$ cells was greater than $CD3^+CD4^-CD8^+$ cells. Of the 5 patients who had a response, 3 had a greater percentage of $CD4^+$ with the remaining 2 having greater numbers of $CD8^+$ cells.

The cytotoxity of the infused cells was minimal as illustrated in Table 9.4. TILs were lytic for autologous tumor in 2/12 patients tested. Interestingly cultured TIL from those two individuals were not lytic for other cells tested, including Daudi, RC-2[19] and a short-term allogeneic renal cell.

The lytic response of patients peripheral blood lymphocytes (PBL) was also monitored before (prestudy) and during (day 8, 15, 22 and 29) therapy using both autologous RCC and Daudi cells as tumor

Table 9.1. Summary of anti-tumor response

Pt. No.	Type	Site of Response	Measured Disease Pretreatment (cm)	Measured Disease Post treatment (cm)	Time to Response (Days)	Duration (Weeks)	Site of Progression
6	MR	Lung	4.0 x 4.0	3.0 x 3.5	56	5	Lymph Node
9	PR	Lung	2.5 x 1.5	1.5 x 1.0	23	116	Lung
13	PR	Chest wall	6.5 x 6.0	0.0 x 0.0	32	16	Bone
19	PR	Lung	2.5 x 2.0	1.0 x1.0	29	41[a]	Brain
20	CR[b]	Liver	3.5 x 3.0	2.0 x 1.5	56	5	–

[a] Patient refused further therapy.
[b] Patient expired due to cardiopulmonary arrest during IL-2 therapy.

targets. In 2/12 instances, PBL had LAK activity, and these two patients were nonresponders. The highest lytic response to Daudi occurred on day 15 in patient 12 (40 LU) and on day 22 in patient 14 (73 LU). These same PBL also had lytic activity against autologous tumor cells (patient 12, 4 LU; patient 14, 57 LU).

From the TILs cultured for this trial, five tumor specific T cell lines were eventually established.[18] These cell lines were tested for their responses to tumor through utilizing cytotoxity, proliferation and IFNγ production. The results are summarized in Table 9.5. One cell line, RC-TIL4 ($CD8^+$) was developed from a patient not involved

Table 9.2. Expansion of TIL infused

	Mean (± S.E.M.)	Median	Range
TIL Infused[a]	$1.88 \times 10^{11} \pm 4.03 \times 10^{10}$	1.86×10^{11}	3.39×10^{9} - 5.29×10^{11}
Fold Increase[b]	8172.0 ± 5357.1	799.0	28.3 - 85517.2

[a] TIL were grown in Aim V medium supplemented with IL2 (1000 U/ml) and IL4 (1000 U/ml) for an average of 34 days prior to infusion.
[b] Fold increases were calculated by dividing the starting number of cells into the final number of cells infused.

Table 9.3. Phenotyping of the cultured TILs infused on day 1

	Phenotype[a] of TIL Infused Day 1 of Therapy		
Phenotype	Mean	Median	Range
Total $CD3^+$	98.2	99.2	92.8 - 100.0
Total $CD4^+$	66.1	69.0	15.6 - 98.5
Total $CD8^+$	35.6	25.9	2.2 - 99.1
Total $CD56^+$	9.6	5.9	1.4 - 26.6
$CD3^-CD56^+CD2^-$	0.1	0.05	0.0 - 0.6
$CD3^+CD25^-HLA\text{-}DR^+$	61.8	61.7	22.9 - 91.7
$CD3^+CD25^+HLA\text{-}DR^+$	35.4	34.5	2.9 - 76.5

[a] Immunocytometry was performed as described in the materials and method section. n = 16

Table 9.4. Cytolytic assay of TIL infused

	Target Cells[a]				
	Autologous RCC	Daudi	RC-2	Allogeneic	NonRenal
Number of Patients Tested	12	12	12	14	12
LU /1 x10^6 Cells					
Mean	1.9	0.5	0.0	0.0	0.0
Median	0.0	0.0	0.0	0.0	0.0
Range	0.0-21.1	0.0-5.5	0.0-0.0	0.0-0.0	0.0-0.0

[a] TIL were cultured with ^{51}Cr labeled target cells (5×10^3) to achieve effector-to target cell ratios of 25:1 to 0.78:1. Effector and target cells were incubated for 4 hrs at 37°C. Thereafter, supernatant fluid from each well was harvested with the Skatron harvesting system and the amount of released ^{51}Cr was determined in a LKB Gamma 4000 counter. The results were presented as lytic units per 10^6 mononucleur cells ($LU_{15}/10^6$ cells). Targets included short term cultured autologous and allogeneic RCC, the established RCC line RC-2, Daudi cell line and other nonrenal tumors (HT-29).

Table 9.5. Summary of RC-TIL lines that have selective or specific reactivity to autologous RCC

Call Line	Patient	Phenotype	Response to Autologous Tumor Lysis	Proliferation	IFNγ Production
RC-TIL1	6	$CD3^+CD8^+CD4^-\alpha\beta^+$	+	+	+
RC-TIL2	9	$CD3^+CD8^-CD4^+\alpha\beta^+$	_	+	+
RC-TIL3	13	$CD3^+CD8^+CD4^-$	+	_	_
RC-TIL4	R1	$CD3^+CD8^+CD4^-$	+	+	+
RC-TIL5	18	$CD3^+CD8^-CD4^+\alpha\beta^+$	+	_	_
RC-TIL6	17	$CD3^+CD8^-CD4^+\alpha\beta^+$	-	+	+

This table summarizes the phenotype and functional properties of 6 TIL lines that have specificity for autologous RCC tumor or have selective reactivity for RCC. The phenotype of the lines was determined by flow cytometry immediately following cell separation and at regular intervals thereafter. The presence of lytic activity was determined using a 4 hr ^{51}Cr release assay. Proliferation was assessed by the uptake of ^3H-Thymidine after three days of culture. IFNγ production of TIL in response to tumor was examined from supernatant fluid removed 48-72 hours after initiation of culture by the use of an RIA kit (Centocor). RC-TIL1 and RC-TIL6 were derived from IL2 grown TIL whereas RC-TIL2, RC-TIL3, RC-TIL4 and RC-TIL5 were obtained from IL2/IL4 grown cultures. RC-TIL4 was isolated from cells cultured from a patient not on the phase II trial. (Table adapted from Finke et al Characterization of TIL subsets from human renal cell carcinoma: Specific reactivity defined by cytotoxity, IFNγ secretion and proliferation. J of Immunoth In Press.)

in this phase II trial. Two of the six lines [RC-TIL1 ($CD8^+$) and RC-TIL4 ($CD8^+$)] specifically lysed their autologous tumors but not allogeneic RCC, K562, Sk-Mel or HT-29. Two of the lines [RC-TIL3 ($CD8^+$) and RC-TIL5 ($CD4^+$)] displayed selective lysis of RCC in that they lysed one or more allogeneic RCC in addition to the autologous tumor. Of these lines, RC-TIL1 and RC-TIL4, were reactive to their own tumor in all three types of assays, they were able to lyse, proliferate and produce IFNγ to the autologous tumor. The four cell lines that were able to proliferate to their tumor also were able to produce IFNγ to the autologous tumor. These lines did not proliferate or produce IFNγ in response to allogeneic RCC suggesting that the responses were specific. RC-TIL1 and RC-TIL6 were derived from IL-2 grown cultures whereas RC-TIL2, RC-TIL3, RC-TIL4 and RC-TIL5 were derived from IL-2/IL-4 grown cultures.

It is of interest that we detected RCC specific TIL lines from 3 of the patients that demonstrated tumor regression. In addition TIL lines were isolated from one nonresponder, one patient who died prior to therapy, and one patient who was not on this study.

DISCUSSION

IL-4 is a T-cell growth factor[15-17,20] and has been used in combination with IL-2 to modulate IL-2 induced proliferation of TIL from several types of tumor. IL-4 has been found to enhance the IL-2 proliferation of ovarian malignant ascites infiltrating lymphocytes.[21] Belldegrun et al, found IL-4 added to renal cell cultures grown in both high (1000 U/ml) and low (20 U/ml) dose IL-2 augmented the TIL growth and produced cultures enriched in $CD3^+$ cells with few $CD56^+$.[22] Their cells also had minimal cytotoxic activity against the autologous tumor and significantly reduced nonspecific lytic activity. We and others have previously reported that the cytotoxity of TIL grown in IL-2 can be attributed to $CD3^-CD56^+$ cells.[23-25] The combination of IL-2 and IL-4 has also been shown to be effective in promoting the generation of melanoma specific CTL while inhibiting the growth of LAK effectors.[17]

TILs cultured in IL-2 plus IL-4 are composed of cells that are highly enriched for T cells, and these cells along with continuous infusion IL-2 can produce objective clinical responses in patients with renal cell carcinoma. In the previous trial using TILs and IL-2 performed at the Cleveland Clinic, the TIL were cultured with high dose IL-2 (1000 U/ml) and the resulting cell population was very heterogeneous with many of the cultures having a large percentage of NK cells.[14] By combining IL-4 with IL-2 for culturing TILs in the second trial, the cells that were infused were >96% $CD3^+$. In the previous Phase I trial, 0/18 objective responses (95% CI 0 to 19%) were seen, and in the Phase II trial 5/16 patients had a response (95% CI 11 to 59%). There are other notable differences between the trials including the dose and duration of rIL-2 therapy and the schedule of the TIL infusions. It is possible that the TIL cultured in IL-2 and IL-4 produced the increased number of responses in the present trial compared to our previous experience,[14] but the small patient numbers and the preliminary nature of these clinical trials does not permit these conclusions. IL-2 as a single agent can produce tumor regression in 10 to 20% of patients,[26,27] and therefore may be responsible for these results. Additionally, the dose of IL-2 in the present trial was 4.5×10^6 U/m^2, which is substantially higher than in our initial trial in which patients received variable doses of this cytokine.

In the 16 patients treated with TILs, four TIL lines with specificity for the autologous tumor were established. Although specific cells have been readily found in melanoma derived TIL,[6,24] only recently have specific cells been found from RCC. We previously identified a $CD8^+$ cell line that was shown to be specific for the autologous tumor in cytotoxicity, proliferation and production of IFNγ.[28] A $CD4^+$ T cell clone was isolated from renal cell ascitic fluid that was specific for autologous tumor.[29] Schendel et al have a $CD8^+$ cell line derived from renal cell carcinoma that has HLA-A2 restricted recognition of autologous tumor.[30] This $CD8^+$ cell line had enhanced CTL recognition of the autologous tumor when rIL2 was retrovirally transduced into the tumor.[31] Of the three $CD8^+$ TIL lines we isolated with cytolytic activity, two (RC-TIL1 and RC-TIL4) had specific activity for their autologous tumor. These two cell lines were capable of lysing the autologous tumor and not other short term allogeneic RCC or other histological tumor types. These $CD8^+$ cell lines appear to recognize the tumor through the TCR/CD3 receptor and are MHC class I-restricted.[18] The other two cytotoxic lines in our studies lysed allogeneic RCC as well as the autologous tumor but not other histologic tumor types. These TIL lines appear similar to those observed from other types of cancer where T cells preferentially lysed tumor of the same histologic type but not tumors of other histologic types.[32,33]

The fact that specific/selective T cell lines can be found to renal cancer raises the possibility of finding antigens that serve as targets for these cells. Recently peptides have been identified on human melanoma cells that are able to be recognized by Class I restricted tumor infiltrating lymphocytes.[34] The identification of renal cell carcinoma specific response and the possibility of defined RCC antigens recognized by these cells may facilitate the development of new approaches to the treatment of this disease.

References

1. Vose BM, Moore M. Human tumor-infiltrating lymphocytes: A marker of host response. Seminars in Hematology 22:27-35, 1985.
2. Whiteside TL, Miescher S, Hulimann J, Moretta L, Von Fliedner V. Separation, phenotyping and limiting dilution analysis of T-lymphocytes infiltrating human solid tumors. Int J Cancer 37:803-811, 1986.
3. Alexander J, Rayman P, Edinger M, Connelly R, Tubbs R, Bukowski R, Pontes E, Finke J. TIL from renal cell carcinoma: Restimulation with tumor influences proliferation and cytolytic activity. Int J Cancer 45:119-124, 1990.
4. Itoh K, Tilden AB, Balch CM. Interleukin 2 activation of cytotoxic T-lymphocytes infiltrating into human metastatic melanomas. Cancer Res 46:3011-3017, 1986.
5. Kurnick JT, Kradin RL, Blumberg R, Schneeberger EE, Boyle LA. Functional

characterization of T lymphocytes propagated from human lung carcinomas. Cancer Immunol Immunother 38:367-380, 1986.

6. Muul LM, Spiess PJ, Director EP, Rosenberg SA. Identification of specific cytolytic immune responses against autologous tumor in humans bearing malignant melanoma. J Immunol 138:989-995, 1987.
7. Finke JH, Tubbs R, Connelly B, Pontes E, Montie J. Tumor-infiltrating lymphocytes in patients with renal-cell carcinoma. Ann N Y Acad Sci 532:387-394, 1987.
8. Belldegrun A, Muul LM, Rosenberg SA. Interleukin 2 expanded tumor-infiltrating lymphocytes in human renal cell cancer: isolation, characterization and anti-tumor activity. Cancer Res 48:206-214, 1988.
9. Rosenberg SA, Spiess P, Lafreniere R. A new approach to the adoptive immunotherapy of cancer with tumor-infiltrating lymphocytes. Science (Wash DC) 233:1318-1321, 1986.
10. Spiess PJ, Yang JC, Rosenberg SA. In vivo anti-tumor activity of tumor-infiltrating lymphocytes expanded in recombinant interleukin 2. J Natl Cancer Inst. 75:1067-1075, 1987.
11. Topalian SL, Solomon D, Avis FF, Chang AE, Freerksen DL, Linehan WM, Lotze MT, Robertson CN, Seipp CA, Simon P, Simpson CG, Rosenberg SA. Immunotherapy of patients with advanced cancer using tumor-infiltrating lymphocytes and recombinant Interleukin-2: A pilot study. J Clin Oncol 6:839-853, 1988.
12. Kradin RL, Lazarus DS, Dubinett SM, Gifford J, Grove B, Kurnick JT, Pretter FI, Pinto CE, Davison E, Collahan RJ, Strauss HW. Tumor-infiltrating lymphocytes and interleukin-2 in treatment of advanced cancer. The Lancet 1:577-580, 1989.
13. Foon KA, Walther PJ, Bernstein ZP, Vaickus L, Rahman R, Watanabe H, Sweeney J, Park J, Vesper D, Russell D, et al. Renal cell carcinoma treated with continuous-infusion interleukin-2 with ex-vivo-activated killer cells. J of Immunoth 11:184-190, 1992.
14. Bukowski RM, Sharfman W, Murthy S, Rayman P, Tubbs R, Alexander J, Budd GT, Sergi J, Bauer L, Gibson V, Stanley J, Boyett J, Pontes E, Finke J. Clinical results and characterization of tumor-infiltrating lymphocytes with and without recombinant interleukin-2 in human metastatic renal cell carcinoma. Cancer Res 51:4199-4205, 1991.
15. Widmer MB, Acres RB, Sassenfeld HM, Grabstein KH. Regulation of cytolytic cell populations from human peripheral blood by B cell stimulatory factor 1 (Interleukin 4). J Exp Med 166:1447-1455, 1987.
16. Spits H, Yssel H, Takebe Y, Arai N, Yokota T, Lee F, Arai K, Banchereau J, DeVries J. Recombinant interleukin 4 promotes the growth of human T cells. J of Immunol 139:1142-1147, 1987.
17. Kawakami Y, Rosenberg SA, Lotze MT. Interleukin 4 promotes the growth of tumor-infiltrating lymphocytes cytotoxic for human autologous melanoma. J Exp Med 168:2183-2191, 1988.
18. Finke JH, Rayman P, Hart L, Alexander J, Edinger M, Tubbs R, Klein E, Tuason L, Bukowski R. Characterization of TIL subsets from human renal cell carcinoma: Specific reactivity defined by cytotoxity, IFNγ secretion and proliferation. J of Immunoth In Press.
19. Hashimura T, Tubbs R, Connelly R, Trindade SC, McMahon JT, Caulfield M, Prayer-Galetti T, Edinger M, Sandburg A, Dal-Cin P, Sait SPJ, and Pontes E. Characterization of two cell lines with distinct phenotypes and genotypes established from a patient from renal cell carcinoma. Cancer Res 49:7064-7071, 1989.
20. Spits H, Yssel H, Palirard X, Kastelein R, Figdor C, DeVries JE. IL4 inhibits IL2-mediated induction of human lymphokine activated killer cells, but not the generation of antigen specific cytotoxic T lymphocytes in mixed lymphocyte cultures. J Immunol 141:29-36, 1988.
21. Ioannides CG, Rashed S, Fisk B, Fan D, Itoh K, Freedman RS. Lymphocytes infiltrating ovarian malignant ascites: modulation of IL2-induced proliferation by IL4 and selective increase in $CD8^+$ T cells by TNF-alpha. Lympho & Cytokine Res 10:307-315, 1991.
22. Tso CL, Duckett T, deKernion JB, Belldegrun AS. Modulation of tumor-infil-

trating lymphocytes derived from human renal cell carcinoma by interleukin-4. J of Immunoth 12:82-89, 1992.

23. Finke JH, Rayman P, Alexander J, Edinger M, Tubbs R, Connelly R, Pontes E, Bukowski R. Characterization of the cytolytic activity of CD4+ and CD8+ TIL subsets in human renal cell carcinoma. Cancer Res 50:2363-2370, 1990.
24. Itoh K, Platosoucas CD, Balch CM. Autologous tumor-specific cytotoxic T lymphocytes in the infiltrate of human metastatic melanomas. Activation of interleukin 2 and autologous tumor cells, and involvement of the T cell receptor. J Exp Med 168:1419-1441, 1988.
25. Whiteside TL, Heo DS, Takagi S, Johnson JT, Iwatsuki S, Herberman RB. Cytolytic anti-tumor effector cells in long-term cultures of human tumor-infiltrating lymphocytes in recombinant Interleukin-2. Cancer Immunol Immunother 26:1-10, 1988.
26. Rosenberg S, Lotze M, Yang JC, Topalian SL, Chang AE, Schwartzentruber DJ, Aebersold P, Leitman S, Linehan M, Seipp CA, White DE, Steinberg SM. Prospective randomized trial of high-dose interluekin-2 alone or in conjunction with lymphokine-activated killer cells for the treatment of patients with advanced cancer. J Natl Cancer Inst 85:622-632, 1993.
27. Bukowski RM, Goodman P, Crawford ED, Sergi JS, Redman BG, Whitehead RP. Phase II trial of high-dose intermittent interleukin-2 in metastatic renal cell carcinoma: a Southwest Oncology Group study. J Natl Cancer Inst 82:143-146, 1990.
28. Finke JH, Rayman P, Edinger M , Tubbs R, Stanley J, Klein E, Bukowski R. Characterization of a human renal cell carcinomas specific cytotoxic CD8+ T cell line. J of Immunoth 11:1-11, 1992.
29. Belldegrun A, Kasid A, Uppenkamp M, Rosenberg SA. Lymphokine mRNA profile and functional analysis of a human CD4+ clone with unique anti-tumor specificity isolated from renal cell carcinoma ascitic fluid. Cancer Immunol Immunother 31:1-10, 1990.
30. Schendel DJ, Gansbacher B, Oberneder R, Kriegmair M, Hofstetter A, Riethmuller G and Segurado OG. Tumor-specific lysis of human renal cell carcinomas by tumor-infiltrating lymphocytes. I. HLA-A2 restricted recognition of autologous and allogeneic tumor lines. J Immunol 151:4209-4220, 1993.
31. Schendel DJ, Gansbacher B. Tumor-specific lysis of human renal cell carcinomas by tumor-infiltrating lymphocytes: Modulation of recognition through retroviral transduction of tumor cells with Interleukin 2 complementary DNA and exogenous a Interferon treatment. Cancer Res 53:4020-4025, 1993.
32. Letesjier EM, Heo DS, Okarma T, Johnson JT, Herberman RB, Whiteside TL. Enrichment in tumor-reactive CD8+ T-lymphocytes by positive selection from the blood and lymph nodes of patients with head and neck cancer. Cancer Res 51:3891-3899, 1991.
33. Jerome KR, Brand DL, Bendt KM, Boyer C, Taylor-Papadimtriou J, McKenzie I, Bast R, Finn O. Cytotoxic T- lymphocytes derived from patients with breast adenocarcinoma recognize an epitope present on the protein core of a mucin molecule preferentially expressed by malignant cells. Cancer Res 51:2908-2916, 1991.
34. Storkus WJ, Zeh HJ, Maeurer M, Salter RD, Lotze MT. Identification of human melanoma peptides recognized by class I restricted tumor infiltrating T lymphocytes. J Immuno 151:3719-3727, 1993.

CHAPTER 10

Tumor-Infiltrating Lymphocytes in Head and Neck Cancer

Theresa L. Whiteside

INTRODUCTION

Infiltrations of inflammatory cells, which are commonly seen at the tumor margins, in the stroma or within the nests of tumor cells in head and neck carcinoma (HNC), are mainly composed of lymphocytes and granulocytes.[1] The lymphocytic component of the infiltrate consists mostly of T cells, but B cells and plasma cells may be numerous in HNC.[1] The role of these mixed lymphocyte/granulocyte infiltrates in growth and recurrence of HNC and their impact on prognosis have been a subject of much discussion and controversy. In particular, it has been suggested that tumor-infiltrating lymphocytes (TILs) are not just inflammatory cells but immune effector cells, which have been specifically recruited to the tumor as a part of anti-tumor immune surveillance mechanisms.[2] Others have suggested that tumor-infiltrating granulocytes are important in defense against tumors, because they mediate "cross-talk" between various cellular components of the infiltrate.[3]

Whether it is TIL or tumor-associated granulocytes or both that contribute to host defense, it would seem that this prominent presence of inflammatory cells in the tumor should be associated with a better prognosis or longer recurrence-free survival in HNC, as has been suggested for other human tumors.[4,5] To this end, many studies have sought to document a positive relationship between the cellular composition or intensity of tumor infiltrates and survival in HNC.[6-11] The results of these studies, which largely focused on TIL, failed to demonstrate a clear-cut correlation between the presence or composition of TIL infiltrates and prognosis or survival. Nevertheless, some of these studies have suggested

Immunotherapy of Cancer with Sensitized T Lymphocytes, edited by Alfred E. Chang and Suyu Shu.

that the intensity of infiltrates present in squamous cell carcinoma of the head and neck (SCCHN) may positively correlate with disease-free survival.[10] In an immunohistologic study of TIL in over 70 patients with HNC performed in my laboratory, four-year survival correlated neither with the phenotype, nor the localization in the tumor of the infiltrating lymphocytes, but with the intensity of the infiltrate, as determined at the time of surgery (unpublished data). These and similar observations imply that TILs play an active role in tumor progression and that the host's ability to control tumor growth may, at least in part, depend on functional competence of these cells. Similarly, immunocompetence of lymph node lymphocytes (LNL) in HNC has been thought to be important in host-tumor interactions, especially since the cervical lymph nodes are often an initial site of metastasis in this type of cancer.[12]

TIL in HNC and other human tumors have received considerable attention in recent years, because of the possibility that they are enriched in immune effector cells endowed with the ability to mediate antitumor effects. Furthermore, based on preclinical studies in experimental murine tumors and subsequent clinical trials initiated by Rosenberg and collaborators, it appeared that TIL obtained from murine or human solid tumors were more effective anti-tumor effector cells in adoptive transfer experiments than spleen- or peripheral blood-derived, respectively, interleukin-2 (IL-2)-activated lymphocytes.[13,14] The early clinical trials with TIL in patients with metastatic melanoma or renal cell carcinoma (RCC) have indicated that systemic immunotherapy with TIL and IL-2 can lead to long-term responses in about 30-40% of patients unresponsive to conventional therapies.[14,15] These clinical trials generated a great deal of interest and focused attention on TIL as a possible source of therapeutically desirable effector cells. Today, after nearly a decade of work, neither the biologic role of TIL in tumor progression nor their therapeutic advantages have been definitively confirmed.[16] A number of questions about TIL have been generated, which apply as much to TIL in HNC as in other human tumors, and which mainly concern a role of TIL in the control of tumor growth in situ, the presence among TIL of autotumor-specific cytolytic T lymphocytes (CTLs) and the prospects for immune therapy with TIL of a wide range of human tumors, including HNC. While attempting to answer these questions about TIL, I hope to provide the reader with a comprehensive and balanced evaluation of TIL potential both as a source of autotumor-specific CTL and as a key to developing new strategies for locoregional immunotherapy of HNC.

PHENOTYPIC CHARACTERISTICS OF TIL IN SITU

Immunohistologic analyses with monoclonal antibodies (mAbs) specific for surface antigens (Ags) on lymphocytes have shown that primary SCCHN are generally well infiltrated with mononuclear cells (MNC),[9,17] while non-squamous-cell head and neck tumors are only moderately or poorly infiltrated.[18] T lymphocytes (CD3$^+$) are a predominant component of these infiltrates (Fig. 10.1). CD8$^+$ T cells appear to preferentially localize to the tumor parenchyma, while CD4$^+$ T cells are more numerous in the tumor stroma.[17,18] The mean CD4/CD8 ratio was 2.4 in the stroma and 0.6 in the parenchyma in one of our studies, as determined by immunohistology.[18] In another study, including 16 patients with SCCHN, we have obtained evidence that a TIL CD4$^+$/CD8$^+$ ratio of less than 1 at the time of surgery appears to be associated with better prognostic indicators, such as the lack of extracapsular spread or absence of cervical metastases.[17] In a double-staining immunoperoxidase method,[19] using anti-CD2 and anti-HLA-DR mAbs or anti-CD2 and anti-CD71 (anti-transferrin receptor) mAbs applied to the same sections of tumor tissue, we observed that T lymphocytes simultaneously expressing CD2/DR or CD2/CD71 Ags were numerous in SCCHN (Fig. 10.2). This observation

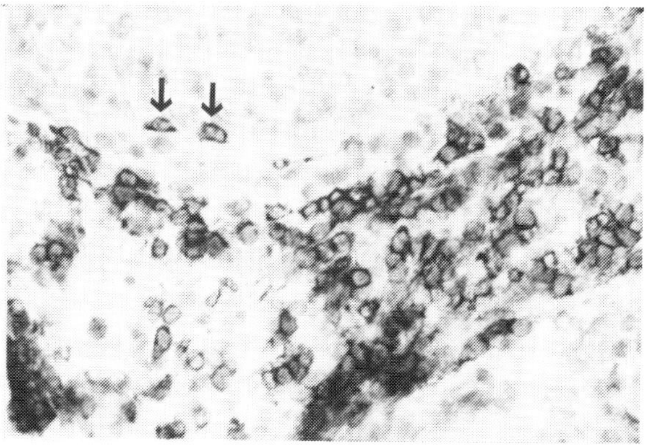

Fig. 10.1. A cryostat section of human SCCHN stained by immunoperoxidase anti-CD3 mAbs. T cells (CD3+) are the main component of the stromal mononuclear cell infiltrate. The arrows indicate CD3+ cells present in the tumor parenchyma. (Mag x400).

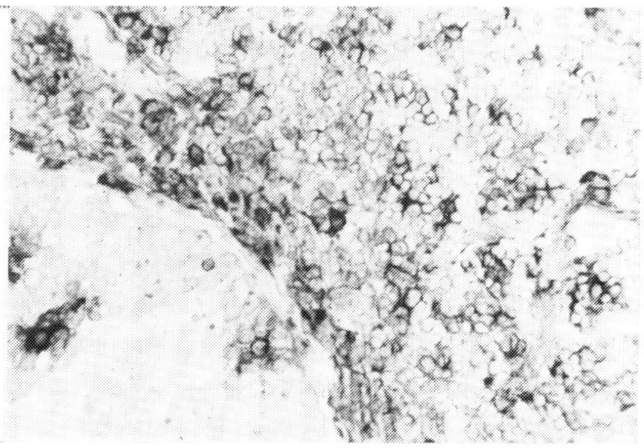

Fig. 10.2. Two-color immunoperoxidase staining was performed in a cryostat section of human SCCHN, using anti-CD2 and anti-HLA-DR mAbs. In this black-and-white photograph, the strongly-stained ells are CD2+DR+ and the faintly-stained cells are CD2+. Many TIL present in the tumor stroma or parenchyma are CD2+DR+, i.e., activated. (Mag x300)

meant that TILs in SCCHN were activated in situ.[20] We also observed that TIL infiltrates were smaller in patients with metastases and those with recurrent tumors than in patients with primary SCCHN.[18]

Newer methods for quantitative recovery of TIL and LNL from tissues[21] have facilitated two-color flow cytometry studies of freshly-isolated TIL in HNC.[17] Phenotypically, such TIL were mixtures of $CD8^+$ and $CD4^+$ T cells ($CD3^+/CD2^+$), many of which also expressed activation Ags, HLA-DR (up to 60%) or CD25 (up to 25%), on the cell surface.[17] TIL obtained from SCCHN contained <5% of $CD3^-CD56^+$ natural killer (NK) cells and generally <5% of $CD3^+CD56^+$ non-MHC-restricted T lymphocytes.[17] The CD4/CD8 ratios were variable, and were often, but not always, greater than 1, indicating that in most TIL isolated from SCCHN, $CD4^+$ T lymphocytes tended to outnumber $CD8^+$ T lymphocytes (Fig. 10.3A and B). Both $CD4^+$ and $CD8^+$ T cells obtained from a limited number of TIL preparations were found by us (unpublished data) to express the primed or memory phenotype ($CD29^+/CD45RO^+$). Although these results need to be confirmed in a greater number of specimens, the data are consistent with the current view that TILs are largely memory or primed T cells.[1] TILs were compared for phenotypic characteristics with autologous peripheral blood lymphocytes (PBL) and found to contain significantly fewer NK cells but more T cells expressing activation Ags (Fig. 10.3A).

When LNL from tumor-involved (I) or -non-involved (NI) LN of patients with SCCHN were compared for phenotypic characteristics with autologous TIL, the only differences observed were a significantly lower content of HLA-DR^+ T cells (<15%) and substantially higher proportion of $CD4^+$ T cells in LNL. No phenotypic differences were detected between I-LNL and NI-LNL,[22] although both TIL and LNL differed from autologous PBL by a significantly lower percentage of $CD8^+CD11b^+$ ("suppressor") lymphocytes ($p < 0.05$) as

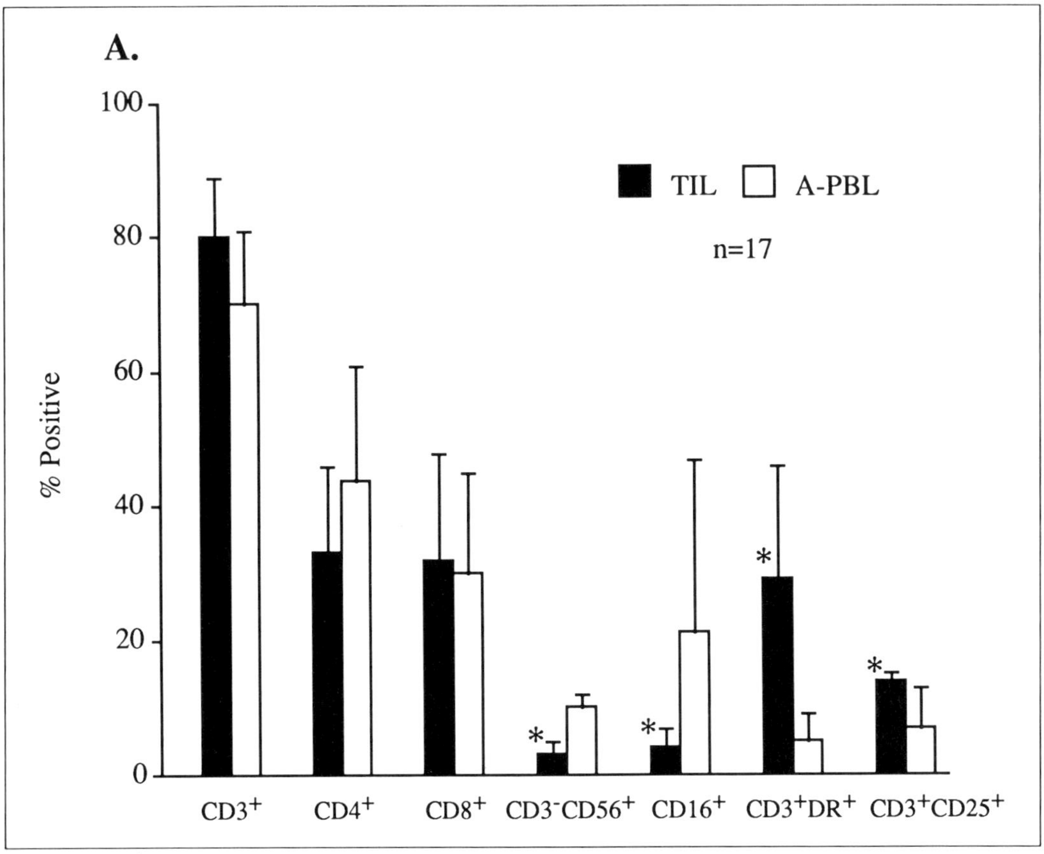

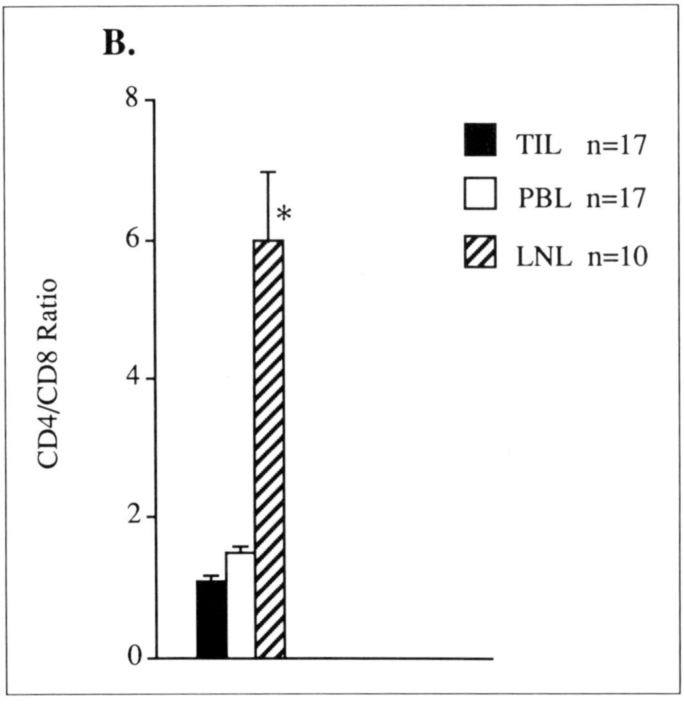

Fig. 10.3. Two-color flow cytometry of TIL and A-PBL obtained from patients with SCCHN. In A, the data are mean percentages of positive cells, with ± 1 SD (see bars). Asterisks indicate significant differences between TIL and PBL at $p < 0.01$. In B, the CD4/CD8 ratios for paired specimens of TIL, PBL and LNL are shown. The asterisk indicates a significantly increased ratio for LNL ($p < 0.001$).

well as a substantially higher proportion of $CD4^+$ than $CD8^+$ T cells in LNL.[22] As a consequence, LNL had a significantly higher CD4/CD8 ratio (mean ± SD of 6 ± 1) than either autologous TIL or PBL (Fig. 10.3B).

Overall, the phenotypic characterization of fresh TILs in suspensions by two-color flow cytometry has allowed for a more precise quantitation of T-cell subsets than earlier immunohistologic studies. These newer data have emphasized the presence of activated and committed or primed T lymphocytes among TILs isolated from HNC as well as other solid tumors.[1]

FUNCTIONAL CHARACTERISTICS OF TIL IN SITU

TIL freshly-obtained from HNC biopsies have not been extensively evaluated for function in the standard immunologic assays, largely due to a limited number of cells recovered from these biopsies.[23] Only more recently, with the availability of micromethods, simultaneous assessments of several functional parameters have become possible with fresh TIL. The main obstacle has been the presence of tumor cells in most TIL preparations obtained from SCCHN, which is undesirable, because of the likely possibility that tumor cells may interfere with the interpretation of results. In SCCHN, it has also been difficult to consistently recover viable tumor cells from enzymatic digests of tumor biopsies for use as targets in cytotoxicity assays or as stimulators in mixed lymphocyte-tumor cultures (MLTC). For these reasons, in situ analysis of the ability of TIL or LNL in biopsy tissue to express mRNA for cytokine genes or IL2 receptor (R) genes appears to be a promising approach, allowing for a partial estimation of the functional potential of TIL or LNL in HNC. Unfortunately, in situ hybridization (ISH) for cytokine gene expression is not only difficult to perform, but by itself, without subsequent demonstration of cytokine production by these cells, it may not be accurate, because genes expressed in pathologic specimens are not always transcribed into functionally-active proteins. Despite of these limitations, ISH for the cytokine gene expression performed with HNC biopsies has been informative and has shown that TIL as well as LNL localized in the immediate proximity of the tumor were activated,[24] as evidenced by the expression of mRNA for IL2, interferon-gamma (IFN-γ), IL1-β, tumor necrosis factor-alpha (TNF-α) and both α- and β-chains of the IL2R (Fig. 10.4A). In addition, many LNL located next to the tumor expressed mRNA for transforming growth factor-beta (TGF-β; see Fig. 10.4B). In contrast, LNL not adjacent to the tumor in I-LN as well as those LNL obtained from tumor-NI-LN, did not express mRNA for cytokines or IL2R. These data suggest that TIL and LNL in tumor-I-LNL of patients with HNC are activated by the tumor to produce mRNA for various cytokines including TGF-β. These data have been subsequently confirmed by us in cytokine production assays, using fresh TIL and LNL isolated from biopsy tissues of patients with HNC (see below).

Following separation of TIL from HNC biopsy tissues by controlled enzymatic digestion as described earlier,[23] preparations enriched for T lymphocytes can be obtained and tested for functional responses in immunologic assays. The LN specimens need not be subjected to enzymatic digestion and can be disaggregated by passage through a wire screen. The method of TIL or LNL separation from tissues is an important aspect of the functional studies of these cells, which appear to have decreased immunocompetence as compared to autologous or normal PBL tested in the same assays.[25] It has been suggested that exposure of TIL to the enzyme cocktail might contribute to their poor functional performance in in vitro assays.[25] However, T lymphocytes obtained from peripheral blood of normal donors and incubated with the same enzyme cocktail as well as T cells separated using enzymes from human spleens responded normally under the same experimental conditions.[25,26] At the same time, LNL of patients with HNC separated

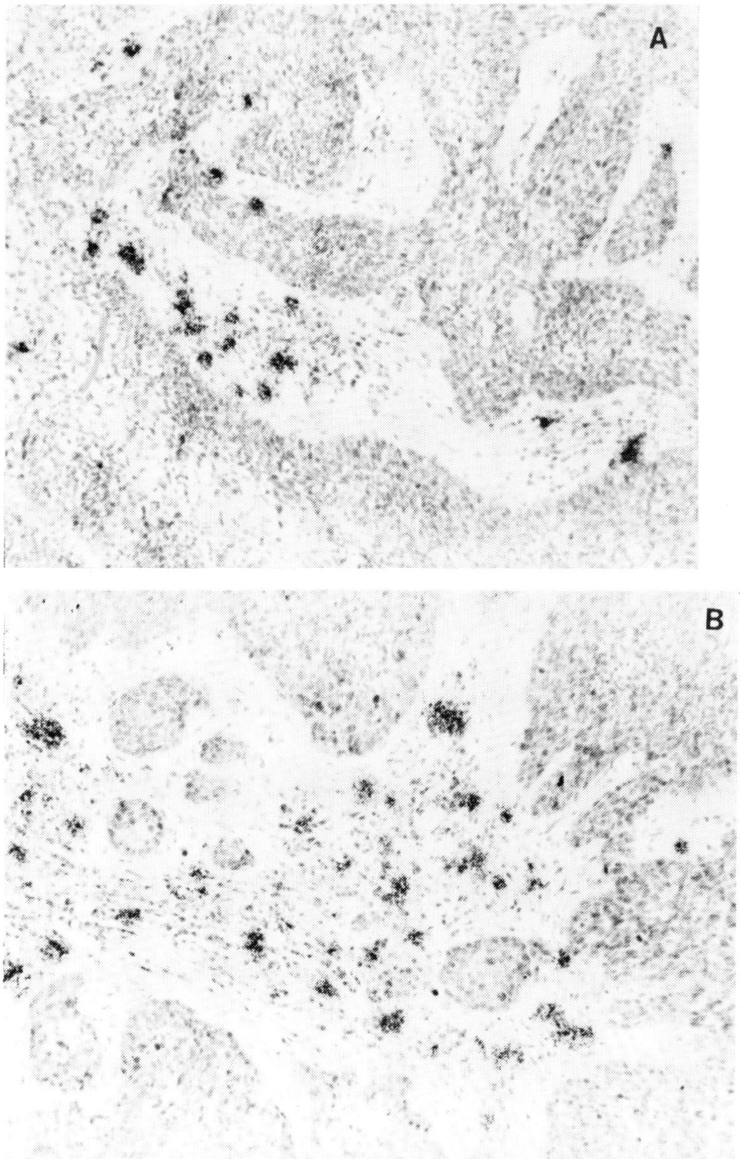

Fig. 10.4. In situ hybridization for the IL2R-α gene (A) and for the TGF-β gene (B) performed on cryostat sections of a SCCHN biopsy. The sections were hybridized with the $^{35}[S]$-labeled cDNA probes for IL2R-α or TGF-β, respectively as described earlier.[24] (Mag x100).

without the use of enzymes were also found to be functionally deficient.[22,27] This type of study ruled out the possibility that poor proliferative or cytotoxic responses of freshly-isolated TIL or LNL in patients with HNC (or other cancers) were in vitro artifacts attributable to tissue processing. These studies confirmed that tumor-derived lymphocytes were, in fact, functionally deficient in situ.[1]

Freshly-isolated TIL, LNL from both tumor I-LNL and NI-LN and autologous (A) PBL obtained from patients with HNC were tested for proliferative responses to a mitogen, PHA, IL2 (6,000 IU/ml) and irradiated autologous tumor (AuTu) cells in 5-day $^{3}[H]$-thymidine incorporation assays.[27] In comparison to A-PBL or normal PBL used as controls, both TIL and LNL were found to be either unresponsive or had proliferative responses that were significantly depressed at $p < 0.001$. In 4 hour ^{51}Cr-release assays, neither TIL nor LNL of patients with HNC were able to lyse NK-sensitive K562 targets or NK-resistant SCCHN cell line (PCI-1) established in our laboratory (Fig. 10.5). On the other hand, in vitro incubation of these lymphoid cells in the presence of IL2 (6,000 IU/ml) for 5 days restored, at least partially, their ability to lyse tumor cell targets in 4 hour ^{51}Cr-release assays (Fig. 10.5). The ability to generate lymphokine activated killer (LAK) cells in the presence of IL2 was significantly decreased ($p<0.05$) in TIL and LNL in comparison to A-PBL (Fig. 10.5). Also, antibody-dependent cellular cytotoxicity (ADCC) of freshly-isolated TIL or LNL was found to be significantly depressed.[27]

The observations described above demonstrated that not only proliferative responses but also anti-tumor cytotoxicity of T cells freshly-isolated from the tumor site or LN of patients with HNC were either depressed or absent.[27] At the same time, freshly-isolated TIL and LNL were able to produce certain cytokines (IL2 and IFN-γ) spontaneously or in response to exogenous activators. As shown in Table 10.1, I-LNL or NI-LNL did not produce measurable levels of TNF-α or IL1-β in vitro. In contrast, PBL obtained from patients with HNC spontaneously produced significantly more ($p < 0.001$) of TNF-α and IL1-β than PBL of normal individuals.[27] TIL spontaneously released TNF-α and IL1-β at levels that were not significantly different from those of normal PBL; however, the LPS-induced production of these cytokines

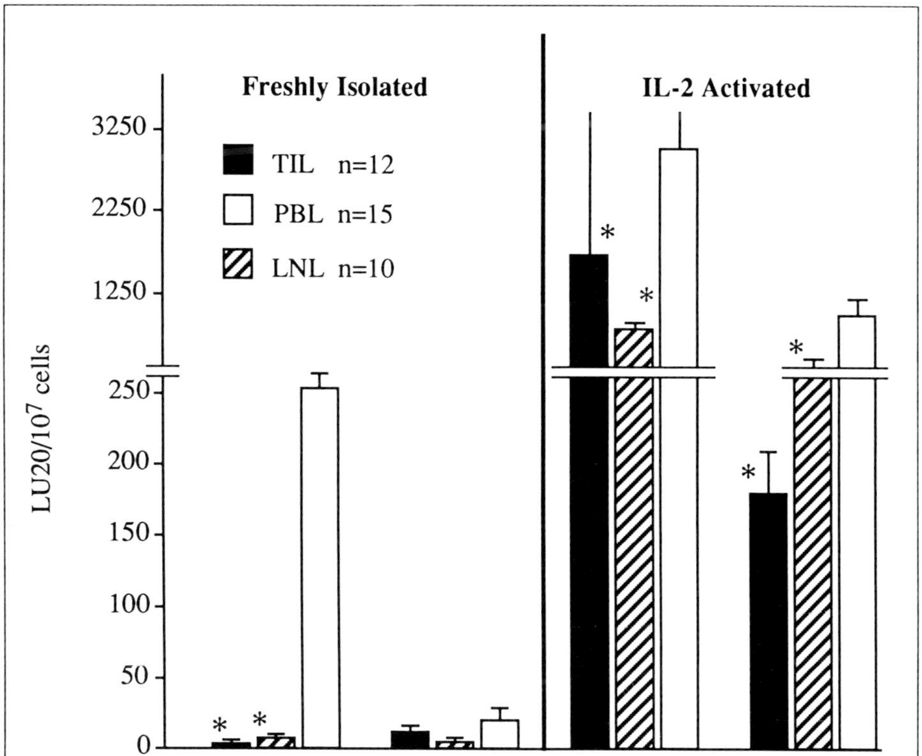

Fig. 10.5. Cytotoxic activity of freshly isolated (left) TIL, PBL and LNL of patients with SCCHN against an NK-sensitive target, K562, and an NK-resistant SCCHN target, PCI-1. On the right, cytotoxic activity of the same lymphocyte preparations tested for cytotoxicity against the two tumor cell targets after 5-day activation of effector cells in the presence of 6,000 IU/ml of IL2. Cytotoxicity was measured in 4 hours ^{51}Cr-release assays. Asterisks indicate significant differences between TIL and LNL versus PBL ($p < 0.001$, left and $p < 0.05$, right).

Table 10.1. Spontaneous and induced in vitro production of cytokines by TIL, LNL or PBL obtained from patients with head and neck cancer[a]

Lymphocytes	n	Spontaneous IL1-β, pg/ml	Induced IL1-β, pg/ml	n	Spontaneous TNF-α, pg/ml	Induced TNF-α, pg/ml
TIL	7	47 ± 26	39 ± 17*	7	36 ± 19	70 ± 35*
I-LN	11	0	0	11	0	0
NI-LN	10	0	0	10	0	0
Patient PBL	11	1036 ± 525*	1472 ± 824	11	370 ± 173*	610 ± 212
Normal PBL	30	32 ± 7	4600 ± 473	30	12 ± 3.5	1550 ± 128
		IL2, U/ml			IFN-γ, U/ml	
TIL	6	2.3 ± 1.6	43 ± 18	6	0	46 ± 23**
I-LN	9	1.7 ± 0.8	65 ± 12	9	0	35 ± 8**
NI-LN	9	2.0 ± 0.8	66 ± 11	9	0	20 ± 10**
Patient PBL	10	2.5 ± 1.8	20 ± 6.8	12	2.1 ± 2.3	76 ± 40**
Normal PBL	33	0.6 ± 0.2	17.3 ± 2.3	37	4.6 ± 1.2	267 ± 31

[a] Fresh or fresh-frozen lymphocytes were incubated in TCM (spontaneous) or in TCM plus either PHA-P or LPS (induced) for 48 hours. Culture supernatants were harvested and assayed for cytokines. Data are means ± SEM.
* p<0.001;
** p<0.01 versus normal PBL.

by TIL was much lower ($p < 0.001$) than that of normal or patient PBL (Table 10.1). TIL or LNL obtained from patients with HNC did not spontaneously produce IFN-γ, and PHA-induced production of IFN-γ by patient's cells was lower than that of normal PBL ($p < 0.01$). On the other hand, PHA-induced IL2 production was normal in these TIL and LNL.[24] Overall, we observed considerable differences between patients' lymphocytes obtained from different compartments in the ability to synthesize cytokines, with LNL being the least responsive, TIL partially responsive and PBL characterized by the higher-than-normal spontaneous release of TNF-α and IL1-β. TIL differed from LNL in that they produced variable, but nearly always detectable, levels of all four cytokines.

The functional deficiencies observed with fresh TIL or LNL obtained from patients with HNC were not an "all or none" phenomenon. On the contrary, some preparations of fresh TIL retained considerable functional activities. Also, not all responses of TIL were equally depressed, with proliferative and cytolytic functions being most consistently affected, and the ability to express mRNA for cytokines and to produce cytokines largely intact.[24,27] This selective functional deficit observed in TIL of patients with HNC appears to be a generalized phenomenon, as TIL from a wide variety of human tumors have been described to have similar characteristics.[1] Recently, Ochoa and his colleagues reported that murine CD8$^+$ T lymphocytes from animals bearing tumors (colon carcinoma MCA-38) for more than 26 days had impaired cytotoxicity, decreased expression of TNF-α and granzyme B genes, decreased ability to mediate anti-tumor responses in vivo after adoptive transfer and clearly demonstrable deficiency in signal transduction.[28] Despite the normal level of surface expression of the T cell receptor (TCR)-CD3 complex, these T lymphocytes completely lacked the CD3 zeta chain and had reduced expression of tyrosine kinases p56^{lck} and p59^{fyn}.[28] Similar changes have been now reported to be present in TIL obtained from patients with renal cell carcinoma (RCC) and colon carcinoma.[29,30] It seems possible that these or similar alterations in the TCR-CD3 and signal transduction pathways associated with this complex of surface molecules are the basis of immune defects observed in TIL and possible in other populations of anti-tumor effector cells in tumor-bearing hosts. The nature of the factors that induce these defects in signal transduction is presently unknown. If, however, these factors are tumor-derived, then functions of TIL in situ are likely to be affected to a greater extent than those of T lymphocytes in peripheral blood.

TIL AND TUMOR-INDUCED IMMUNOMODULATION IN HNC

Current evidence from both animal experiments and clinical studies indicates that various events that take place at the site of tumor progression are regulated by soluble products, cytokines, released in part by tumor cells, in part by infiltrating mononuclear cells and in part by stromal or other tissue cells present in the tumor microenvironment. These mutual interactions probably determine the ability of TIL to function in situ and, consequently, both the prognosis and disease outcome. While emphasizing the importance of the tumor microenvironment on anti-tumor effectiveness of TIL in situ, it is necessary to recall that HNC may secrete immunosuppressive as well as immunostimulatory factors.[31-34] Tumor-induced immunosuppression is a well-described phenomenon in HNC.[35,36] Of more than 60 SCCHN cell lines established in my laboratory, many have been shown to produce prostaglandin E_2 (PGE_2) spontaneously, as determined by assaying their supernatants in a radioimmunoassay.[37] Furthermore, such PGE_2-containing supernatants of SCCHN cell lines were shown to inhibit generation of LAK cells in vitro from normal PBL in the presence of IL2.[37] Although SCCHN cell lines produce significantly less PGE_2 than normal keratinocytes in primary cultures,[37] TIL at the tumor site are likely to be exposed continuously to PGE_2, which has been identified as an immunosuppressive factor in patients with SCCHN.[37] These tumors are known to also produce other immunosuppressive factors, such as p15E.[38,39] In addition, MNC which accumulate in or around the tumor, and which have been shown to express activation markers and produce cytokines in the tumor microenvironment (see above), may themselves be a source of immunosuppressive cytokines such as TGF-β.[24] Indeed, our ISH for TGF-β gene expression in SCCHN has indicated that the cells infiltrating the tumor stroma or those accumulating around tumor in I-LN,[40] express the message for this cytokine (Fig. 10.4B). It is thus likely that soluble factors produced either by the tumor or by TIL contribute to the immunosuppressive environment present in or around the tumor.

T lymphocytes which accumulate at the site of tumor growth may be initially activated by tumor-associated antigens (TAA). To demonstrate that SCCHN are capable of inducing activation of human immune effector cells, we used an in vitro model, in which freshly-isolated human NK cells were co-incubated with irradiated human SCCHN cell line, PCI-1, with or without the presence of IL-2. Expression of mRNA for IL-2R, perforin, and various cytokines in NK cells was observed within 5h.[41] Contact with the tumor cells stimulated NK cells to proliferate, secrete IFN-γ, TNF-α and soluble IL-2R, upregulate cell surface expression of IL-2R p55 and p75 as well as FcγRIII (CD16), and mediate higher levels of anti-tumor activity in ^{51}Cr-release assays. These observations indicated that human SCCHN could indeed induce NK-cell activation, as measured by many different parameters, as well as proliferation of NK cells and augmentation of their anti-tumor function.[41] The SCCHN-induced effects were observed in the absence of IL2, although exogenous IL2 greatly augmented proliferation and up-regulated cytolytic function of NK cells.[41] If similar events take place in vivo, then it is possible that before activated TIL have a chance to develop into anti-tumor effector cells, the tumor intervenes by means of immunosuppressive factors which inhibit lymphocyte functions. This inhibition might be quite selective, depending on the tumor environment, and/or the type of infiltrating lymphocyte. For example, CD8⁺ T lymphocytes were found to be particularly sensitive to tumor-induced inhibition, and their proliferation was found to be inhibited to a significantly greater extent than that of CD4⁺ TIL obtained from various human tumors.[42] In patients with HNC, tumor-related selective activation by the tumor of lymphoid "suppressor" cells has been proposed as a major mechanism of immunosuppression.[43,44] However, in our own studies, we have failed to identify "suppressor" T lymphocytes among effector cells separated from I-LNL, NI-LNL or PBL of patients with HNC or obtain support for selective activation of tumor-specific suppressor cells by SCCHN cell lines.[27] Another mechanism of immunosuppression might operate at the level of signaling or signal transduction, as recently proposed by Ochoa and colleagues.[28,30] Such alterations in TCR-mediated signal transduction pathway may be more obvious in TIL than PBL, and certain subpopulations of effector cells may be more susceptible than others to tumor-induced immunosuppression.[1] The result may be that SCCHN are intensely infiltrated with lymphocytes, most of which are functionally paralyzed in the tumor microenvironment. Additionally, tumor-derived immunosuppressive factors present in the circulation are probably responsible for decreased systemic immune responses commonly seen in patients with HNC.[35,45-47]

While tumor-mediated immunosuppression has been well-documented in the HNC literature,[35,36,39] the ability of these tumors to activate and promote proliferation of immune cells has received relatively little attention. In vitro evidence for this phenomenon comes largely from MLTC studies with freshly-isolated human TIL, LNL or PBL co-cultured in the presence of AuTu cells, and with or without the addition of IL-2, in order to outgrow autotumor-specific T lymphocytes.[34,48,49] Using MLTC, in which autologous or allogeneic SCCHN cell lines served as stimulators, we have obtained evidence that many of these lines are able to produce soluble factors stimulatory for human T cells, specifically, CD4⁺ T lymphocytes and human NK cells.[34] Incubation of purified CD4⁺ cells in the presence of such factors, partially-purified recently from supernatants of a SCCHN cell line (PCI-50), and in the absence of IL2, has led to activation, proliferation, and up-regulation of anti-tumor cytotoxicity and cytokine production in these T cells.[34] While purification of the SCCHN-derived T-cell stimulatory factor(s) is in progress, our preliminary results indicate that HNC are capable of producing immunostimulatory factors, which might play an important role in modulating functional responses of MNC present at the tumor site. Studies of others also provide evidence that SCCHN are capable of producing immunostimulatory cytokines.[32,33]

Functional studies with TIL obtained from HNC indicate that a variety of factors, including the intrinsic property of each tumor to produce immunomodulating cytokines, contribute to phenotypic and functional properties of these cells at the tumor site. As TIL have normal expression of activation and memory surface markers, it is possible that the functional impairments are acquired by TIL after they reach the activated state at the tumor site. With a better understanding of the nature of functional deficits detectable in freshly-isolated TIL, it is now possible to explain the apparent contradiction between phenotypic markers of activation expressed on these cells and their decreased immunocompetence. Interactions between TIL and tumor cells are complex and may result not only in selective immunosuppression but also immunostimulation of infiltrating cells. Hence, correlations of the phenotypic characteristics of TIL or the intensity of TIL infiltrates with prognosis or survival are bound to be inaccurate. Instead, the outcome might depend on the level of anti-tumor responses TIL are capable of mediating in a given tumor microenvironment. With respect to immunotherapy of HNC, it would be, therefore, important to prevent undesirable inhibition of immune function and to augment anti-tumor responses of TIL in situ. Little can be done about the former, until the nature of inhibitory factors produced by HNC and the mechanism of their immunosuppressive activity are understood. On the other hand, efforts to activate TIL and use them for therapy have been ongoing, with the focus on (a) generation of autotumor-specific CTL in patients with HNC and (b) up-regulation of locoregional responses of TIL with cytokines delivered perilesionally.

GENERATION OF ANTI-TUMOR EFFECTOR CELLS FROM TIL

TIL isolated from HNC generally, but not always, proliferate well in the presence of high concentration of IL2 (6,000 IU/ml). Several years ago, we compared TIL and A-PBL for the ability to respond to IL2 and proliferate in long-term cultures.[18,50] As shown in Table 10.2, TIL achieved a higher-fold proliferation in these cultures than A-PBL, although the median number of days these cells proliferated in vitro was comparable for TIL and A-PBL. In our experience, proliferation of TIL from HNC was highly variable, and in some cases, TIL would not proliferate at all.[18,50] TIL frequently, but not always, showed a delayed proliferative response relative to A-PBL (Fig. 10.6), and TIL from primary SCCHN did not begin proliferating until day 15-20, while TIL from recurrent tumors had a lag time of 20-40 days, as compared to 4-5 days for A-PBL.[18] Although delayed in response, TIL proliferated at a rapid rate, achieving in some cases extremely high fold-proliferation late in cultures.

Anti-tumor cytotoxicity of TIL expanded in the presence of IL2 was compared at various time periods in culture with that of A-PBL (Fig. 10.6). The main issue addressed by these experiments has been to determine whether TIL obtained from patients with HNC are a better source of anti-tumor, and especially, of AuTu-specific effector cells. Generation of non-MHC-restricted cytotoxic effector cells with broad anti-tumor reactivity can be successfully accomplished using unseparated TIL and TIL or LNL enriched in $CD8^+$ T cells by panning on anti-CD8 antibody-coated surfaces.[51] In many instances, TIL were a better source of non-MHC-restricted effector cells than A-PBL, as shown in Table 10.3. When cultured $CD8^+$ and $CD4^+$ T cells obtained from LNL of patients with HNC and separated by panning on the anti-CD8 or anti-CD4 antibody-coated flasks were tested for anti-tumor cytotoxicity using a panel of SCCHN cell lines established in our laboratory (Table 10.4), a modest degree of enrichment in cytotoxicity against SCCHN cell lines, but not K562 or melanoma cell line, was obtained in the captured $CD8^+$ T cells.[51] However, repeated attempts to obtain AuTu-specific $CD3^+CD8^+$ CTL from TIL of SCCHN have been unsuccessful in our hands. In vitro sensitization of TIL with irradiated AuTu cells (fresh or available as cell lines) in long-term culture in the presence of IL2 invariably resulted in outgrowth of broadly-reactive anti-tumor effector cells.[49] Specific

Table 10.2. Interleukin 2-induced proliferation of TIL and A-PBL obtained from patients with HNC[a]

	TIL	A-PBL	TIL versus A-PBL[b] p Value
Fold Expansion	69 (0-35 x 10^4)	27 (0-1200)	< 0.01
Days in Culture	56 (0-88)	50 (0-80)	NS[c]

[a] Data presented as medians. Ranges given in parenthesis. Paired samples from 17 patients were tested.
[b] Wilcoxon's signed rank test.
[c] NS = not significant.

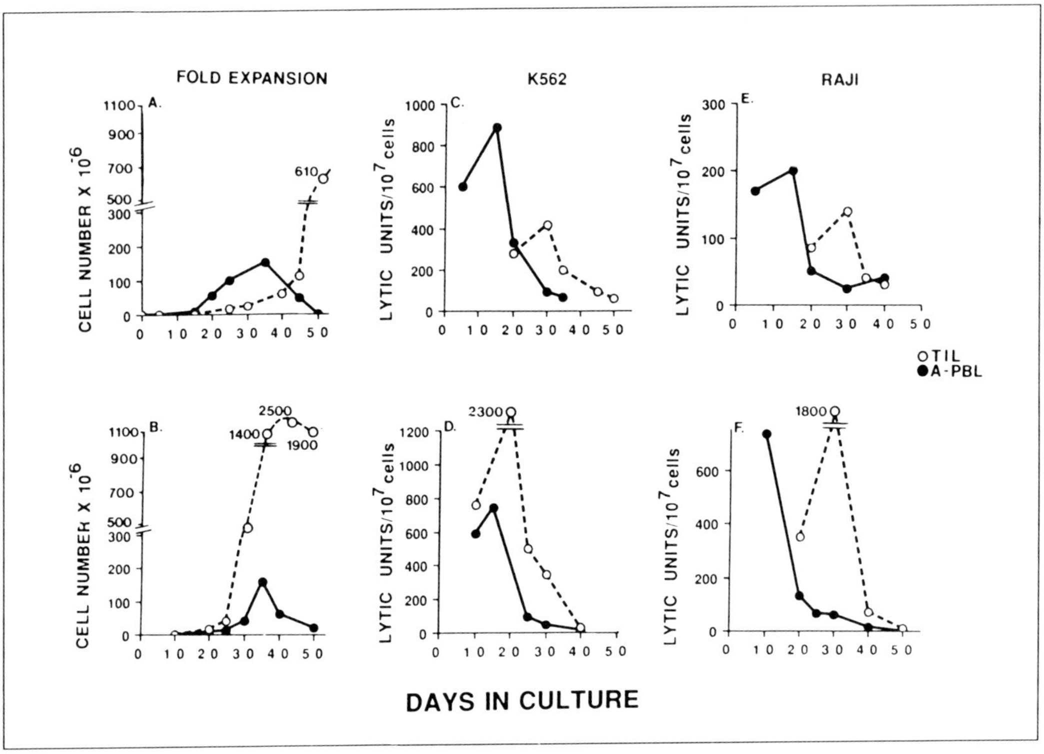

Fig. 10.6. Proliferation and anti-tumor cytotoxicity measured serially in representative cultures of paired TIL and A-PBL grown in the presence of 6,000 IU/ml of rIL2. Panels A, C and E show fold expansion (A), and cytotoxicity against K562 targets (C) and against Raji targets (E) for TIL-A-PBL obtained from a patient with primary, untreated squamous cell carcinoma of the head and neck. Panels B, D and F show similar data for TIL/A-PBL obtained from a patient with squamous cell carcinoma of the head and neck treated with radiation prior to surgery.

T-cell mediated responses to autologous SCCHN have been difficult to demonstrate in general, although a large body of evidence exists for the ability of these tumors to induce humoral responses[52,53] and to induce non-MHC-restricted effector mechanisms.[18]

Recently, we have succeeded in generation of autotumor-reactive CTL lines from PBL of a patient with SCC of the tongue.[48] The cultured CTL were $CD3^+CD8^+CD11b^-$ $HLA\text{-}DR^+$ $TCRa/\beta^+$ (Fig. 10.7). When tested in 4h ^{51}Cr-release assays against various SCCHN lines (n = 11) and a variety of non-squamous human tumor (n = 9) and normal (n = 5) cell targets, the CTL were found to lyse the autologous SCCHN cell line (PCI-50) and seven allogeneic SCCHN lines: PCI-1, -2, -4A, -4B, 13, -30 and -38 (Fig. 10.8). Of these tumor cell lines, PCI-13, -30 and -38 shared HLA-A2 locus with the AuTu, PCI-50, while PCI-4A and -4B shared HLA-B44 with AuTu. Lysis of AuTu ($A2^+B44^+$), PCI-13 ($A2^+B44^-$) and PCI-4b ($A2^-B44^+$) by the CTL was efficiently inhibited by mAbs to CD3, CD8, TCR-α/β or the class I major histocompatibility complex (MHC) Ags. The mAbs to HLA-A2 Ags inhibited lysis of PCI-50 or PCI-13 targets by the CTL. In cold target inhibition assays, unlabeled PCI-4B or PCI-13 cells inhibited CTL lysis of AuTu targets. The CTL incubated in the presence of the $HLA\text{-}A2^+$ SCCHN PCI-50 or -13, but not an $HLA\text{-}A2^+$ gastric carcinoma, produced TNF-α, IFN-γ and GM-CSF. The CTL were tested for their TCR Vβ gene expression by polymerase chain reaction (PCR). At week 10 in culture, the time of the highest AuTu cytotoxicity mediated by

Table 10.3. Anti-tumor cytotoxicity in IL-2-expanded cultures of TIL and A-PBL obtained from patients with HNC[a]

	TIL	A-PBL	TIL versus A-PBL[b]p Value
LU/10^3 cells	26 (0-184)	39 (0-313)	<0.05
TLU	900 (0-75 x 10^{-3})	175 (–15 x 10^3)	p<0.01

[a] TLU = LU per culture x cell number. Data are the highest median cytotoxicity achieved in culture and measured against NK-cell resistant fresh tumor cell targets against fresh ovarian carcinoma cells (ranges in parenthesis). Paired samples from 22 patients were tested.
[b] Wilcoxon's signed rank test.

Table 10.4. Enrichment in anti-tumor cytotoxicity against SCCHN cell lines mediated by positively selected CD8⁺ lymph node lymphocytes obtained from patients with SCCHN and tested against various tumor cell targets

Tumor cell target[a]	Captured $CD8^+$ (n = 10)	Captured $CD4^+$ (n = 6)
K562	880 ± 490	630 ± 230
PCI-1	4420 ± 2100[b]	760 ± 520
PCI-13	3980 ± 2120[b]	1070 ± 720
PCI-4A	3100 ± 1500[b]	80 ± 40
FEMX	350 ± 310	100 ± 90

[a] Cytotoxicity was determined in 4 hour ^{51}Cr-release assays performed with a panel of tumor cell targets including Daudi and the targets listed. PCI cell lines are NK cell-resistant SCCHN cell lines established in our laboratory.[79] FEMX is an NK-resistant melanoma cell line. Effector cells were $CD8^+$ or $CD4^+$ LNLs captured on antibody-coated surfaces and expanded in the presence of IL-2 for 15 days as described earlier.[51]
[b] Significant ($p < 0.05$) differences between cytotoxicity mediated by $CD8^+$ versus $CD4^+$ effectors.

the CTL line, Vβ6 was expressed by 26% of T cells. Three clones, obtained by limiting dilution from 10-week CTL and selected for high cytotoxicity against AuTu, were found to be Vβ6⁺. Further analysis of the specificity of these clones indicated lytic activity against PCI-13 ($A2^+B44^-$), but not PCI-4B ($A2^-B44^+$) targets. In 16-week cultures, which retained AuTu cytotoxicity, as well as Vβ6 expression, TCR Vβ2 was also expressed at high frequency (29%), and AuTu-reactive clones were found to be Vβ2⁺. Our results indicate that at least two different CTL populations (Vβ6⁺ and Vβ2⁺) are able to recognize a SCCHN-associated Ag(s) and that the Vβ6⁺ T cells are HLA-A2 restricted, while Vβ2⁺ T cells may be HLA-B44 restricted.[48]

The results described above clearly indicate that it is possible to generate and culture in vitro AuTu-reactive CTL in some patients with HNC, but they also raise questions about difficulties encountered in obtaining these effector cells more consistently. The one intriguing aspect of the process of CTL generation in the patient described above has been that all three separate attempts to establish CTL from peripheral blood over a period of 2 years after surgery were successful, while we failed to obtain CTL under the same culture conditions from TIL of this patient or from TIL or PBL of at least 10 other patients with SCCHN for whom AuTu cell lines were established. It might be that in those patients with HNC who have circulating CTL precursors, PBL are a better source of CTL than TIL, which are likely to be functionally compromised due to immunosuppressive effects encountered in the tumor microenvironment. In view of considerable difficulties encountered in generation of CTL from TIL or LNL of patients with HNC, we and others have considered an alternative approach of in situ activation of TIL with exogenous cytokines as a means for up-regulating local anti-tumor responses.[54]

LOCOREGIONAL THERAPY OF HNC WITH TIL AND/OR CYTOKINES

Previous results from my laboratory have indicated that locoregional immunotherapy of SCCHN with effector cells and/or cytokines such as IL2 or IFN-γ or supernatants of in vitro activated NK cells are effective in the control of tumor growth and lead to regression of established tumors

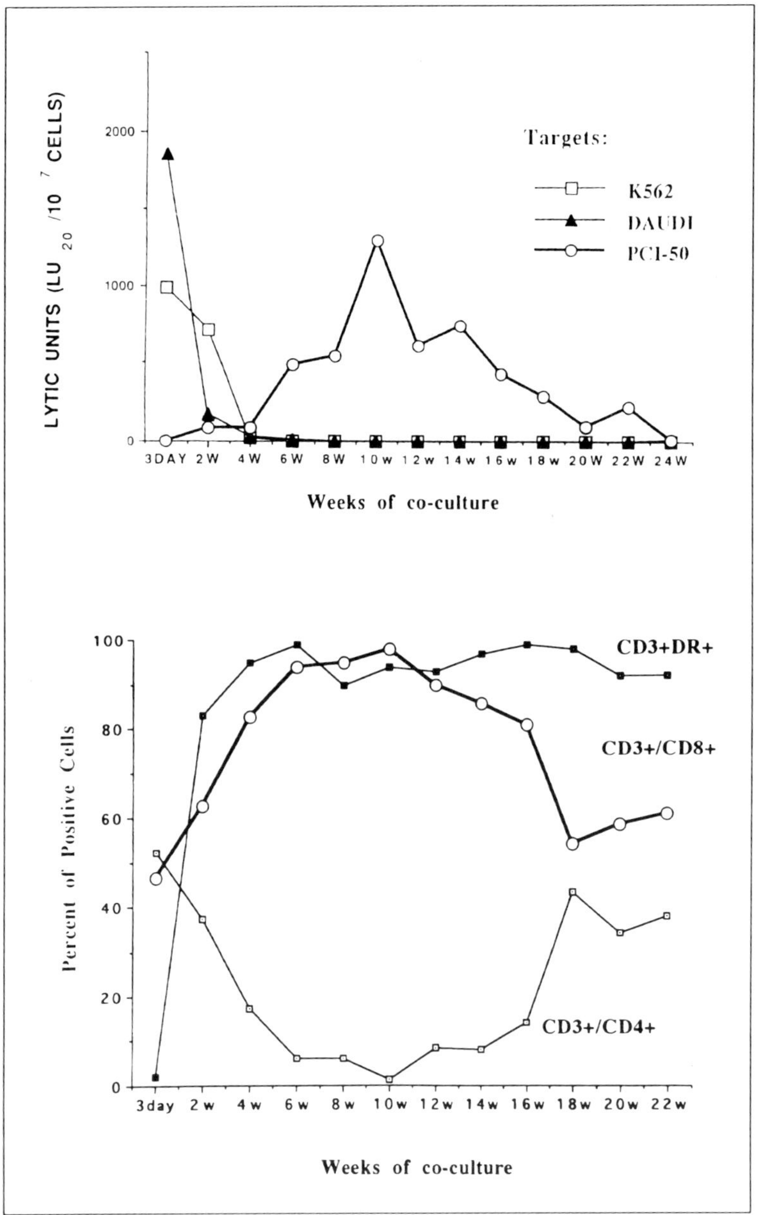

Fig. 10.7. Changes in cytotoxicity against K562, Daudi or autologous SCCHN cell line (PCI-50) of PBL obtained from a patient with SCC of the tongue and co-cultured with AuTu in the presence of IL2 (300 IU/ml) and IL4 (300 U/ml) are shown in A. In B, changes in the phenotype of the cultured cells over 22 weeks are shown. At the time of optimal AuTu cytotoxicity (weeks 8 to 16), the culture contained primarily CD3⁺CD8⁺DR⁺ T lymphocytes. Reproduced with permission from Yasumura et al, Cancer Res. 53:1461, 1993.

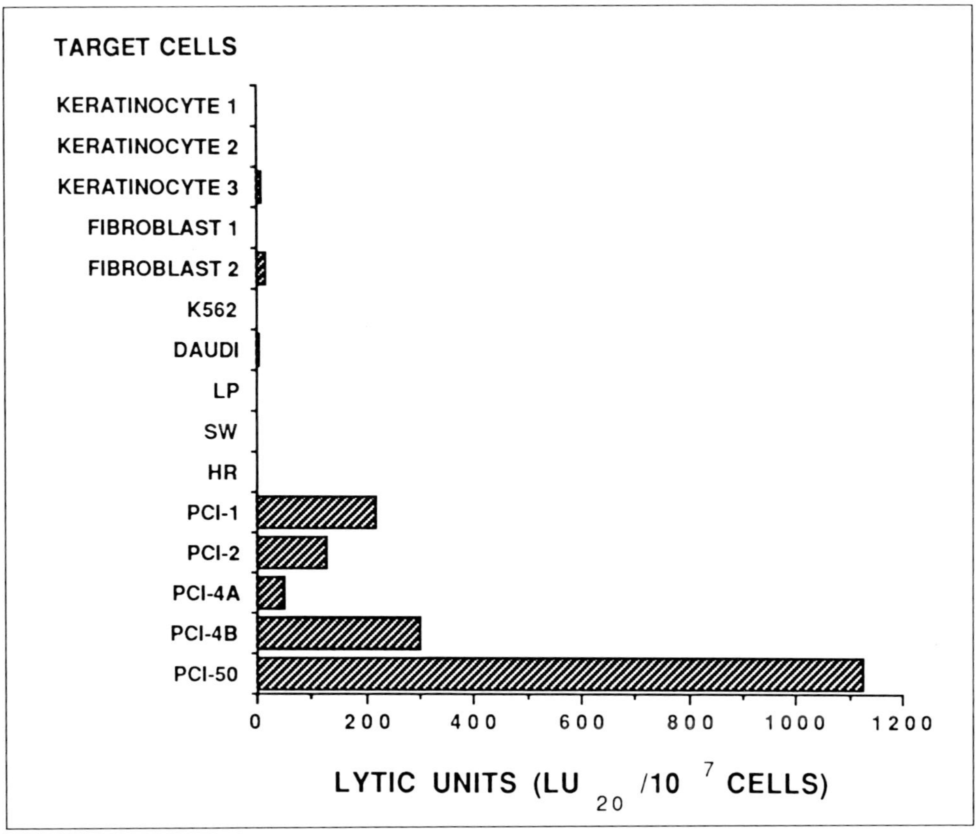

Fig. 10.8. Cytotoxicity of the AuTu-reactive CTL line established in MLTC from PBL of a patient with a SCC of the tongue. PCI-50 is the autologous tumor cell line. PCI targets are allogeneic SCCHN cell lines; HR is a gastric carcinoma, LP and SW are cholangiocarcinomas; fibroblasts and keratinocytes are from primary cultures. All cell lines were established and cultured in our laboratory. Cytotoxicity was tested in one assay Reproduced with permission from Yasumura et al, Cancer Res. 53:1461, 1993.

in a xenograft model of SCCHN in immunosuppressed nude mice.[55,56] Experiments now in progress attempt to evaluate anti-tumor activities of the available CTL lines both in vitro in a spheroid model of SCCHN[57] and in vivo in the xenograft SCCHN model established by us and described earlier.[55,56] At the same time, it would be important to compare in vivo effectiveness of CTL versus non-MHC restricted effector cells such as human IL2-activated NK cells against established SCCHN in this experimental model. The availability of well-characterized effector cells and of AuTu cell lines is obviously a prerequisite for these in vivo studies, aimed at obtaining further insights into effector-tumor cell interactions. At the same time, AuTu-specific T cells we have generated are being used as probes for the identification of TAA, which initiate and sustain effector-tumor cell interactions in vivo.

Clinical trials evaluating effectiveness of locoregional delivery of biologic agents, whether cytokines administered alone or together with effector cells, to patients with advanced HNC have been in progress in the U.S. and in Europe.[58-63] HNC represent a logical choice for locoregional therapy with biologics, because they tend to grow and recur locally, are generally well infiltrated with immune effector cells, are surrounded by an extensive lymph node network, and are well vascularized and accessible to the local delivery of therapeutic agents. An argument can also be made that patients with advanced HNC often have cellular immune defects, and that locoregional administration of biologic agents with known up-regulatory effects on functions of immune cells might be expected to be beneficial in these individuals. The vast majority of HNC patients with advanced, recurrent disease fail to respond to surgery and/or radiotherapy, and chemotherapy has been shown to have no significant impact on survival.[64] It appears that novel therapeutic approaches, including locoregional administration of cytokines, with the intent to up-regulate antitumor activities of TIL in situ, offer an opportunity for improving survival in this group of patients.

With this rationale in mind and based on our in vivo studies in animal models, we have performed a phase Ib clinical trial in patients with inoperable SCCHN who received perilesional and/or intranodal injections of IL2.[54,63] This trial provided us with an opportunity to monitor local and systemic immune responses of patients treated with escalating doses (2×10^2, 2×10^3, 2×10^4, 2×10^5, 2×10^6 and 4×10^6 U) of IL2 daily 5 times/week for 2 weeks. Tumor biopsies were obtained before and after IL2 therapy. Tumor tissue was provided for histology, and the remaining fresh tissue was divided for snap-freezing in -75°C and for separation of TIL and tumor cells. Immunophenotyping of TIL performed on cryostat sections of paired pre- and post-IL2 biopsy tissues showed increases after IL2 therapy in the number of T cells ($p = 0.005$), NK ($CD16^+$) cells ($p = 0.0001$), $CD25^+$ cells ($p = 0.004$), and HLA-DR^+ cells ($p = 0.001$) accumulating in the tumor stroma. In the tumor parenchyma, NK cells ($p = 0.0001$) and HLA-DR^+ cells ($p = 0.003$) were increased after IL2 therapy. The T:NK cell ratios in the tumor stroma and parenchyma were decreased after therapy, suggesting selective accumulation of NK cells. By flow cytometry, TIL recovered from post-IL2 biopsy tissues were enriched ($p < 0.05$) in $CD3^-CD56^+$ (NK) cells. ISH with [^{35}S] cDNA probes for cytokines and IL2R indicated that the numbers of cells expressing mRNA for IL-2, TNF-α, IL-1-β, IFN-γ, TGF-β, and IL2R p55 or p70 were increased in post-IL2 biopsy tissues as compared to pre-IL2 tissues. Cytolytic activity of TIL isolated from post-IL-2 tissues was also increased, as determined in 4h ^{51}Cr-release assays against K562 targets (12 ± 3 mean lytic units (LU)/10^7 cells ± SEM pre-IL-2 versus 46 ± 13 post-IL2; n = 16) and against AuTu (13 ± 8 versus 68 ± 26; n = 9). Fresh TIL of one clinical responder showed relatively high levels (195 LU) of autotumor cytotoxicity after IL2 therapy versus no activity prior to therapy. In the blood, NK and LAK cell activity, and percentages of $CD3^-$ $CD56^+$ NK cells and of activated ($CD25^+$) T-lymphocytes were increased for all doses of IL2. A significant dose-response effect was observed for the percentage of $CD3^-$ $CD56^+$ NK cells and LAK cell cytotoxicity against AuTu, with the highest values observed at the two highest doses of IL-2. Our data have indicated that local as well as systemic activation of anti-tumor effector cells occurred during local administration of IL-2 in patients with SCCHN.[54] We have demonstrated significant accumulation of activated MNC and up-regulation of their anti-tumor activity as a result of IL-2 therapy. Increases in the number of TIL-T which expressed activation antigens, as well as higher cytotoxicity of fresh TIL recovered from post-treatment tissue specimens that we have observed, clearly indicate that local cell-mediated responses have improved following two short cycles of daily locoregional IL2 therapy. Increased and selective accumulation during therapy with IL2 of activated NK cells in the tumor stroma and parenchyma further indicates that IL2 not only had effects on the number of infiltrating cells but also altered the composition of MNC infiltrates in the tumor.

A variety of other therapeutic approaches targeted at up-regulation of local or locoregional responses of TIL are being currently considered. Among them are strategies based on transduction of cytokine genes into AuTu cells[65,66] or fibroblasts[67] with an intent to implant such genetically engineered cells as a local source of cytokines. In SCCHN, transfer of fibroblasts transduced with IFN-γ genes may be particularly attractive in view of in vitro evidence that this cytokine has direct growth inhibiting effects on these tumors.[68]

Transduction of cytokine receptor genes into tumor cells could also be explored as a therapeutic option in HNC. In this respect, we have demonstrated that genetic modification of IL-2R expression on IL-2R$^+$ SCCHN significantly altered proliferative responses of the tumor to IL-2, resulting in a significant growth inhibition of tumor growth.[69] Similarly, our recent observations that IL-4 promotes growth of SCCHN cell lines and that these tumors express IL-4R[70] suggest that the administration of anti-IL-4 reagents or attempts to prevent IL-4 production by TIL may be therapeutically important.

Adoptive transfer of effector cell subsets activated in vitro and selected for their ability to eliminate tumor cells in vivo is another therapeutic option in HNC. The cells can be delivered to the tumor area, either perilesionally, intratumorally or intralymphatically, alone or together with a cytokine or a combination of cytokines.[58] For example, subsets of NK cells have been recently generated in our laboratory and tested for anti-tumor effects in vitro using SCCHN spheroids and in vivo in SCCHN xenografts established in nude mice.[57] Human SCCHN contain few NK cells, and it could be argued that their locoregional delivery might not only provide anti-tumor effector cells but also a source of many cytokines which these cells are known to produce.[71] In fact, the supernatant of IL2-activated human NK cells has been shown to have potent anti-tumor effects both in vitro on SCCHN cell lines and in vivo in the SCCHN xenograft nude mouse model.[41]

Another therapeutic strategy takes advantage of the current availability of mAbs to SCCHN Ags.[72-74] Such mAbs are being currently explored not only for delivery of radionucleotides to the tumor but also for arming of effector cells such as NK cells, in order to target them more efficiently to the tumor.

To up-regulate in vivo activities of T cells present in or around the tumor, it might be possible to resort to vaccination with natural or synthetic tumor vaccines. This approach is particularly promising today, because of recent advances made in purification of SCCHN-associated Ags[75] and in understanding of the Ag presentation process to T cells.[76] Since SCCHN might express shared TAA,[49] vaccination of patients with tumor cells transduced with genes for such shared TAA could be possible in the future. The rationale behind this strategy is the augmentation of sites on the tumor capable of inducing specific T-cell response in vivo. Since several cellular adhesion cellular adhesion molecules (CAMs) have been shown to be involved in T-cell activation,[77,78] it might be possible to further augment T-cell responses in vivo by transducing tumor cells with ligands for CAM genes. In the future, these and other therapeutic approaches should be particularly vigorously tested in HNC, as many of these tumors are easily accessible and thus amenable to local or locoregional immunologic intervention.

References

1. Whiteside TL. Tumor-Infiltrating Lymphocytes in Human Malignancies. Austin: RG Landes Co, 1993.
2. Vose BM, Moore M. Human tumor-infiltrating lymphocytes: A marker of host response. Sem Hematol 22:27-40, 1985.
3. Colombo P, Modesti A, Parmiani G, Forni G. Local cytokine availability elicits tumor rejection and systemic immunity through granulocyte-T lymphocyte cross talk. Cancer Res 52:4853-4857, 1992.
4. Underwood JCE. Lymphoreticular infiltration in human tumors: Prognostic and biological implications. A review. Br J Cancer 30:538-548, 1974.
5. Ioachim HL. The stromal reaction of tumors: An expression of immune surveillance. JNCI 57:465-475, 1976.
6. Hiratsuka H, Imamura M, Ishii Y, Kohama GI, Kikuchi K. Immunohistologic detection of lymphocyte subpopulations infiltrating in human oral cancer with special ref-

erence to its clinical significance. Cancer 53:2456-2466, 1984.

7. Zeromski J, Szmeja Z, Rewers A, Kruk-Zagajewska A. Immunofluorescent assessment of tumor-infiltrating cells in laryngeal carcinoma. Application of monoclonal antibodies. Acta Otolaryngol 102:325-332, 1986.
8. Guo H, Rabin BS, Johnson JT, Paradis IL. Lymphocyte phenotypes at tumor margins in patients with head and neck cancer 1986(UnPub)
9. Wolf GT, Hudson JL, Peterson KA, Miller HL, McClatchey KD. Lymphocyte subpopulations infiltrating squamous carcinomas of the head and neck: Correlations with extent of tumor and prognosis. Arch Otolaryngol Head Neck Surg 95:142-152, 1986.
10. Bennet SH, Futrell JW, Roth JA, Hoye RC, Ketcham AS. Prognostic significance of histological host response in cancer of the larynx or hypopharynx. Cancer 28:1255-1265, 1971.
11. Hirota J, Veta E, Osaki T, Ogawa Y. Immunohistologic study of mononuclear cell infiltrates in oral squamous cell carcinomas. Head Neck Surg 12:118-125, 1990.
12. Wanebo HJ. Immunobiology of head and neck cancer: Basic concepts. Head Neck Surg 2:42-55, 1979.
13. Rosenberg SA, Spiess P, Lafreniere R. A new approach to adoptive immunotherapy of cancer with tumor-infiltrating lymphocytes. Science 233:1318-1321, 1986.
14. Rosenberg SA, Packard BS, Aebersold PM, Solomon D, Topalian SL, Toy ST, Simon P, Lotze MT, Yang JC, Seipp CA, Simpson C, Carter C, Bock S, Schwartzentruber D, Wei JP, White DE. Use of tumor-infiltrating lymphocytes and interleukin-2 in the immunotherapy of patients with metastatic melanoma. A preliminary report. N Engl J Med 319:1676-1680, 1988.
15. Aebersold P, Hyatt C, Johnson S, Hines K, Korcak L, Sanders M, Lotze M, Topalian S, Yang J, Rosenberg SA. Lysis of autologous melanoma cells by tumor-infiltrating lymphocytes: Association with clinical response. JNCI 83:932-937, 1991.
16. Whiteside TL, Jost LM, Herberman RB. Tumor-infiltrating lymphocytes: Potential and limitations to their use for cancer therapy. Crit Rev Oncol Hematol 25-47, 1992.
17. Snyderman CH, Heo DS, Chen K, Whiteside TL, Johnson JT. T-cell markers in tumor-infiltrating lymphocytes of head and neck cancer. Head Neck Surg 11:331-336, 1989.
18. Heo DS, Whiteside TL, Johnson JT, Chen K, Barnes EL, Herberman RB. Long-term interleukin 2-dependent growth and cytotoxic activity of tumor-infiltrating lymphocytes (TIL) from human squamous cell carcinomas of the head and neck. Cancer Res 47:6353-6362, 1987.
19. Chen K, Demetris AJ, Van Thiel DH, Whiteside TL. Double immunoenzyme staining method for analysis of tissue and blood lymphocyte subsets with monoclonal antibodies. Lab Invest 56:114-119, 1987.
20. Whiteside TL, Heo DS, Chen K, Adler A, Johnson JT, Herberman RB. Expansion of tumor-infiltrating lymphocytes from human solid tumors in interleukin 2. In: Truitt RL, Gale RP, Bortin MM, eds. Progress in Clinical and Biological Research Volume 244. New York: Alan R Liss Inc, 1987:213-222.
21. Whiteside TL, Miescher S, MacDonald RH, Von Fliedner V. Separation of tumor-infiltrating lymphocytes from tumor cells in human solid tumors. A comparison between velocity sedimentation and discontinuous density gradients. J Immunol Methods 90:221-233, 1986.
22. Snyderman CH, Heo DS, Johnson JT, d'Amico F, Barnes L, Whiteside TL. Functional and phenotypic analysis of lymphocytes isolated from tumors and lymph nodes of patients with head and neck cancer. Arch Otolaryngol Head Neck Surg 117:899-905, 1991.
23. Whiteside TL, Miescher S, Hurlimann J, Von Fliedner V. Separation phenotyping and limiting-dilution analysis of T-lymphocytes infiltrating human solid tumors. Int J Cancer 37:803-811, 1986.
24. Vitolo D, Letessier EM, Johnson JT, Whiteside TL. Immunologic effector cells in head and neck cancer. JNCI Monographs 13:203-208, 1992.

25. Whiteside TL, Miescher S, Hurlimann J, Moretta L, Von Fliedner V. Clonal analysis and in situ characterization of lymphocytes infiltrating human breast carcinomas. Cancer Immunol Immunother 23:169-178, 1986.
26. Miescher S, Whiteside TL, Carrel S, Von Fliedner V. Functional properties of tumor-infiltrating and blood lymphocytes in patients with solid tumors: Effects of tumor cells and their supernatants on proliferative responses of lymphocytes. J Immunol 136:1899-1907, 1986.
27. Letessier EM, Sacchi M, Johnson JT, Herberman RB, Whiteside TL. The absence of lymphoid suppressor cells in tumor-involved lymph nodes of patients with head and neck cancer. Cell Immunol 130:446-458, 1990.
28. Mizoguchi H, O'Shea JJ, Longo DL, Loeffler CM, McVicar DW, Ochoa AC. Alterations in signal transduction molecules in T lymphocytes from tumor-bearing mice. Science 258:1795-1798, 1992.
29. Nakagomi H, Petersson M, Magnusson I, Juhlin C, Matsuda M, Mellstedt H, Taupin J-L, Vivier E, Anderson P, Kiessling R. Decreased expression of the signal-transducing zeta chains in tumor-infiltrating T-cells and NK cells of patients with colorectal carcinoma. Cancer Res 53:5610-5612, 1993.
30. Finke JH, Zea AH, Stanley J, Longo DL, Mizoguchi H, Tubbs RR, Wiltrout RH, O'Shea JJ, Kudoh S, Klein E, Bukowski RM, Ochoa AC. Loss of T-cell receptor zeta chain and $p56^{lck}$ in T-cells infiltrating human renal cell carcinoma. Cancer Res 53:5613-5616, 1993.
31. Johnson JT, Rabin BS, Wagner RL. Prostaglandin E2 of the upper aerodigestive tract. Ann Otol Rhinol Laryngol 96:213-216, 1987.
32. Luger TA, Uchida A, Kock A, Colot M, Micksche M. Human epidermal cell and squamous carcinoma cells synthesize a cytokine that augments natural killer cell activity. J Immunol 134:2477-2483, 1985.
33. Luger TA, Stadler BM, Luger BM, Sztein M, Schmidt JA, Hawley-Nelson P, Grabner G, Oppenheim JJ. Characteristic of an epidermal cell thymocyte-activating factor (ETAF) by human epidermal cells and a human squamous cell carcinoma cell line. J Invest Dermatol 81:187-93, 1983.
34. Hirabayashi H, Yasumura S, Lin W-c, Amoscato A, Johnson JT, Herberman RB, Whiteside TL. Production by human squamous cell carcinomas of a factor inducing activation and proliferation of immune cells. Arch Otolaryngol Head Neck Surg, In press 1994.
35. Berlinger NT. Deficient immunity in head and neck cancer is due to excessive monocyte production of prostaglandins. Laryngoscope 94:1407-1410, 1984.
36. Lapointe H, Lampe H, Banerjee D. Head and neck squamous cell line-induced suppression of in vitro lymphocyte proliferation responses. Arch Otolaryngol Head Neck Surg 106:149-158, 1992.
37. Snyderman CH, Klapan I, Heo DS, Wagner R, Johnson JT, Whiteside TL. In vitro production of prostaglandin E2 by squamous cell carcinoma of the head and neck. Arch Otolaryngol Head Neck Surg, In press 1994.
38. Snyderman R, Cianciolo GJ. Immunosuppressive activity of the retroviral envelope protein p15E and its possible relationship to neoplasia. Immunol Today 5:240-242, 1984.
39. Tan IB, Drexhage HA, Mullink R, Hensen-Logmans S, DeHaan-Meulman M, Snow GB, Balm AJM. Immunohistochemical detection of retroviral-p15E-related material in carcinomas of the head and neck. Arch Otolaryngol Head Neck Surg 96:251-255, 1987.
40. Vitolo D, Kanbour A, Johnson JT, Herberman RB, Whiteside TL. In situ hybridization for cytokine gene transcripts in the solid tumor microenvironment. Eur J Cancer 3:371-377, 1993.
41. Rabinowich H, Vitolo D, Altarac S, Herberman RB, Whiteside TL. Role of cytokines in the adoptive immunotherapy of an experimental model of human head and neck cancer by human IL2-activated natural killer cells. J Immunol 149:340-349, 1992.
42. Miescher S, Stoeck M, Qiao L, Barras C, Barrelet L, Von Fliedner V. Preferential clonogenic deficit of CD8+ T lymphocytes

infiltrating human solid tumors. Cancer Res 48:6992-6998, 1988.

43. Cozzolino F, Torcia M, Carossino AM, Giordani R, Selli C, Talini G, Reali E, Novelli A, Pistoia V, Ferrarini M. Characterization of cells from invaded lymph nodes in patients with solid tumors. J Exp Med 166:303-318, 1987.
44. Cozzolino F, Torcia M, Castigli E, Selli C, Giordani R, Carossino AM, Squadrelli M, Cagnoni M, Pistoia V, Ferrarini M. Presence of activated T-cells with a T8+ M1+ Leu 7+ surface phenotype in invaded lymph nodes from patients with solid tumors. JNCI 77:637-641, 1986.
45. Veltri RW, Rodman SM, Maxim PE, Baseler MW, Sprinkle PM. Immune complexes serum proteins cell-mediated immunity and immune regulation in patients with squamous cell carcinoma of the head and neck. Cancer 57:2295-2308, 1986.
46. Mickel RA, Kessler DJ, Taylor JM, Lichtenstein A. Natural killer cell cytotoxicity in the peripheral blood cervical lymph nodes and tumor of head and neck cancer patients. Cancer Res 48:5017-5022, 1988.
47. Schantz SV, Brown BW, Lira E, Taylor DL, Beddingfield N. Evidence for the role of natural immunity in the control of metastatic spread of head and neck cancer. Cancer Immunol Immunother 141-145, 1987.
48. Yasumura S, Weidmann E, Hirabayashi H, Johnson JT, Herberman RB, Whiteside TL. HLA restriction and T-cell receptor Vβ gene expression of cytotoxic T lymphocytes reactive with human squamous cell carcinoma of the head and neck. Int J Cancer 1994.
49. Yasumura S, Hirabayashi H, Schwartz DR, Toso JF, Johnson JT, Herberman RB, Whiteside TL. Human cytotoxic T-cell lines with restricted specificity for squamous cell carcinoma of the head and neck. Cancer Res 53:1461-1468, 1993.
50. Whiteside TL, Heo DS, Takagi S, Johnson JT, Iwatsuki S, Herberman RB. Cytolytic anti-tumor effector cells in long-term cultures of human tumor-infiltrating lymphocytes in recombinant interleukin 2. Cancer Immunol Immunother 26:1-10, 1988.
51. Letessier E, Heo DS, Okarma T, Johnson JT, Herberman RB, Whiteside TL. Enrichment in tumor-reactive CD8+ T lymphocytes by positive selection from the blood and lymph nodes of patients with head and neck cancer. Cancer Res 51:3891-3899, 1991.
52. Vlock DR, Arnold B, Humpierres J, Schwartz DR, Baker SR, Krause CJ, Swanson N, Carey TE. Serial studies of autologous antibody reactivity to SCCHN. Cancer Immunol Immunother 34:329-336, 1992.
53. Vlock DR, Scalise D, Schwartz DR, Richter DE, Krause CJ, Baker SR, Carey TE. Incidence of serum antibody reactivity to autologous head and neck cancer cell lines and augmentation of antibody reactivity following acid dissociation and ultrafiltration. Cancer Res 49:1361-1365, 1989.
54. Whiteside TL, Letessier E, Hirabayashi H, Vitolo D, Bryant J, Barnes L, Snyderman C, Johnson JT, Myers E, Herberman RB, Rubin J, Kirkwood JM, Vlock DR. Evidence for local and systemic activation of immune cells by peritumoral injections of interleukin 2 in patients with advanced squamous cell carcinoma of the head and neck. Cancer Res 53:5654-5662, 1993.
55. Sacchi M, Snyderman CH, Heo DS, Johnson JT, d'Amico F, Herberman RB, Whiteside TL. Local adoptive immunotherapy of human head and neck cancer xenografts in nude mice with lymphokine activated killer cells and interleukin 2. Cancer Res 50:3113-3118, 1990.
56. Sacchi M, Vitolo D, Sedlmayr P, Rabinowich H, Johnson JT, Herberman RB, Whiteside TL. Induction of tumor regression in experimental model of human head and neck cancer by human A-LAK cells and IL2. Int J Cancer 47:784-791, 1991.
57. Vujanovic NL, Yasumura S, Hirabayashi H, Lin WC, Watkins S, Herberman RB, Whiteside TL. Anti-tumor activities of human IL2-activated natural killer (A-NK) cells in solid tumor tissues. No Journal 1993.
58. Squdrelli-Saraceno M, Rivoltini L, Cantu G, Ravagni F, Parmiani G, Molinari R. Local adoptive immunotherapy of advanced head and neck tumors with LAK cells and interleukin 2. Tumori 76:566-571, 1991.

59. Rivoltini L, Gambacorti-Passerini C, Squadrelli-Saraceno M, Grosso MI, Cantu G, Molinari R, Orazi A, Parmiani G. In vivo interleukin 2-induced activation of lymphocyte-activated killer cells and tumor cytotoxic-T cells in cervical lymph nodes of patients with head and neck tumors. Cancer Res 50:5551-5557, 1990.
60. Musiani P, De Campora P, Valitutti S, Castellino F, Calearo CV, Jemma C, De Stefani A, Forni G. Effect of low doses of interleukin 2 injected perilymphatically and peritumorally in patients with advanced primary head and neck squamous cell carcinoma. J Biol Resp Mod 8:571-578, 1989.
61. Cortesina G, DeStefani A, Giovarelli M, Barioglio MG, Cavallo GP, Jemma C, Forni G. Treatment of recurrent squamous cell carcinoma of head and neck with low dose of interleukin-2 (IL2) injected perilymphatically. Cancer 62:2482-2487, 1988.
62. Mattijssen V, De Mulder PH, Schornagel JH, Verweij J, Van den Broek P, Galazka A, Roy S, Ruiter DJ. Clinical and immunopathological results of a Phase II study of perilymphatically injected interleukin 2 in locally far advanced non-pretreated head and neck squamous cell carcinoma J. Immunother 10:163-168, 1991.
63. Vlock DR, Snyderman C, Johnson J, Myers E, Rubin J, Dutcher J, Adams G. Phase 1b trial of the effect of peritumoral and intranodal injections of interleukin 2 in patients with advanced squamous cell carcinoma of the head and neck: An Eastern Cooperative Oncology Group Trial. J Immunother 1994.
64. Tannock IF, Browman G. Lack of evidence for a role of chemotherapy in the routine management of locally advanced head and neck cancer. J Clin Oncol 4:1121-1126, 1986.
65. Ogasawara M, Rosenberg SA. Enhanced expression of HLA molecules and stimulation of autologous human tumor-infiltrating lymphocytes following transduction of melanoma cells with gamma interferon genes. Cancer Res 53:3561-3568, 1993.
66. Jaffee EM, Dranoff G, Cohen LK, Hauda KM, Clift S, Marshall FF, Mulligan RC, Pardoll DM. High efficiency gene transfer into primary human tumor explants without cell selection. Cancer Res 53:2221-2226, 1993.
67. Scharfmann R, Axelrod JH, Verma IM. Long-term in vivo expression of retrovirus-mediated gene transfer in mouse fibroblast implants. PNAS 88:4626-4630, 1991.
68. Sacchi M, Klapan I, Johnson JT, Whiteside TL. Antiproliferative effects of cytokines on squamous cell carcinoma. Arch Otolaryngol Head Neck Surg 117:321-326, 1991.
69. Lin W-c, Yasumura S, Whiteside TL. Transfer of interleukin 2 receptor genes into squamous cell carcinoma: Modification of tumor cell growth. Arch Otolaryngol Head Neck Surg 119:1229-1235, 1993.
70. Myers JN, Yasumura S, Hirabayashi H, Lin W-c, Johnson JT, Whiteside TL. Paracrine growth stimulation of human head and neck squamous cell carcinoma cell lines by interleukin 4. AACR Proc 1994(Abstract)
71. Vitolo D, Vujanovic N, Rabinowich H, Schlesinger M, Herberman RB, Whiteside TL. Rapid interleukin-2 induced adherence of human natural killer (NK) cells: II. Expression of mRNA for cytokines and IL2 receptors in adherent NK cells. J Immunol 151:1926-1937, 1993.
72. Quak JJ, Balm AJ, Van Dongen GA, Brakkee JG, Scheper RJ, Snow GB, Meijer CJ. A 22-kd surface antigen detected by monoclonal antibody E48 is exclusively expressed in stratified squamous and transitional epithelia. Am J Path 136:191-197, 1990.
73. Quak JJ, Balm FJ, Braklee JGP, Scheper RJ, Meijer CJL, Snow GB. Production of monoclonal antibodies to squamous cell carcinoma antigens. Arch Otolaryngol Head Neck Surg 116:181-185, 1990.
74. Quak JJ, Van Dongen GAMS, Brakkee JGP, Yoshida DJ, Balm AJM, Snow GB, Meijer CJLM. Production of a monoclonal antibody (K931) to squamousd cell carcinoma associated antigen identified as the 17-1A antigen. Hybridoma 9:377-387, 1990.
75. Vlock DR, Toporowicz A, Arnold B, Aul D, McCoy Jr JP, Carey TE, Brown WE. Isolation and purification of a squamous cell carcinoma of the head and neck-associated antigen identified by autologous antibody.

Biochim Biophys Acta 1181:174-182, 1993.

76. Geppert TD, Davis LS, Gur H, Wacholtz MC, Lipsky PE. Accessory cell signals involved in T cell activation. Immunol Rev 117:5-66, 1990.

77. van Seventer GA, Shimizu Y, Shaw S. Role of multiple accessory molecules in T cell activation. Curr Opin Immunol 3:294-303, 1991.

78. van Seventer GA, Shimizu Y, Horgan KJ, Shaw S. The LFA 1 ligand ICAM 1 provides an important costimulatory signal for T cell receptor mediated activation of resting T cells. J Immunol 144:4579-4586, 1990.

79. Heo DS, Snyderman CH, Gollin SM, Pan S, Walker E, Deka R, Barnes EL, Johnson JT, Herberman RB, Whiteside TL. Biology cytogenetics and sensitivity of immunological effector cells of new head and neck squamous cell carcinoma lines. Cancer Res 49:5167-5175, 1989.

CHAPTER 11

Immunotherapy of Renal Cell Carcinoma with Sensitized T-Lymphocytes: The UCLA Experience

William C. Pierce, Robert A Figlin, Arie S. Belldegrun

INTRODUCTION

In spite of impressive advances in technology and supportive care, the principal modalities of cancer therapy including surgery, radiation therapy, and chemotherapy fail to cure a large percentage of cancer patients. The past two decades have seen early steps in the evolution of a fourth modality of therapy known as biologic therapy. Biologic therapy attempts to enhance host systems, principally the immune system, in an attempt to mediate tumor regression.

Two biologically active substances, interferon-α (IFN-α) and interleukin-2 (IL-2) have demonstrated activity in the treatment of metastatic renal cell carcinoma. Interferons are naturally occurring immunoregulatory proteins with protean effects upon the immune system. Animal and human studies[1] suggest that IFN-α mediated renal cell carcinoma tumor regression may in part occur due to increased major histocompatibility complex (MHC) class I expression on tumor cells enhancing cytotoxic T cell recognition and cell-mediated destruction. In addition, IFN-α augments natural killer cell activity and has a demonstrable anti-proliferative effect upon tumor cells which may augment tumor regression.[2,3]

IL-2 is a cytokine secreted by activated lymphocytes with diverse immunoregulatory functions.[4] IL-2 modulates the secretion of the inflammatory cytokines tumor necrosis factor-α (TNF-α) and interleukin-1

Immunotherapy of Cancer with Sensitized T Lymphocytes, edited by Alfred E. Chang and Suyu Shu.

(IL-1). It stimulates the proliferation and activity of cytotoxic T lymphocytes, natural killer (NK) cells, and lymphokine activated killer (LAK) cells. High dose IL-2 administered as a single agent at a dose of 6.0 or 7.2 x 10^5 IU/kg every eight hours for a maximum of 14 doses has received FDA approval for the treatment of metastatic renal cell carcinoma.[5] The response rate has been modest with 4% complete responses (CR), 11% partial responses (PR), and a median duration of response of 23 months in patients with ECOG performance status 0.

The modest but reproducible responses obtained with IL-2 in a disease previously refractory to therapy has stimulated great interest in identifying means by which to enhance the response rate of IL-2 based therapy. The effect of IL-2 upon cellular components of the immune system has lead to therapies which have combined cellular elements expanded in vitro together with IL-2. Murine studies demonstrate that peripheral blood monocytes termed lymphokine activated killer cells (LAK) which have been expanded in vitro in the presence of IL-2 can be infused in tumor-bearing animals together with IL-2 leading to the regression of experimental tumors previously refractory to IL-2 monotherapy.[6] LAK cells have been further defined[7] as components of the immune system which are able to destroy targets in the absence of major histocompatibility complex (MHC) recognition. LAK cells have been utilized in combination with interleukin-2 in the treatment of immunoresponsive tumors such as renal cell carcinoma and melanoma although it has not been proven that response rates are greater than those achieved with IL-2 alone.[8]

Tumor-infiltrating lymphocytes (TIL) are obtained from solid tumors when single cell suspensions of homogenized tumor are cultured in the presence of IL-2.[9,10] TIL are 50-100 times more potent than LAK in mediating three-day lung and liver metastases in murine models. Due to these promising preclinical studies researchers at University of California at Los Angeles (UCLA) have now treated 40 evaluable patients who presented with measurable metastatic renal cell carcinoma with therapy which has included TIL in combination with IL-2. This chapter will review the UCLA experience of the treatment of metastatic renal cell carcinoma utilizing therapy which has combined low dose outpatient based continuous infusion IL-2 in combination with adoptive cellular immunotherapy with TIL.

MATERIALS AND METHODS

PATIENT POPULATION

Forty-six patients with histologically confirmed metastatic renal cell carcinoma were consecutively entered into a series of four phase II trials. All patients presented with bi-dimensionally measurable metastatic disease and adequate hematopoeitic, renal, and hepatic function to allow the safe administration of low dose interleukin-2. This included adequate blood counts (hemoglobin > 10 g/dl, granulocytes > 1500/ul, and platelets > 100,00/ul), serum creatinine < 2 mg/dl, serum bilirubin 1.6 mg/dl, transaminases < 4 x nl, and PT/PTT within 50% of normal values. Patients required a Karnofsky performance status of greater than 70 to be eligible and an expected survival of more than 3 months without active cancer therapy. Exclusion criteria for the trials included prior therapy with IL-2 or IFN-α, anticancer therapy within 4 weeks of the initiation of therapy, clinically significant pulmonary dysfunction, pleural effusion, ascites, cardiac disease (e.g., congestive heart failure, symptomatic coronary artery disease, cardiac arrhythmias, prior myocardial infarction, or hypertension requiring β-adrenergic or calcium channel blockers), active infection, serum calcium level greater than 12 mg/dl not controlled by diphosphonates, major surgery within the preceding 3 weeks, prior malignancy, active peptic ulcer disease, corticosteroids use, and CNS disease (e.g., brain metastasis, psychiatric illness, or seizure disorder). Patients were provided with and signed an informed consent approved by the UCLA Human Subject Protection Committee.

IL-2

The recombinant human IL-2 (rIL-2; Teceleukin; Ro 23-6019) was provided by Hoffman-La Roche, Inc, Nutley, NJ, as a lyophilized powder in sterile 5-ml vials. The vials contained approximately 1 x 10^6 to 5 x 10^6 U of rIL-2 and were reconstituted with 1 ml of sterile preservative-free isotonic saline. The specific activity of rIL-2 was 1.5 x 10^7 to 2.0 x 10^7 U/mg protein based on an rIL-2 bioassay using a calorimetric determination of cell growth.

IFN-α

The recombinant IFN-α (rIFN-α Roferon-A; Ro22-8181/002) was provided by Hoffman-La Roche, Inc as a lyophilized powder in sterile 5-ml vials. The vials containing approximately 3 x 10^6 or 18 x 10^6 Iu of rIFN-α were reconstituted with sterile water. The specific activity of rIFN-α-2A was 2 x 10^8 IU/mg protein.

Bulk TIL Cell Generation

Renal cell carcinoma (RCC) specimens were obtained from resected kidneys directly from the operating room in sterile fashion. The tumor samples were minced into 8 mm^3 fragments and digested for 16 hours in RPMI 1640 containing 0.01% hyaluronidase type V (1500 U/g), 0.1 % collagenase type IV (163-230 U/g) and 0.002% deoxyribonuclease type I (100 U/mg) (Sigma Chemical Co., St. Louis, MO). Cells were washed twice with Hank's Balanced Salt Solution without Ca^{2+} and Mg^{2+}, and the cells were separated on a Ficoll/Hypaque gradient (LSM, Litton Bionetics, Kensington, MD) at 900 x g for 15 minutes to concentrate the viable cells. These cells were washed (x3) in PBS and finally re-suspended in serum free medium (AIM-V, GIBCO, Chagrin Falls, OH) containing recombinant IL-2 (Hoffmann-LaRoche Inc., Nutley, NJ). Cultured TIL were initially plated into standard tissue culture flasks and upon further expansion were transferred to gas permeable bags (Terumo Medical Co., Elkton, MD) at a total concentration of 1 x 10^6 U/ml supplemented with 400 units/ml of rIL-2 and incubated at 37°C in 5% CO_2 and 95% humidity. Cell concentration was readjusted with fresh medium when necessary. TIL cells were expanded to approximately 10^{11} cells prior to collection. TIL cells were filtered through sterile Nytex (110 mesh; Lawsh Instrument Co., Rockville, MD) and transferred to a stericell machine prior to infusion. Final TIL cell preparations were carefully tested for contamination prior to intravenous infusion.

CD8⁺ TIL Generation

$CD8^+$ TIL were prepared in an identical fashion to bulk TIL except that selection for $CD8^+$ TIL was performed when 20% of TIL cells in bulk culture were $CD8^+$ by FACS analysis (usually 2-3 weeks into culture). 5 x 10^8 bulk TIL cells were collected into T150 T-CELLector CD8 capture flasks (AIS, Menlo Park, CA). Following incubation, non-adherent cells were removed by washing the flask gently 5 times with PBS. After the final wash with PBS, each flask was incubated (activated side down) with 25 ml of RPMI 1640 medium (GIBCO) supplemented with 10% human AB positive serum (NABI, Miami, FL), 0.1 μg/ml phytohemagglutin (PHA-P; Wellcome Diagnostics, Research Triangle, NC), and rIL-2 at a concentration of 400 U/ml for 72 hours. After spontaneous release into the culture medium, $CD8^+$ TIL were expanded in a manner analagous to bulk TIL. Collection into Stericell (Dupont) collection system was performed following expansion to approximately 10^{10} cells.

In Vitro Analysis of TIL Cultures

Cytoxicity of the TIL cells (bulk and $CD8^+$ selected) were determined in vitro by a 4 hour ^{51}Cr-release assay.[11] Lytic activity against a variety of fresh and non renal tumor targets was normalized by expressing the data in (LU) which are defined as the number of effector cells capable of inducing 30% lysis. The resulting data were expressed as the LU per 10^6 effector cells. Phenotypic expression of TIL was determined by two-color fluorescence, using flourescein or phycoerythrin-conjugated monoclonal antibodies. Antibodies used were: anti-Leu-4 (CD3, pan-T cell)-FITC + anti-Leu-19 (CD56, NK cells, LAK cells, T cell subsets)-PE, and anti-Leu-3a (CD4, T helper/inducer cells)-FITC + anti-Leu-2a (CD8, T cytotoxic/T suppressor cells)-PE, respectively. All antibodies were purchased from Becton Dickinson, San Jose, CA, USA. FITC-IgG1 and PE-IgG2a (Simultest Control, Becton Dickinson, San Jose, USA) were used as negative controls. 5 x 10^5 TIL in 50 ul of staining buffer (1 x PBS without Ca^{2+} and Mg^{2+} plus 2% fetal calf serum plus 0.1% sodium azide, pH 7.3) were incubated with 10 ul of each antibody for 30 min. at 4° C. Cells were then washed twice, fixed in 1% paraformaldehyde and resuspended in 0.5 ml of staining buffer. Cell surface antigens were detected using a FACS 440 scan flow cytometer (Becton Dickinson, Mountain View, CA, USA). All TIL cell cultures were characterized by in vitro cytotoxicity testing and flow cytometry performed on the third week of culture and on the day of infusion. TIL cells were tested for their ability to kill fresh (cryopreserved) autologous tumor, allogeneic tumors of the same and different histologic types, and the cultured M14 (natural killer (NK) resistant melanoma) and K-562 (NK sensitive) tumor lines. In addition, the lytic capacity of TIL cells were compared with that of lymphokine activated killer (LAK) cells tested against the same tumor targets in a simultaneous assay. Fluorescence analysis of cultured TIL cells were performed simultaneously with the cytotoxicity assays.

Treatment Regimen

Patients treated with bulk TIL (n = 27) received cytokine priming prior to undergoing nephrectomy. Ten patients received IFN-α (Roferon-A, Hoffman-La Roche, Nutley, NJ) at a dose of 3 MU/M^2 injected subcutaneously each day for five consecutive days prior to surgery. Four patients received IFN-α SQ at a dose of 3 MU/M^2 on days -16 to -3 prior to nephrectomy. Three patients received recombinant IFN-γ (Genetech) at a dose of 100 mcg/M^2/d SQ on days -15 to -2 prior to nephrectomy. Four patients received recombinant tumor necrosis factor-α (TNF-α Genetech) 25 mcg/M^2/d SQ on days -16 to -3 prior to nephrectomy. Three patients received recombinant IL-2 (Hoffman-La Roche) 2 MU/M^2/d via continuous intravenous infusion on days -13 to -10 and on days -6 to -3 prior to nephrectomy. Three patients received no cytokine priming prior to nephrectomy.

Thirteen (13) patients treated with $CD8^+$ selected TIL received no cytokine priming prior to nephrectomy.

Following nephrectomy, all patients were untreated and allowed to recover during TIL cell expansion (4-8 weeks). Prior to treatment, all patients underwent indwelling double lumen central venous Hickman catheter (Davol Inc., Cranston RI) placement. Recombinant human interleukin-2 (rIL-2; teceleukin, Ro 23-6019, Hoffman-La Roche, Inc., Nutley, NJ) was administered for 4 consecutive days 1 through 4 of each treatment week as a continuous intravenous (IV) infusion (96 hrs) in 100 cc of normal saline via the Strato micropump (Strato Medical Corporation, Beverly, MA) at a dose of 2 x 10^6 u/M^2/d (40 patients). rIFN-α-2A was administered as an intramuscular or subcutaneous injection on days 1 and 4 of each treatment week, in the evening, at a dose of 6 x 10^6/M^2/d (33 patients). No treatment with either agent was administered on days 5,6, and 7 of each treatment week (one treatment cycle). One treatment course included 3 weeks of treatment followed by a 3-week rest (10 patients) or 4 weeks of treatment followed by a 2-week rest (30 patients). On the first day of the first treatment cycle patients received their TIL cells as an intravenous infusion over 60-90 minutes. Five of the patients received one additional infusion of fresh TIL cells 9 to 15 days after the first infusion depending on the availability of cells. During the first 4 days of treatment (cycle 1 only), patients were hospitalized to permit close monitoring of any adverse effects. Thereafter, patients were treated in the outpatient setting. Dose escalation was at no time permitted. Patients were closely monitored for changes in clinical status, including vital signs, body weight, and physical examination on a weekly basis while receiving therapy. Patients with grade III toxicity (WHO classification) had treatment withheld until symptoms improved and treatment was resumed at a lower dosage of rIL-2 (75% of starting dose) with no modification of the rIFN-α-2A dose. Patients with a second grade III toxicity had their treatment withheld until symptoms improved and treatment was resumed at a lower dosage of rIL-2 (75% of starting dose) and rIFN-α-2A (50% of starting dose). Development of any grade IV non-hematologic toxicity required the discontinuation of therapy. Courses of rIL-2 and rIFN-α-2A were continued until either disease progression, unacceptable toxicity, or a maximum of four (24 weeks) or six (36 weeks) courses. Patients received acetaminophen 650 mg orally every four hours as needed for fever, indomethacin 25 to 50 mg orally 30 minutes prior and four hours following the rIFN-α-2A injection, meperdine 50 mg orally 30 minutes following the rIFN-α-2A injection as needed to control rigors throughout the course of treatment, diphenhydramine 25 to 50 mg orally as needed for rash and pruritis, dephenozylate hydrochloride with atropine sulfate 2.5 to 5.0 mg orally to control diarrhea and prochloroperazine 10 mg orally as needed for nausea and vomiting. Postural hypotension and volume depletion between cycles were managed with fluid administration.

Patients progressing following immunotherapy with low dose IL-2 and adoptive immunotherapy were able to receive additional therapy with single agent IFN-α, FUdR, or velban.

Response Criteria

A complete response (CR) was defined as the complete disappearance of all clinically detectable disease for a minimum of four weeks. A partial response (PR) was defined as a 50% or greater decrease in the sum of the products of the two longest perpendicular diameters of all measurable lesions for at least 4 weeks with no simultaneous progression of evaluable disease, or the appearance of new lesions. Stable disease (S) was defined as a less than 25% increase or a less than 50% decrease in tumor size with no simultaneous progression of evaluable disease, or the appearance of new lesions. Progressive disease was defined as an increase of greater than 25% in measurable lesions, or the appearance of new lesions. A complete surgical remission (sCR) was defined as a clinical partial remission which, upon surgical resection, rendered the patient clinically free of disease but which contained renal cell carcinoma in the pathologic specimen. A pathologic complete remission (pCR) was defined as a clinical partial remission which, upon surgical resection, rendered the patient clinically free of disease and contained no viable renal cell carcinoma in the pathologic specimen. Patients were evaluated for response after each six-week course of treatment. Response duration was calculated from the date of the initial response to the most recent evaluation of that response or the documentation of progression. Survival duration was calculated as the length of survival from the initiation of treatment.

RESULTS

Response to Therapy

Forty-six patients with metastatic renal cell carcinoma with measurable metastatic disease and primary tumors in place were entered in adoptive cellular immunotherapy trials. Forty patients ultimately received therapy with TIL- and IL-2-based therapy. Reasons that patients failed to receive treatment included transient ischemic attack prior to nephrectomy (1 pt.), myocardial infarction following nephrectomy (1 pt.), diagnosis other than renal cell carcinoma upon pathologic evaluation of nephrectomy specimen (1 pt.), no TIL growth (3 pts.). Thirty-five patients were men and five were women. The median age was 56 years (range 34-75 years). The pretreatment Karnofsky performance status of patients entered into these trials were as follows: 100%-5 pts., 80-90%-20 pts., and 70%-15 pts. Fifteen (38%) patients had measurable metastatic disease in the lung parenchyma while only 25 (62%) had multiple sites of metastases which included lung parenchyma (40%), bone (20%), contralateral adrenal (20%), lymph nodes outside the field of radical nephrectomy (17%), or soft tissue masses (8%). None of the patients had received biologic therapy with IL-2 or IFN-α.

Forty patients received a total of 102 six week courses of therapy (median 3; range 1-4 courses). All patients were hospitalized for nephrectomy and for the first 4 days of immunotherapy on cycle one, week 1 only. All remaining weeks of immunotherapy were administered in the outpatient setting except for emergency admissions.

Four (10%) of 40 patients continue to receive treatment with IL-2 and IFN-α. Seven (17%) of 40 patients have had complete responses (5 CR, 2 sCR) and 6 (15%) of 40 patients have had partial responses for an overall objective response rate of 32% (95% confidence interval, 18.6% to 49.1%, Fisher exact). Responses have been noted in metastatic disease to lung, liver, bone, non-renal lymph nodes, contralateral adrenal, and soft tissue.

The median duration of response for the complete responders is 19+ months (range 13+–37+ months). The median survival from nephrectomy for the complete responders is 24+ months (range 16+–42+ months) and no complete responder has relapsed. The median duration of response for the 6 partial responders is 4+ months (range 2+–14 months) and 3 partial responders have relapsed. The median survival of the partial responders is 10+ months (range 5+–19+) and no partial responder has yet died. In summary, the median survival of 13 responders is 18+ months (range 5+–42+ months) and all remain alive.

A Kaplan-Meier estimate of survival from nephrectomy for the 40 patients with metastatic RCC treated with nephrectomy, adoptive cellular immunotherapy, and IL-2-based therapy was performed. The one-year survival is 73% ± 8%, and the estimated 21-month survival is 61% ± 11%.

Biology of Unselected TIL

The number of lymphocytes obtained from the twenty-seven nephrectomy specimens was 6.7 ± 2.9 x 10^8 and the percentage of lymphocytes in the single cell suspensions ranged from 20-72% with a mean of 60% ± 9.0%. The average duration in culture prior to reinfusion into the patient was 39 ± 3.5 days (range 26-55 days). All twenty-seven TIL cell cultures were successfully expanded to large scale. The average number of TIL cells infused was 0.73 x 10^{11} ± 2.6 (range 0.04-16 x 10^{10}) cells.

The expression of surface lymphocyte markers CD3, CD4, CD8, CD25, CD56, CD4/CD8, and CD3/CD56 were analyzed in infused TIL. In 18/27 cultures greater than 75% of TIL cells were T cells with either a $CD3^+$ or a $CD3^+/CD56^+$ phenotype. There was considerable variation in the ratio of $CD3^+/CD4^+$ to $CD3^+/CD8^+$ within a given culture although the mean percentage of cells expressing $CD8^+$ (56.5% ± 18.8%) was greater than those expressing $CD4^+$ (16.7% ± 10%). A correlation between phenotype of the infused cells and response was identified as responders (n = 8) to adoptive cellular immunotherapy and IL-2 had a higher percentage of cells expressing the phenotype $CD56^+/CD3^-$ (38.1% ± 17.5%) than did nonresponders (n = 19; $CD56^+/CD3^-$ 10.5% ± 7.6%). No other tested phenotype correlated with response.

The cytolytic activity of the twenty-seven unselected TIL cell cultures were analyzed on the day of infusion against a variety of cellular targets including NK sensitive and resistant tumor cell lines, and freshly cultured autologous and allogeneic tumor in 4 hour ^{51}Cr release assays. Twenty-five of twenty-seven cultures demonstrated significant lytic activity against at least one of the cellular targets. However, neither the level of lytic activity nor the ability to lyse autologous tumor correlated with clinical response.

Biology of CD8⁺ Selected TIL

The number of lymphocytes obtained from the thirteen nephrectomy specimens and placed into single cell suspension culture was $5.6 \pm 2.3 \times 10^8$ cells. The percentage of lymphocytes in the initial suspensions was 66% ± 7% (range 48-75%). Including the 2-3 week period of time in culture prior to $CD8^+$ selection, the average duration in culture was 45 ± 5 days (range 39-54 days) prior to patient infusion. All thirteen $CD8^+$ TIL cell cultures were successfully expanded to large scale. The average number of TIL cells infused was $7.5 \pm 5.0 \times 10^9$ (range $0.47\text{-}17 \times 10^9$) cells. The expression of surface lymphocyte markers CD3, CD4, CD8, CD56, CD3/CD8, CD4/CD8, and CD3/CD56 were analyzed in infused $CD8^+$ TIL. The phenotype of the infused $CD8^+$ TIL was 94% (range 79%-100%) $CD8^+$. There was no correlation between surface phenotype marker expression and response.

The cytolytic activity of the 13 $CD8^+$ TIL cell cultures were analyzed on the day of infusion against a variety of cellular targets including NK sensitive and resistant tumor cell lines, and freshly cultured autologous and allogeneic tumor in four-hour ^{51}Cr release assays. Eleven of 13 cultures displayed significant autologous lytic activity against at least one target tissue, although only 5 of 13 cultures displayed significant lytic activity against autologous tumor. Neither the level of lytic activity nor the ability to lyse autologous tumor correlated with clinical response.

Toxicity of Therapy

All patients experienced mild to moderate fever, chills, fatigue and anorexia. All patients developed an erythematous, pruritic maculopapular rash usually beginning on day three of cycle one, week one, and resolving and not returning by the completion of cycle one, week two. All patients experienced mild nausea, vomiting, and diarrhea which was not dose limiting; three of the patients experience grade III nausea and vomiting, and one patient experienced grade III diarrhea. Eight patients (20%) developed reversible thyroid dysfunction. Low dose dopamine at less than 5 µg/kg was used for systolic blood pressure of less than 90 during the first infusion of IL-2 (in hospital). Three of the patients developed severe hypotension requiring pressor support and hospital admission. There was a single episode of ventricular arrhythmia associated with pressor support for hypotension and two episodes of brief supraventricular tachycardia. Neurologic toxicity consisting of somnolence and episodes of disorientation occurred in 7 patients. Dyspnea at rest occurred in two patients. The serum creatinine increased to 2-5 times normal in 6 of the patients and > 5 times normal in three of the patients although none required dialysis. There was a single grade IV electrolyte abnormality as one patient developed a sodium of 109. Five of the patients required blood transfusions during therapy. There was a single grade IV thrombocytopenia requiring a platelet transfusion and neutropenia with a WBC of less than 1000/µl did not occur during therapy. Aspartate aminotransferase (AST) elevations were mild and less than 4 times normal in all patients; the bilirubin increased to 1.7-5 times normal in 3 of the patients. No treatment related deaths occurred during therapy and the majority of IL-2 therapy was administered on an outpatient basis.

DISCUSSION

Prior to the advent of biologic therapy metastatic renal cell carcinoma was considered a universally fatal illness with little or no response to chemotherapy. The majority of patients who presented with metastatic disease died within one year of diagnosis.[12] Interleukin-2 treatment of metastatic renal cell carcinoma represents a breakthrough in that durable and complete remissions have been obtained in a metastatic solid tumor previously refractory to therapy.

Unfortunately, IL-2 fails to benefit the majority of patients with renal cell carcinoma for two principal reasons. First, IL-2 in high dose bolus fashion can only be administered to high performance status patients rendering many patients unable to receive therapy. Second, the low response rate of 15% in high performance status patients demonstrates that even the majority of high performance status patients fail to derive benefit from therapy.

At UCLA we have attempted to enhance the benefit of IL-2 therapy through the addition of adoptive immunotherapy with TIL. Although we have not performed a randomized clinical trial, several important observations have been noted. First, treatment which consisted of nephrectomy followed by immunotherapy was safely administered to patients with lower Karnofsky scores. Fifteen (37%) of 40 patients treated had a Karnofsky performance of 70%. We noted that in patients with large, bulky primary tumors nephrectomy often enhanced performance status when performed prior to the initiation of IL-2 therapy. Second, the Kaplan-Meier survival analysis estimates a 73% one year and 60% 21 month survival for the 40 patients treated in these trials. It has been previously reported that patients presenting with metastatic renal cell carcinoma have had poor survival with the majority of patients dying within one year of diagnosis. Although not proven, this data suggests that therapy consisting of nephrectomy and immunotherapy may result in statistical and clinically significant improvement in both the duration and quality of life.

Extensive in vitro analysis of TIL cell growth characteristics, phenotype, and in vitro cytotoxicity were performed. TIL cells were successfully expanded to large numbers from 40/43 nephrectomy specimens. The utilization of $CD8^+$ selection resulted in an approximate one log decrease in the yield of TIL cells for infusion. Unselected TIL cell cultures were heterogeneous in phenotype although TIL cell cultures from responding patients contained a high percentage of $CD56^+/CD3^-$ cells which suggests a role for natural killer cells in mediating metastatic tumor regression. In vitro cytotoxicity failed to correlate with clinical response.

Due to the small number of patients treated and the lack of control groups in these phase II trials, the benefit of the addition of TIL cells and/or nephrectomy to immunotherapy with IL-2 remain unproven in patients with metastatic renal cell carcinoma. However, the impressive survival data and good response rate suggests that it may be time to begin phase III clinical trials.

References

1. Wan YJ, Orrison BM, Lieberman R, et al. Induction of major histocompatibility class I antigens by interferons in undifferentiated F9 cells. J Cell Physiol 130:276-283, 1987.
2. Lindahl P, Leary P, Gresser I. Enhancement by interferon of the specific toxicity of sensitized lymphocytes. Proc Natl Acad Sci USA 69:721-725, 1972
3. Nanus DM, Pfeffer LM, Bander NH, et al. Antiproliferative and antitumor effects of α-interferon in renal cell carcinomas: Correlation with the expression of a kidney-associated differentiation glycoprotein. Cancer Res 50:4190-4194, 1990
4. Rosenberg SA, Grimm EA, McGrofan M, et al. Biological activity of recombinant human interleukin-2 produced in *Escherichia coli*. Science 223:1412-1415, 1984
5. Rosenberg SA, Lotze MT, Yang JC, et al. Experience with the use of high-dose interleukin-2 in the treatment of 652 cancer patients. Ann Surg 210:474-485, 1989
6. Mulé JJ, Shu S, Schwarz SL, et al. Adoptive immunotherapy of established pulmonary metastases with LAK cells and recombinant interleukin-2. Science 225:1487-1489, 1984
7. Grimm EA, Ramsey KM, Mazumder A, et al. Lymphokine-activated killer cell phenomenon. II. Precursor phenotype is serologically distinct from peripheral T lymphocytes, memory cytoxic thymus-derived lymphocytes, and natural killer cells. J Exp Med 157:884-897, 1983
8. Rosenberg SA, Lotze MT, Muul LM, et al. A progress report on the treatment of 157 patients with advanced cancer using lymphokine activated killer cells and inter-

leukin-2 or high dose interleukin-2 alone. N Engl J Med 316:889-905, 1987

9. Spiess PF, Yang JC, Rosenberg SA. In vivo antitumor activity of tumor-infiltrating lymphocytes expanded in recombinant interleukin-2. J Natl Cancer Inst 79:1067-1075, 1987
10. Rosenberg SA, Spiess P, Lafrenier R. A new approach to the adoptive immunotherapy of cancer with tumor infiltrating lymphocytes. Science 233:1318-1321, 1986
11. Belldegrun A, Pierce W, Kaboor R, et al. Interferon-, primed tumor infiltrating lymphocytes combined with interleukin-2 and interferon-, as therapy for metastatic renal cell carcinoma. J Urol 150:1384-1390, 1993
12. Linehan WM, Shipley WU, Parkinson DR. Cancer of the kidney and ureter. V.T. DeVita, S. Hellman and S.A. Rosenberg (eds.) Cancer Principles & Practice of Oncology, Philadelphia: J.B. Lippencott Co., 1:1023-1051, 1993.

CHAPTER 12

Activated Lymph Node Cells in the Treatment of Human Cancer

Alfred E. Chang, Atsushi Aruga,
Mark J. Cameron, Suyu Shu

INTRODUCTION

The feasibility of adoptive immunotherapy of cancer is based on two fundamental observations derived from experimental animal studies. The first of these observations is that tumor cells express unique antigens that can elicit an immune response in the syngeneic host. The other is that the immune rejection of tumors can be mediated by the adoptive transfer of appropriately sensitized lymphoid cells to the tumor bearing host. One of the significant obstacles in the application of adoptive immunotherapy to human malignancies has been the lack of reliable methods to isolate tumor-reactive lymphoid cells from the tumor-bearing patient and to expand them ex vivo without loss of function. Additionally, human malignancies have been considered non-immunogenic by virtue of their spontaneous origins and thought to be incapable of eliciting a T cell immune response. These latter misconceptions have been proven incorrect by the recent molecular characterization of tumor antigens expressed on different human malignancies and their ability to act as recognition structures for sensitized T cells.[1,2]

Earlier attempts by investigators to derive sensitized T cells in cancer patients were performed with peripheral blood lymphocytes. Methods to sensitize these peripheral blood lymphocytes (PBL) were generally unsuccessful in identifying tumor-reactive lymphoid cells for potential therapy. With the discovery of interleukin-2 (IL-2), the phenomenon of lymphokine-activated killer (LAK) cells was described by Rosenberg and co-workers to react and lyse tumor cells in a nonspecific fashion.[3] Moreover,

Immunotherapy of Cancer with Sensitized T Lymphocytes, edited by Alfred E. Chang and Suyu Shu.

animal studies demonstrated that LAK cells mediated significant regression of micrometastatic tumor upon adoptive transfer.[4] Based upon these observations, LAK cells in combination with IL-2 therapy were utilized in therapeutic trials mainly in patients with advanced melanoma and renal cell carcinoma. The significance of these trials is the demonstration that autologous LAK cells can be produced on a large scale with infusions of up to 2 x 10^{11} cells per patient and that a subset of these patients went on to have durable complete responses. Subsequent randomized trials evaluating IL-2 alone versus LAK cells plus IL-2 have reported that there were minimal outcome differences between these two treatment arms.[5,6] Nevertheless, the concept of cellular therapy for malignancy has stimulated other efforts to identify alternative effector cells for adoptive transfer.

Another source for potential tumor-reactive T lymphocytes has been derived from progressively growing tumors. These T lymphoid cells have been termed tumor infiltrating lymphocytes (TIL) and have been characterized to be more specific in their immunological reactivity to tumor cells in in vitro cytotoxicity assays.[7] Unlike LAK cells, TIL reactivity to tumor is class I major histocompatibility (MHC)-restricted. Moreover, in animal studies, TIL have been demonstrated to be significantly more potent than LAK cells in mediating regression of established tumor on a per cell basis.[8] Clinical trials with TIL cells have demonstrated up to 40% tumor responses in patients with advanced melanoma suggestive of improved activity relative to LAK cells[9,10] with response rates of approximately 15-20%. There is less experience with TIL therapy in the treatment of patients with metastatic renal cell cancer (RCC), and has not been as efficacious in the treatment of this group of patients as compared to patients with melanoma.[11] From murine studies, one of the limitations in the use of TIL has been the inability to generate therapeutic effector cells from non-immunogenic tumors.[8]

We have examined an alternate source of T lymphoid cells for the generation of tumor-reactive effector cells. This involves the use of lymph nodes draining sites of progressively growing tumor or draining sites of tumor vaccination. Based on animal models, we have been able to develop methodologies to generate tumor-reactive lymphoid cells for adoptive immunotherapy against non-immunogenic or poorly immunogenic tumors. These methodologies have been utilized in clinical studies of vaccine-primed lymph node cells for the treatment of advanced malignancies. This chapter will summarize our animal studies defining the principles by which we have based our methods of T cell activation in clinical studies. In addition, this chapter will also update the results of our clinical studies.

PRINCIPLES ESTABLISHED FROM ANIMAL MODELS

During the last several years, we observed that tumor-draining lymph node harbor lymphoid cells that are not functionally capable of mediating tumor rejection in adoptive transfer experiments; however, further in vitro activation of these cells resulted in the generation of tumor-specific T cells that were therapeutically efficacious in adoptive immunotherapy. One approach to the activation of these lymph node cells involved in vitro sensitization (IVS) with irradiated tumor cells in the presence of low concentrations of IL-2.[12,13] During IVS culture, tumor-draining lymph node cells numerically expand and differentiate into potent effector cells and when adoptively transferred to tumor-bearing hosts can mediate the regression of advanced, macroscopic tumors established in visceral organs. Of importance was the ability to generate therapeutic IVS cells against a defined poorly immunogenic tumor. It has been postulated that human tumors are poorly immunogenic based on their spontaneous origins and that many animal tumors are not relevant for study because they are chemically or virally induced and hence are significantly immunogenic. Therefore, we examined the ability to generate immune T cells reactive to a defined poorly immunogenic tumor, the MCA 102 sarcoma. Animals cannot develop systemic immunity to these tumors with several conventional vaccination procedures, and therapeutic TIL cannot be generated with standard techniques from these tumors.[8] In accordance with these observations, we found that tumor-draining lymph node cells could not be successfully stimulated by the IVS culture method to develop into immune T cells. However, we discovered that the subcutaneous inoculation of MCA 102 tumor cells admixed with the bacterial adjuvant, *Corynebacterium parvum* (*C. parvum*), resulted in reactive lymph node cells that differentiated into therapeutic effector T cells upon culture in IVS.[14] Moreover, only lymph nodes draining the tumor "vaccination" site were capable of differentiating into immune T cells during IVS culture; PBL, splenocytes, distant lymph nodes and bone marrow cells did not have this capability. Besides the regional restriction of the development of sensitized cells within the immediate draining lymph node cells, our studies also indicated that the cellular response within the draining lymph node cells was critically dependent upon the time of retrieval of the lymph node cells. After inoculation with tumor cells admixed with *C. parvum*, sensitized cells could be retrieved from the draining lymph node by 7 days after inoculation, but diminished by 21 days after tumor inoculation. This suggested that during progressive tumor growth there may be the development of tumor-induced suppression within the host inhibiting the immune response in the draining lymph node.

We have also developed an alternate in vitro method to activate lymph node cells without the use of tumor stimulator cells which are required by the IVS culture method. In this regard, we found that antibodies that bind to the T cell receptor/CD3 complex (anti-CD3) can mimic antigen in the stimulation of tumor-sensitized T cells.[14-16] Even though anti-CD3 can activate all T cells nonspecifically, the sequential culture of tumor-draining lymph node cells with anti-CD3 and low concentration IL-2 resulted in an expanded population of tumor-reactive T cells with exquisite immunologic specificity. Application of this anti-CD3/IL-2 activation procedure was examined with the poorly immunogenic murine B16-BL6 melanoma, a highly invasive tumor of spontaneous origin. Because of its non-immunogenicity, anti-CD3/IL-2 activation of lymph node cells draining this tumor did not result in the generation of therapeutically effective cells. However, similar to the generation of therapeutic IVS cells reactive to MCA 102 tumor, we found that therapeutic anti-CD3/IL-2 activated cells could be reliably generated from lymph node draining inoculation sites of B16-BL6 tumor admixed with *C. parvum.*[17] In addition to the ability to mediate regression of experimentally induced pulmonary metastases, these activated cells were effective in the treatment of spontaneous visceral metastases originating from a primary tumor, a condition that more closely approximates human malignancies. As previously demonstrated with IVS culture of MCA 102 tumor-primed lymph node cells, the activation of B16-BL6 draining lymph node cells with anti-CD3/IL-2 was dependent upon the timing of lymph node harvest after inoculation of tumor cells and *C. parvum*. T cell sensitization within the B16-BL6 draining lymph node cells was evident by day 7 after tumor inoculation and decreased after day 14.[17]

As indicated by our animal models, tumor-draining or tumor-primed lymph node cells contain sensitized but functionally deficient cells. These "preeffector" cells however, can differentiate into potent therapeutic effector cells after activation by either the IVS or the anti-CD3/IL-2 activation procedures. We have previously reported that IVS cells mediate cytolysis of tumor during standard 4 hr. chromium release assay.[13] By contrast, anti-CD3/IL-2 activated lymph node cells are non-cytolytic in similar in vitro assays.[16] These findings underscore previous observations by other investigators that in vitro cytotoxicity assays have not been reliable in determining whether activated cell populations will mediate in vivo anti-tumor effects. Recent studies have demonstrated that tumor-specific cytokine release may offer a better method to determine functional therapeutic activity of activated lymphoid cells.[18] We therefore investigated the cytokine release of IVS cells derived from tumor-draining lymph node as well as other lymphoid sites in order to characterize their in vitro immunologic reactivity. Granulocyte-macrophage colony stimulating factor (GM-CSF) was examined because it is secreted by immune cells and promotes the activation of inflammatory cells. In animal studies, C57BL/6 mice were inoculated with 10^6 syngeneic MCA 207 tumor cells subcutaneously in the lower flank. Ten days later, cells from several different lymphoic organs were harvested and cultured by the IVS method with irradiated MCA 207 tumor cells and IL-2 (10 υ/ml). Splenocytes from non-tumor bearing mice were used as an additional control. After culture, the cells were restimulated in vitro with MCA 207 or the immunologically distinct MCA 205 tumor, and GM-CSF measured in the culture supernatant 24 h. later. A GM-CSF specific release ratio (SRR) was calculated for each IVS population by dividing the GM-CSF concentration stimulated with MCA 207 by the GM-CSF concentration stimulated with the immunologically distinct MCA 205. An SRR of greater than 1 should indicate relative tumor-specific release of GM-CSF (Table 12.1). Although all IVS cell populations from the tumor-bearing

Table 12.1. Tumor-specific GM-CSF release of MCA 207 draining lymph node cells

Source of Lymphoid Cells[a]	GM-CSF Release (pg/ml)[b] MCA 207	MCA 205	Specific Release Ratio
Inguinal LN	247	15	17.2
Axillary LN	149	119	1.3
Mesenteric LN	69	154	0.5
Spleen	180	210	0.9
Bone marrow	147	390	0.4
Thymus	491	794	0.6
PBL	222	737	0.3
Nl spleen	152	305	0.5

[a] MCA 207 inoculated s.c. in lower flank. Lymphoid cells harvested 9 days later and cultured in IVS with irradiated MCA 207 and IL-2 (10 μ/ml).
[b] Release of GM-CSF in the culture supernatant after 24 hours by restimulation with irradiated tumor.

Table 12.2. Kinetics of tumor-specific GM-CSF release of MCA 207 draining lymph node cells

Day after Tumor Inoculation[a]	GM-CSF Release (pg/ml)[b] MCA 207	MCA 205	Specific Release Ratio
0	136	166	0.3
4	1151	1719	0.6
7	726	156	4.7
10	516	206	2.4
14	416	156	2.6
21	230	147	1.1

[a] MCA 207 inoculated s.c. in flank and inguinal lymphoid cells harvested at different times after inoculation. Cells were cultured in IVS with irradiated MCA 207 and IL-2 (10 μ/ml).
[b] Release of GM-CSF in the culture supernatant after 24 hours by restimulation with irradiated tumor.

and normal host secreted GM-CSF in response to MCA 207 stimulation, only the immediate draining inguinal lymph node had significant tumor-specific release of the cytokine with an SRR of 17.2. The only other site with an SRR > 1 was axillary lymph node. In order to examine the kinetics of the tumor-specific release of GM-CSF from inguinal lymph node, mice were inoculated with MCA 207 tumor as before at different time intervals prior to lymph node harvest. lymph node cells were harvested on the same day for culture by the IVS method and subsequently re-stimulated with MCA 207 or MCA 205 to assess GM-CSF release as previously described (Table 12.2). Mesenteric lymph node from non-tumor bearing animals were used as day 0 lymph node. The GM-CSF SRR for inguinal lymph node draining day 0, 4, 7, 10, 14, and 21 tumors was 0.3, 0.6, 4.7, 2.4, 2.6, and 1.1, respectively. This indicated that tumor-specific release of GM-CSF was observed only with 7, 10 and 14 draining IVS-lymph node cells with a peak response on day 7. This correlated with what we defined as the preeffector cell response in our previously reported animal models.[12,17] Based on these studies, tumor-specific GM-CSF release may predict which lymphoid population will be therapeutically effective in adoptive immunotherapy. Further studies are being conducted to determine if this correlation exists.

CLINICAL STUDIES WITH VACCINE-PRIMED LYMPH NODE CELLS

Based on our animal experimental observations, we have been investigating the immune function of vaccine-primed lymph node cells in the treatment of patients with advanced cancers. Patients with RCC or melanoma received two intradermal inoculations of 1-2 x 10^7 irradiated (2,500 cGy) autologous tumor cells admixed with 10^7 cfu of BCG as a vaccine. BCG was chosen because of its documented efficacy as an immune adjuvant in clinical studies using autologous tumor cells. As per our animal models, lymph nodes draining the vaccine sites were harvested 7-10 days later and cultured by the IVS method in our initial clinical study.[19] Approximately 10^9 vaccine-primed lymph node were retrieved from nodal regions draining two vaccine sites. During IVS culture, lymph node cells expanded up to 14-fold and a mean of 7 x 10^9 cells were infused in 10 patients (7 melanoma, 3 RCC) along with the concomitant intravenous administration of IL-2 (180,000 IU/kg every 8 hrs. for 5 days). Phenotype analysis of the IVS-lymph node cells revealed 78 ± 4% $CD3^+$ T cells which were predominantly $CD4^+$ (67 ± 5%) with expression of HLA-DR and IL-2 receptors. IVS-lymph node cells displayed relative specificity of autologous tumor lysis in 4 of 10 cases compared to 0 of 7 IVS-PBL derived from the same patients as measured by the chromium release assay. Among the 3 RCC patients, 2 of the 3 demonstrated specific tumor lysis when comparing autologous tumor targets versus an allogeneic renal cell cancer target. One month after therapy, 7 of the 9 patients treated with IVS-lymph node cells developed delayed-type hypersensitivity (DTH) reactivity to autologous tumor compared to 0 of 9 patient treated with tumor vaccination and IL-2 only ($p < 0.002$). The latter group of patients were not anergic since DTH reactivity to old tuberculin developed in all patients after vaccination. These observations suggested that anti-tumor reactivity was passively transferred with the IVS-lymph node cells. Among the 10 patients treated with IVS-lymph node cells and IL-2, there was 1 partial (melanoma) and 1 minor (RCC) response. In addition, 1 patient has had stable disease at 36+ months. By contrast, there was no evidence of tumor response in the patients treated with tumor vaccination and IL-2 only. It was concluded that one of the major restrictions in this approach was the inability to generate larger numbers of IVS-lymph node cells. This was directly related to the limited number of tumor cells that were necessary for stimulation in the IVS culture system. Nevertheless, the vaccine-primed lymph node cells were able to transfer tumor immunity as demonstrated by the development of DTH reactivity to autologous tumor after treatment.

Due to the limited number of IVS-lymph node cells which could be generated in our clinical studies, we proceeded to examine the immunological reactivity of vaccine-primed lymph node cells which were activated by the anti-CD3/IL-2 method. As before, eligible patients included those with advanced RCC and melanoma. Tumor vaccination consisted of intradermal inoculations of irradiated autologous tumor cells admixed with BCG. Vaccine primed lymph node cells were harvested 7 days later. lymph node cells were activated in 150 cm² culture flasks pretreated with 10 µg/ml OKT3 in borate buffer for 12 hrs at 4°C. Plates were washed with PBS and cells were plated at 2 x 10^6 cells/ml of complete media. After 48 hrs, the cells were harvested from the plates and cultured in Lifecell 3000 tissue culture bags in complete media plus 10 u/ml IL-2 at 3 x 10^5 cells/ml at 37°C in 5% CO_2. The cells were split when the density was greater than 10^6 cells/ml. After approximately 6 days, this activation cycle was repeated. To date, a total of 18 patients have undergone this procedure. The initial lymph node number placed in anti-CD3/IL-2 activation represented a mean of 5.3 x 10^8 cells. After approximately 15 days of activation, a mean of 7.5 x 10^{10} cells were harvested representing an overall 141-fold expansion (Table 12.3). The anti-CD3/IL-2 activation procedure was found to preferentially activate and expand

Table 12.3. Anti-CD3/IL-2 activation of vaccine-primed lymph node cells

Tumor Histology	No. of Patients	Initial #LN	Days of Activation	Final # Cell	Fold Expansion
Melanoma	11	5.2 x 10^8	15	3.5 x 10^{10}	67
Renal cell	7	6.3 x 10^8	16	10.5 x 10^{10}	166
Total	18	x = 5.3 x 10^8	15	7.5 x 10^{10}	141

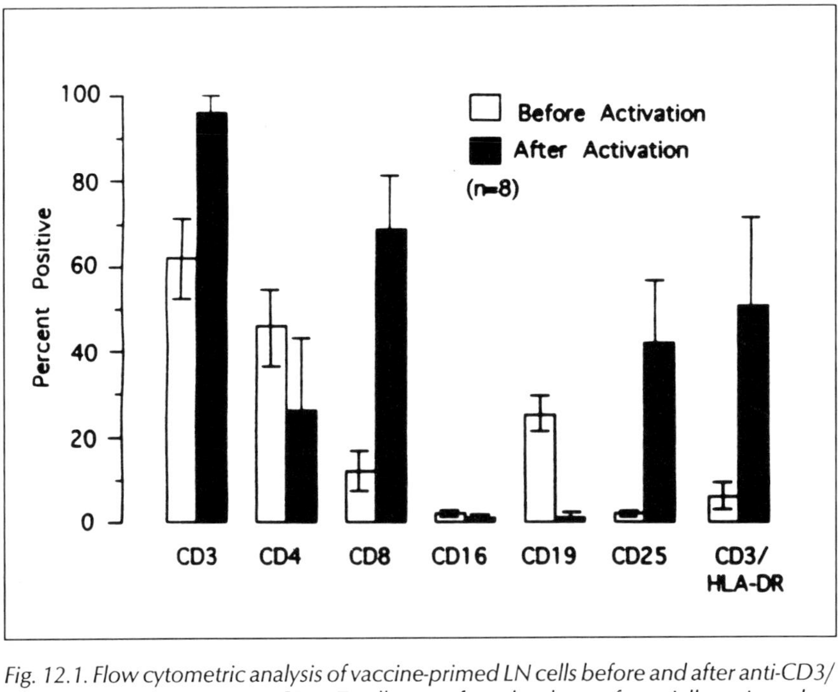

Fig. 12.1. Flow cytometric analysis of vaccine-primed LN cells before and after anti-CD3/IL-2 activation in 8 patients. CD8⁺ T cells were found to be preferentially activated.

CD8⁺ cells (Fig. 12.1). The cytolytic activity of the activated cells were analyzed using the standard 4 hr. chromium release assay which included an autologous tumor target as well as 2 allogeneic targets and the Daudi cell line as a LAK target. The cytolytic profile of these activated cells differed between the different tumor histologies. Among the 11 melanoma patients studied, there was 0 to minimal cytolytic activity against autologous tumor as noted in Table 12.4. This nonlytic profile was also seen with the allogeneic melanoma targets; however, Daudi cells appeared to be lysed among the majority of the targets tested indicating some LAK-like activity. By contrast, 4 of 7 RCC patients demonstrated significant autologous tumor killing in the cytotoxicity assay as illustrated in Table 12.5. Three out of 4 of these RCC patients had relative tumor-specific autologous tumor cytotoxicity when compared to lysis of the allogeneic targets.

Among the 11 melanoma patients treated, a mean of 3.5 x 10^{10} cells were infused. One of 11 melanoma patients demonstrated a partial tumor response which lasted 8 months. Two of the 11 melanoma patients which included the patient who responded developed DTH reactivity to autologous tumor after treatment (Table 12.6). Among the 7 RCC patients treated, 5 are currently evaluable for response. Among those 5 patients, 3 have

Table 12.4. Cytotoxicity of anti-CD3/IL-2 activated lymph node cells from melanoma patients

Patient		Lytic Units[a]			
		Autologous	Allo 1	Allo 2	Daudi
1.	JS	0	0	0	-
2.	SB	6	0	2	-
3.	AP[b]	0	0	0	0
4.	RC	0	0	0	14
5.	MR	5	2	2	13
6.	JM	0	0	0	0
7.	NV	0	0	12	16
8.	DC	0	0	-	18
9.	GA	0	0	0	7
10.	LT	0	0	-	25
11.	SI	0	0	-	50

[a]20% lysis per 10^7 effector cells; all targets were of melanoma origin.
[b]Responder to therapy

Table 12.5. Cytotoxicity of anti-CD3/IL-2 activated lymph node cells from renal cell cancer patients

Patient		Lytic Units[a]			
		Autologous	Allo 1	Allo 2	Daudi
1.	JB[b]	14	2	0	3
2.	SW[b]	33	12	12	-
3.	JH[b]	2	10	10	6
4.	AC	0	0	0	25
5.	WS	33	40	36	33
6.	RR	50	0	-	0
7.	RD	5	100	-	125

[a] 20% lysis per 107 effector cells; all targets were of RCC origin.
[b] Responder to therapy.

had a response (1 complete and 2 partial). Among the 5 evaluable patients, 2 have developed DTH reactivity to autologous tumor, both of whom have demonstrated response to treatment.

As previously indicated, cytolytic activity does not appear to be a reflection of the potential therapeutic efficacy of adoptively transferred cells. Utilizing the cytokine release protocol described in our animal models, we have performed preliminary analyses of the GM-CSF release of vaccine-primed lymph node cells derived from RCC patients. In Table 12.7, two patients with renal cell carcinoma underwent activation of their vaccine-primed lymph node cells using the IVS method as well as the anti-CD3/IL-2 activation procedure. After activation was completed, these effector cells were restimulated with autologous tumor or an allogeneic RCC (allo 1) or a melanoma tumor (allo 2). Twenty-four hours later, the supernatants were collected and GM-CSF concentration determined by ELISA. As noted in Table 12.7, both IVS cultured cells as well as anti-CD3/IL-2 activated cells released GM-CSF upon stimulation with autologous tumor cells. This release was immunologically specific when compared to the stimulation with the other allogeneic tumors. Based on our animal models, these data would suggest that vaccine-primed lymph node cells harbor tumor-reactive lymphoid cells which respond in an immunologically specific manner to autologous tumor and have therapeutic potential in adoptive immunotherapy.

FUTURE DIRECTIONS

Alternate approaches to the generation of primed lymph node cells are being explored by our laboratory. One area of investigation has been to selectively stimulate primed lymph node cells with microbial superantigens. Superantigens are bacterial toxins which cause many severe clinical syndromes which are most likely a result of massive T cell activation within the

Table 12.6. Tumor responses and DTH reactivity to autologous tumor after transfer of anti-CD3/IL-2 activated Cells

Tumor Histology	No. of Evaluable Patients	Response		DTH	
		CR	PR	Before	After
Melanoma	11	0	1	0/11	2/11
Renal cell	5	1	2	0/4	2/5

Table 12.7. Tumor-specific GM-CSF release of vaccine-primed lymph node cells

Patient	In Vitro Diagnosis	Tumor Activation	GM-CSF (pg/ml) Restimulation	Release
RR	Renal cell	IVS	Autologous	1988
		IVS	Allo 1	0
		IVS	Allo 2	0
		αCD3/IL-2	Autologous	126
		αCD3/IL-2	Allo 1	0
		αCD3/IL-2	Allo 2	0
RD	Renal cell	IVS	Autologous	258
		IVS	Allo 1	0
		IVS	Allo 2	0
		αCD3/IL-2	Autologous	255
		αCD3/IL-2	Allo 1	16
		αCD3/IL-2	Allo 2	0

host. Bacterial superantigens bind to MHC class II molecules to form ligands that interact with distinct Vβ elements of the T cell receptor. This permits the preferential stimulation of T cell subsets which may potentially promote the selective activation of tumor-reactive preeffector cells. In animal studies, we have found that stimulation of tumor-draining lymph node cells with staphylococcal enterotoxins A (SEA) or B (SEB) followed by cultured in IL-2 resulted in selective activation and expansion of Vβ 3 and Vβ 11 or Vβ 3 and Vβ 8 T cells, respectively.[20] However, in adoptive immunotherapy, SEB but not SEA-activated cells mediated the regression of established pulmonary metastases. To define the relative anti-tumor effects of Vβ 3 and Vβ 8 T cells, SEB-activated cells were depleted of either Vβ 3 or Vβ 8 T cells with monoclonal antibodies and magnetic beads. The anti-tumor effects were demonstrably diminished after Vβ 8 cell depletion but enhanced after Vβ 3 cell depletion. The ability of SEB to stimulate induction of therapeutically effective T cells has implications to clinical applications. Sequence analyses of Vβ genes from mice and humans have shown some homologies both by primary sequence and by their relative locations in the Vβ gene complex. Similar to mouse T cells, Vβ selective stimulation by staphylococcal toxins has been defined in humans. This would suggest that the use of bacterial superantigens may be advantageous for propagating large numbers of human T cells of selected Vβ elements for adoptive immunotherapy.

Another approach to the induction of preeffector lymph node cells to tumor antigen is the use of genetically modified tumor cells as vaccines. Utilizing poorly immunogenic tumors such as the B16BL6 melanoma, we have begun to explore the in vivo priming of draining lymph node cells with tumors genetically modified to secrete cytokines or express other immunoregulatory proteins. For example, we have found that the in vivo transfection of B16BL6 melanoma with DNA/liposomes or naked DNA encoding for an allogeneic MHC class I protein can upregulate the induction of preeffector cells in the draining lymph node.[21] In other studies, we have demonstrated that the transduction of the B16BL6 melanoma with the human IL-4 gene resulted in reduced tumorigenicity of transduced tumors secreting IL-4. These IL-4 transduced tumor cell clones were also found to upregulate the induction of preeffector cells sensitized to parental tumor antigens in the draining lymph node.[22] Further investigations with the use of genetically modified tumor cells are in progress to determine optimal approaches to induce preeffector cells in vaccine-primed lymph node cells.

SUMMARY

From extensive animal studies, we have demonstrated that tumor-draining or vaccine-primed lymph node contain lymphoid cells sensitized to tumor antigen. However, these preeffector lymph node cells are incapable of mediating tumor regression in adoptive immunotherapy experiments unless they are secondarily stimulated in vitro to differentiate into effector cells. We have defined a number of in vitro methodologies for this secondary stimulation. One method involves the in vitro sensitization of preeffector cells with irradiated autologous tumor cells in the presence of low concentrations of IL-2 which we have termed IVS. Another approach which avoids the need for irradiated autologous tumor cells for in vitro stimulation is the use of anti-CD3 mAb for initial T cell activation followed by expansion in low concentrations of IL-2. The use of anti-CD3 obviates the need for tumor stimulator cells. More recently, we have identified that bacterial superantigens which activate T cells by binding to MHC class II molecules and distinct Vβ elements can also activate preeffector lymph node cells for adoptive immunotherapy. Moreover, this may provide a more selective method to stimulate tumor-reactive preeffector cells.

Our clinical studies have substantiated the hypothesis that vaccine-primed lymph node contain sensitized T cells capable of transferring tumor immunity. Our initial studies with vaccine-primed IVS-lymph node cells in the treatment of patients with RCC and melanoma indicated that the techniques of vaccine-priming and secondary in vitro sensitization of lymph node cells were feasible. The transfer of these IVS-lymph node cells resulted in the transfer of DTH reactivity to autologous tumor in the majority of patients that were treated. Because of the limited number of IVS-lymph node cells which could be generated, we are currently conducting a study of anti-CD3/IL-2 activated vaccine-primed lymph node cells. To date, we have been able to generate significantly larger numbers of activated lymph node cells utilizing the anti-CD3/IL-2 method. The activation method preferentially stimulates $CD8^+$ T cells. Preliminary data indicates that the vaccine-primed lymph node cells secrete GM-CSF upon specific tumor stimulation in vitro. The adoptive transfer of anti-CD3/IL-2 activated, vaccine-primed lymph node cells appears to be promising for patients with RCC, and this protocol is continuing as a phase II study.

Acknowledgments

This study was supported in part by NIH grant RO1 CA51220 and MO1 RR00042. Dr. A.E. Chang is a recipient of a Faculty Research Award from the American Cancer Society. We thank Debbie Birdsall for her skillful administrative and secretarial assistance.

References

1. Van Der Bruggen P, Traversari C, Chomez P, et al. A gene encoding an antigen recognized by cytolytic T lymphocytes on a human melanoma. Science 254:1643-1647, 1991.
2. Kawakami Y, Zakut R, Topalian SL, Stotter H, Rosenberg SA. Shared human melanoma antigens. Recognition by tumor-infiltrating lymphocytes in HLA-A2.1 transfected melanomas. J Immunol 148:638-643, 1992.
3. Mule JJ, Shu S, Schwarz SL, Rosenberg SA. Adoptive immunotherapy of established pulmonary metastases with LAK cells and recombinant interleukin-2. Science 225:1487-1489, 1984.
4. Mule JJ, Shu S, Rosenberg SA. The antitumor efficacy of lymphokine-activated killer cells and recombinant interleukin-2 in vivo. J Immunol 135:646-652, 1985.
5. Rosenberg SA, Lotze MT, Yang JC, et al. Prospective randomized trial of high-dose interleukin-2 alone or in conjunction with lymphokine-activated killer cells for the treatment of patients with advanced cancer. J Natl Cancer Inst 85:622-632, 1993.
6. McCabe MS, Stablein D, Hawkins MJ. The modified group C experience-Phase III randomized trials of IL-2 versus IL-2/LAK in advanced renal cell carcinoma and advanced melanoma. Proc Am Soc Clin Oncol 10:213, 1991.
7. Rosenberg SA, Spiess P, Lafreniere R. A new approach to the adoptive immunotherapy of cancer with tumor-infiltrating lymphocytes. Science 233:1318-1321, 1986.
8. Spiess PJ, Yang JC, Rosenberg SA. In vivo anti-tumor activity of tumor-infiltrating lymphocytes expanded in recombinant interleukin-2. J Natl Cancer Inst 79:1067-1075, 1987.
9. Rosenberg SA, Packard BS, Aebersold PM, et al. Use of tumor-infiltrating lymphocytes and interleukin-2 in the immunotherapy of patients with metastatic melanoma. NEJM 319:1676-1680, 1988.
10. Aebersold P, Hyatt C, Johnson S, et al. Lysis of autologous melanoma cells by tumor-infiltrating lymphocytes: Association with clinical response. J Natl Cancer Inst 83:932-937, 1991.
11. Bukowski RM, Sharfman W, Murthy S, et al. Clinical results and characterization of tumor-infiltrating lymphocytes with or without recombinant interleukin-2 in human metastatic renal cell carcinoma. Cancer Res 51:4199-4205, 1991.
12. Shu S, Chou T, Rosenberg SA. Generation from tumor-bearing mice of lymphocytes with in vivo therapeutic efficacy. J Immunol 139:295-304, 1987.
13. Chou T, Chang AE, Shu S. Generation of therapeutic T lymphocytes from tumor-bearing mice by in vitro sensitization. Culture requirements and characterization of immu-

nologic specificity. J Immunol 140:2453-2461, 1988.

14. Yoshizawa H, Chang AE, Shu S. Cellular interactions in effector cell generation and tumor regression mediated by anti-CD3/interleukin-2 activated tumor draining lymph node cells. Cancer Res 52:1129-1136, 1992.
15. Yoshizawa H, Sakai K, Chang AE, Shu S. Activation by anti-CD3 of tumor-draining lymph node cells for specific adoptive immunotherapy. Cellular Immunol 134:473-479, 1991.
16. Yoshizawa H, Chang AE, Shu S. Specific adoptive immunotherapy mediated by tumor-draining lymph node cells sequentially activated with anti-CD3 and IL-2. J Immunol 147:729-737, 1991.
17. Geiger JD, Wagner PD, Cameron MJ, Shu S, Chang AE. Generation of T cells reactive to the poorly immunogenic B16-BL6 melanoma with efficacy in the treatment of spontaneous metastases. J Immunother 13:153-165, 1993.
18. Barth RJ, Mule JJ, Spiess PJ, Rosenberg SA. Interferon γ and tumor necrosis factor have a role in tumor regressions mediated by murine CD8+ tumor-infiltrating lymphocytes. J Exp Med 173:647-658, 1991.
19. Chang AE, Yoshizawa H, Sakai K, Cameron MJ, Sondak VK, Shu S. Clinical observations on adoptive immunotherapy with vaccine-primed T lymphocytes secondarily sensitized to tumor in vitro. Cancer Res 53:1043-1050, 1993.
20. Shu S, Krinock RA, Matsumura T, et al. Stimulation of tumor-draining lymph node cells with superantigenic staphylococcal toxins leads to the generation of tumor-specific effector T cells. J Immunol 152:1277-1288, 1994.
21. Wahl WL, Strome SE, Nabel GJ, et al. Generation of therapeutic T lymphocytes after in vivo tumor transfection with an allogeneic class I major histocompatibility complex gene (in preparation).
22. Krauss JC, Strome SE, Chang AE, Shu S. Characteristics of the poorly immunogenic B16 melanoma genetically engineered to secrete IL-2 and IL-4(Abst. #2235). Proc Am Assoc Canc Res 35: 375, 1994.

INDEX

E

F

G

H

I

J

K

L

M